BOVINE BRUCELLOSIS
An International Symposium

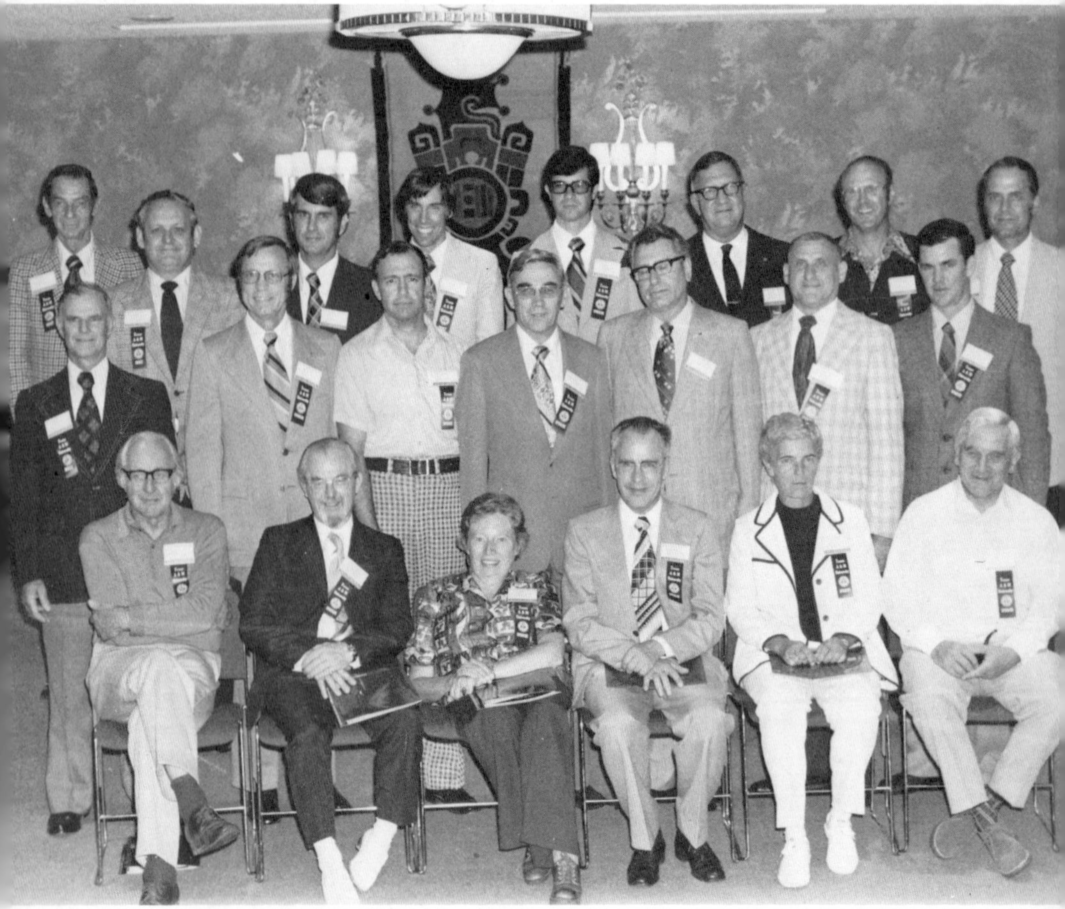

Symposium participants, l. to r., front row: Godfrey Alton, W. J. Brinley Morgan, Lois M. Jones, Michel Plommet, Margaret Meyer, Brendan Cunningham; second row: Charles Boyd, Donald Pietz, Paul Nicoletti, Paul Becton, G. R. McKeown, Winthrop C. Ray, William Slatter; third row: Archie I. Flowers, Leon H. Russell, Richard J. Hidalgo, Richard Hall, Jaime Arturo del Rio, Frank A. Hayes, Richard P. Crawford, Neville P. Clarke. Not pictured—Claude Nelson.

Ltd.) in devising a system for "taking over" the chores of doing the RBP test so as to reduce to a minimum (if not altogether) errors in doing, interpreting and extrapolating the results (Gower et al. 1974).

The ADAM system uses 35 mm, transparent plastic tape on which to conduct the tests during the reaction period. The tape moves at a constant speed with the sample tubes moving in a chain alongside. Metered volumes of antigen are dispensed from a reservoir onto the tape in discrete droplets of specific shape and size. A rotating sampling device transfers a similar volume of serum from the sample tube into the antigen already on the tape. The section of nylon tube used for the sampling procedure is automatically discarded and a new section is used for each successive sample. This procedure eliminates carry-over from sample to sample. The discrete droplets of combined serum and antigen move into an enclosed section where they are incubated and thoroughly mixed by fine jets of humidified air. Cross contamination of samples cannot occur during the mixing procedure.

After a predetermined period of incubation, each test is scanned by a fixed optical reading system for the presence of agglutination. A narrow beam of light is passed through the centre of each test and the emergent light is collected by a photomultiplier. This converts the light signal into an electrical signal which is then analysed electronically to detect and count agglutinates larger than 10 μm. Each sample result is recorded on either a teletype or printer unit and includes the following information: a sample reference number (1 to 999); the total count of detected particles or agglutinates; the validity of the test and a coloured indication as to the positive or negative status of the sample as determined by a preset threshold value. A viewing screen is mounted to enable visual observation of the tests and agglutinates may be seen clearly within the test profile. An automatic tube marking system identifies all positive samples, allowing for double identification of positive samples. On completion of the test the used tape is wound-up in a plastic cassette containing a suitable bactericidal agent to minimise infective risk. The Autotape System has a nominal throughput rate of 1200 samples per hour.

We have also been using the SATAS machines developed in France for conducting the serum agglutination test. In this machine, fixed volumes (usually 0.2 ml) of serum are placed in the 1st tube of a five tube test, with four tests in each rack. The racks which can be identified photoelectrically are placed in baskets, each basket containing 12 racks. The first machine adds diluent to the tubes, makes serial two-fold dilutions of serum and adds antigen. The baskets are incubated for 18-20 hours at 37°C and then presented to the second (reading) machine. The degree of agglutination in each tube is recorded photoelectrically against pre-determined standards and a print-out is given identifying the rack number and the degree of agglutination (-, 1+ through to 4+) for each tube. These machines have been in almost daily use at the CVL for the last five years and, with one reading and two diluting machines 2500 sera can be tested daily with a minimum of supervision.

Therefore, with the ADAM machine capable of testing 6000 sera per day and the SATAS machines capable of testing 2500 sera per day we have been able to achieve a significant breakthrough in automating these two tests. Because of the greater complexity of the CF test, we have not yet been able to achieve the same degree of automation. However, the use of automatic dispensing has enabled a much greater throughput of testing.

To summarize with specific emphasis on the questions posed:

1. The standard reference for defining an animal infected with Brucella is either bacteriological recovery of the causal

BOVINE BRUCELLOSIS

An International Symposium

Edited by RICHARD P. CRAWFORD

and RICHARD J. HIDALGO

TEXAS A&M UNIVERSITY PRESS

College Station and London

Library of Congress Cataloging in Publication Data

Main entry under title:

Bovine brucellosis.

Includes bibliographical references.
1. Brucellosis in cattle—Congresses.
I. Crawford, Richard P., 1934- II. Hidalgo, Richard J., 1938-
SP967.B7B68 636.2'08'94565' 76-51649
ISBN 0-89096-032-1

Manufactured in the United States of America
First edition

Contents

Foreword

The problems of bovine brucellosis are a very well known concern to all industries involved with production of cattle and their products, particularly in the Southern and Gulf Coast states, including Texas, since much of the recognized infection in the United States is located in these regions. The Texas Agricultural Experiment Station, a part of the Texas A&M University System, entered into an active program of research on bovine brucellosis approximately two years ago. The objectives of the research are to seek improved methods of detecting and preventing the disease and to develop methods to more economically and effectively clean up infection in high prevalence areas.

As one of the steps in initiating this research program, the Texas Agricultural Experiment Station and the College of Veterinary Medicine conducted a symposium on bovine brucellosis at the campus of Texas A&M University in College Station in July, 1976. The symposium was organized to specifically address the issues of most acute concern to producers and scientists dealing with brucellosis. Participants registered for the symposium represented 30 states in the United States plus eight other countries.

The symposium produced the following general results:

1. The need for additional research on the disease, including development of improved methods of detection, immunization and management was clearly established.

2. State regulatory officials and key leaders of producer groups now feel there has been a thorough examination of current knowledge about the disease and that, short of acquiring new information from research, we have pulled together what is known so it can be considered in making immediate decisions on regulatory procedures.
3. The symposium was the technical basis for recommended modifications of current brucellosis regulatory programs which were presented by the Texas Animal Health Commission to the U. S. Animal Health Association annual meeting in November, 1976. The recommendations were accepted by the Association and are being endorsed by them to USDA. If approved by USDA, the changes would open up several new flexibilities in the present regulatory program for use by Texas producers, such as selected use of adult vaccination for brucellosis in problem herds.
4. The symposium was important in establishing a state, national and international awareness of the commitment of the Texas Agricultural Experiment Station to develop productive research on brucellosis.
5. The symposium is furnishing an authoritative basis for communicating with producer groups to convince them that proposed changes in the state-federal regulatory programs are justified and worthy of their support.

By any measure, the symposium would have to be considered an unqualified success. The organization of the program focused attention on the issues that needed to be addressed. The speakers were informative and thorough in their treatment of the material they covered. The discussions were candid and factual. This document, containing the proceedings of the symposium, should prove to be a classical reference on the subject of bovine brucellosis. I would like to express my appreciation to everyone involved in preparing, conducting and recording this symposium. My particular thanks are extended to those scientists who came from other countries to participate in this meeting.

Clyde H. Wells

CLYDE H. WELLS, Chairman
Board of Regents
The Texas A&M University System
February 1, 1977

Editors' Summary of the Symposium

An International Symposium on Bovine Brucellosis was hosted at Texas A&M University on July 13-15, 1976. This symposium was sponsored by several groups in the Texas A&M University system, namely the Texas Agricultural Experiment Station, the Office of University Research and the College of Veterinary Medicine. Participants that registered for the symposium represented 30 states in the United States plus 8 foreign countries. The foreign countries represented were Ireland, England, France, Mexico, Argentina, Canada, Columbia, and Australia.

Dean George C. Shelton of the College of Veterinary Medicine welcomed the group in the J. Earl Rudder Conference Tower on Tuesday morning, July 13. Dr. Shelton indicated that there are areas in Texas in which much frustration and much concern has been voiced about the disease, bovine brucellosis. Dr. Shelton indicated that the group was assembled to assess the current state of scientific knowledge about the disease. Dr. Neville Clarke, the General Chairman for the Symposium and Associate Dean for Research in the College of Veterinary Medicine, reiterated Dr. Shelton's acknowledgement of the level of concern here in the State of Texas. Dr. Clarke told the participants that the symposium had been designed to answer a series of questions about bovine brucellosis that had been formulated by the research group here at Texas A&M University.

The questions concerned the areas of diagnosis, epidemiology, immunization, management and prevention of the disease and national programs currently followed in the countries represented. There were 15 invited speakers - one each from Ireland, England, Mexico, Canada, France, California, Florida, Wisconsin, Iowa, and Georgia; two from Australia and three from Maryland.

Dr. Brendan Cunningham, Chairman of Pathology, Bacteriology and Parasitology at the Veterinary College in Dublin, Ireland, indicated that brucellosis is a fairly straight forward disease from a textbook. "It is only when one becomes involved in working with the disease in the field that one realizes it is anything but a simple disease". Dr. Cunningham made the following remarks about the difficult disease we call brucellosis: Although cattle have been infected experimentally by a number of different routes, the only route of any real and practical importance in the field is the oral route; therefore, most cattle acquire infection by eating, licking or drinking infected contaminated materials. When an infected cow gives birth, whether the calf is premature or full term the fetal tissues and fluids are grossly infected and from them an enormous number of organisms are shed into the environment. The disease is very contagious and the only frequent clinical sign in cattle is abortion. The exposure of non-immunized pregnant heifers or cows almost certainly leads to abortion and this fact underlines the importance of completely segregating pregnant animals from any possible sources of exposure. Non-pregnant immature animals are not very susceptible to infection. The definitive diagnosis for brucellosis requires the recovery of the organism; however, it is not always possible to recover *Brucella* from the live infected animal. Therefore, most diagnoses are made on the results of serological tests.

Dr. Cunningham indicated that the disease would not be as difficult to manage if exposure to infection led to either:

1) prompt abortion within a few days or even a few weeks; 2) the regular and early development of blood antibodies or 3) a positive reaction to any other type of test. Unfortunately, none of these things happen with any great degree of regularity so that diagnosis at all times can be problematical and sometimes extremely difficult. In Ireland the most common source of exposure is an aborting female and under the conditions of intensive management in Ireland close daily inspection of pregnant stock is essential. Any animal showing signs of impending parturition is isolated from the remaining pregnant animals. Dr. Cunningham is also of the opinion that the fetus in an infected cow is grossly exposed while in the uterus to *Brucella abortus*. The aborted fetus contains viable organisms in the stomach contents, lungs, brain, and other organs. It would appear that calves may suffer at least a *Brucella* bacteriemia prior to birth. Dr. Cunningham indicated that in the young calf, colostrum antibodies appear to be highly protective and are capable of neutralizing an injection of *Brucella abortus* strain 19 vaccine administered up to about four and one half months of age.

Dr. Brinley Morgan, Deputy Director of the Central Veterinary Laboratory in Weybridge, England, in speaking to the diagnosis of *Brucella abortus* infection in the United Kingdom stated that no single test satisfies all the criteria of an ideal test for diagnosis. The response of the individual animal and the interpretation of the various tests are affected by a number of factors. However, a great deal is known about the various test, and certain statements can be made about the usefulness and limitations of each. In Dr. Morgan's opinion it is important to have sequential tests at properly spaced intervals, preferably during the whole stage of pregnancy, for serologic detection of infection. The tests must be interpreted in light of the overall disease status of the herd. In England, a combination of the rose bengal test (similar to the card test), along with the serum agglutination test (SAT) and complement-fixation test (CFT) is used. Results on nearly 11,000 serum samples from 158 herds in which no evidence of *Brucella* infection could be found indicated that 1.2 percent of the serums reacted positively to the rose bengal test (RBT). Conversely, on a group of cattle considered to be infected, 0.8 percent of the cattle were negative to the RBT. In the United Kingdom the RBT is considered to be overly sensitive, especially in the areas that have practiced extensive use of vaccines, and therefore, the RBT is used as a screening test and those serums that are positive are tested by the supplemental SAT or CFT. According to Dr. Morgan, false positive RBT reactions may be the result of vaccines (either strain 19 or strain 45/20), the ingestion of colostrum, *Yersinia enterocolitica* type 9 bacteria, certain strains of *Salmonella* bacteria, and/or human error. On the other hand, false negative reactions may result when the animal is in the early incubative stages of the disease, or immediately after abortion because there is a variation in the rate at which test results reach positive levels, and/or human error. Dr. Morgan feels that the CFT comes nearest to being the ideal test but this would be a rather expensive test procedure when large numbers of tests are conducted.

In England some strain 45/20 bacterin is being used at the present time. The use of this bacterin in areas that have previously practiced strain 19 vaccination is creating problems in the interpretation of serologic test results. The use of strain 45/20 bacterin confuses the interpretation of serological results and makes it rather difficult to differentiate between vaccine reactions and field infections.

Dr. Lois Jones from the University of Wisconsin agreed with Dr. Morgan that the ideal test that is 100 percent accurate in all cases has not been developed. Dr. Jones said that "although a number of tests are employed in the serologic diagnosis of bovine brucellosis, we are still looking for the perfect test - a simple rapid test which will detect an infected animal early in the incubation period as well as at all subsequent stages of the disease. Furthermore, this test should not react to serums from vaccinated animals as it is now evident that vaccination of cattle will have to continue and increase in certain heavily infected areas. Until such an ideal test is devised, we will have to make the best possible use of those presently available". She also indicated that the sensitivity of the various agglutination tests used in the United States can be changed by adjusting the density of the Brucella cells in the test antigen.

Dr. Donald Pietz, Chief of the Diagnostic Reagents and the Veterinary Services Laboratory in Ames, Iowa, indicated that interpretation of titers should be entrusted to persons familiar with all aspects of the disease before a diagnosis of brucellosis is made. He also indicated that the supplemental tests (e.g. mercaptoethanol, rivanol) and their interpretations make it even more important for persons to be familiar with all aspects of the disease. The card test (CT) detects infection earlier than the other agglutination tests, and in the field fewer herd tests are necessary using the CT to eliminate infection from the herd than when other agglutination tests are used. In addressing the over-sensitivity (false positive reactions) that occurs with the CT, Dr. Pietz indicated that this varied depending on the conditions that exist in the herd or the area. More false positives occur in infected herds than in those in which there is no evidence of infection. In areas with a relatively low prevalence of infection the number of CT false positive results vary with the amount of vaccination that is practiced and the age at which calves were vaccinated with strain 19 vaccine. In his opinion, the CT should not be used as the sole diagnostic test in areas with low prevalence of brucellosis but only as a screening test. In these areas that have a low level of infection other supplemental tests should be used to support the CT positive reactions. The mercaptoethanol and the rivanol tests are the most commonly used supplemental tests in this country. The CFT is a good test but very little information can be provided that is not already available with some of the other tests that are easier to perform. Various biologic products such as shipping fever, leptospirosis, and mastitis bacterins have been incriminated as creating problems in the diagnosis of brucellosis, but in the laboratory, workers have not been able to duplicate these results by inoculating the products under experimental conditions. The supplemental tests can be used to differentiate between antibody responses to vaccination, non-Brucella antigens and brucellosis. However, Dr. Pietz emphasized that the test themselves do not make the differentiation - the individual must conduct an epidemiological investigation, perform a battery of serologic tests which include a serial dilution milk ring test, culture the milk or tissues, and use the pattern of the results together with the epidemiology and culture information to make a diagnosis.

Dr. Pietz indicated that the probability of detecting a single infected cow in a lactating dairy herd with the milk ring test depends on the size of the herd when the milk is collected in bulk tanks. As the herd gets larger the probability decreases. In several states variations in the test to increase the sensitivity are being performed as the size of the milking herd increases. The milk ring test is a highly effective test in detecting brucellosis infection in dairy herds and should be performed a least three times a year and preferably four times.

Dr. Godfrey Alton, From the Animal Health Research Laboratory in Parkville, Victoria, Australia, indicated that research in differentiating between vaccine reactions and infection would be of great benefit to any eradication program. He agreed with the previous speakers that supplemental tests can be utilized to differentiate vaccine titers from infection titers. Dr. Alton indicated that the buffered brucella antigens (card test or rose bengal antigens) are used in Australia primarily in a screening test and any positives are tested by complement fixation. In their particular laboratory approximately one out of every three RBT positives are CFT positive but this varies with the amount of strain 19 that is used in the area. For example, increased use of strain 19 increases the number of RBT positives that are CFT negative. Dr. Alton also indicated that in Australia it is quite common to find culture positive cows that are serologically negative. At least 11 percent of the time in their laboratory, culture positive cows have less than diagnostic titers to serum agglutination. There are some parts of Australia that are using strain 45/20 bacterins, and in his spinion, these bacterins affect the agglutination reaction less than strain 19 vaccine.

Dr. Paul Nicoletti, Regional Epidemiologist for the United States Department of Agriculture, Gainesville, Florida, discussed the use of strain 45/20 bacterin for detecting latent infection of cattle that had been exposed to Brucella and are undergoing a long period of incubation. In other words, animals that are infected but are serologically negative. Under experimental conditions a high percentage of cattle that are sensitized to Brucella by either strain 19 vaccination or exposure to a field strain gave increased titers at six weeks to Coombs (CAT) and CFT following an injection of strain 45/20 bacterin (anamnestic response). The conventional complete agglutinating antibodies were not affected by the injection of strain 45/20 bacterin. Under field conditions lower percentages of strain 19 vaccinated calves gave an increased response to an injection with strain 45/20 bacterin. Approximately 20 percent of vaccinated calves had CFT titers and 25 percent had CAT positive reactions. This compares with the experimental results in the field in Australia. Dr. Nicoletti quoted Dr. Cunningham who used strain 45/20 in 53 herds in Ireland whereby 31 percent of the animals were removed from the herds because they were responders to the anamnestic test. Dr. Cunningham's statement was that this procedure was highly successful in eliminating infections from these problem herds. No *Brucella* isolations were attempted from the cattle that were slaughtered. In the use of strain 45/20 bacterin as a diagnostic antigen in four herds in the United States, the cattle were first tested using the rivanol test (RT) and the animals with RT antibodies removed. The remainder of the animals were injected with strain 45/20 and CFT and CAT positive cows were purchased for study. There were 64 cattle (20 percent of the total) that were CAT positive and 50 cattle (16 percent) that were CFT positive. There were no isolation facilities that were available and it is possible that *Brucella* transmission did occur from cow to cow after they were removed from the herd. There were 12 of the cattle that were CFT and CAT positive that were demonstrated to be excreting *Brucella* organisms. These cattle were slaughtered and the organism was again recovered at slaughter. There were an additional six cattle that were found to be infected for periods up to six months later. There were 19 percent of the CAT positive cattle and 24 percent of the CFT positive cattle that were demonstrated to be excreting *Brucella* at the time of the first test. In Dr. Nicoletti's opinion, controlled breeding is necessary to achieve at least a 12 week period where no natural exposure can occur in the herd in order for the strain 45/20 anamnestic test to have any benefit. In his opinion, the RT is the best indicator of the ability to recover the organism from an infected cow. Data presented by Dr. Dave Berman of the

Veterinary Science Department, University of Wisconsin, indicated that his past studies revealed that in infected herds that had been vaccinated with strain 19, the CFT was a better prognosticator of the ability to recover Brucella than were the agglutination tests.

Dr. Pietz and Dr. Morgan agreed that although a better test for diagnosis would be desirable and worth pursuing, the present tests and methods, if properly utilized, are adequate and that we have the capability of eradicating brucellosis with what is now available.

Dr. Winthrop Ray, Chief Staff Veterinarian for the National Brucellosis Eradication Program in Hyattsville, Maryland, in speaking to the epidemiology of brucellosis indicated that this is not a static problem and that changes in agent, host, or the environment effect the complex relationships in brucellosis epidemiology. The factors that have influenced the change in the epidemiology of brucellosis are the reduction in the overall prevalence of infection by the National Eradication Program and the increase in the percentage of problem herds. Modernization of farms with increased cattle density and increased stress and management of cattle have created a change in the epidemiology of brucellosis. The survival of Brucella in nature was discussed and the conclusion was reached that Brucella do not survive for very long periods in soil or water especially where warm temperatures are involved. Generally, Brucella survive for a matter of days and maybe even hours when sunlight and higher temperatures are involved. Field evidence indicates that with minimal cleaning and disinfection of buildings that susceptible cattle added after 30 days do not acquire the infection from the environment.

Dr. Michel Plommet, Director of Pathology of Reproduction Laboratory in Nouzilly, France, reported that Brucella survived in liquid manure in underground holding tanks for eight months in France which was the longest time examined. All speakers agreed that proper disposal of fetuses and fetal membranes are important in eliminating the environmental sources of infection.

Young calves are normally considered resistant to pathogenic *Brucella*. Dr. Plommet presented the results of experiments that described the latent form of the infection that sometimes occurs in calves born to infected cows. These calves show very little detectable evidence of infection until they become pregnant and abort or calve and then excrete the virulent *Brucella* into the environment. Several speakers acknowledged the fact that some herds that are apparently free of infection will have relapses that appear to be related to first calf heifers raised or purchased as calves.

There appears to be no natural reservoir of infection that threatens the cattle industry other than infected cattle or swine. Horses and wildlife are occassionally found to be infected but no evidence was presented that these animals were dangerous to cattle. *Brucella* tend to localize in horses in areas other than the reproductive tissue. Most equine infections involve the joints, tendons and bursa and many times can be traced to association of the horses with infected cattle or swine.

Nearly all countries that have attempted a national brucellosis program have employed vaccination at some time in their program. Many different products have been employed to increase the resistance of cattle but most of the literature supports the fact that no vaccine developed to date develops 100 percent protection. Vaccination is but one of the tools we have at our disposal in fighting brucellosis. Dr. Claude Nelson of Hyattsville, Maryland, explained that the level of circulating antibody cannot be relied on as an indicator of immunity, because the immunity to brucellosis appears to be a cell-mediated immunity located in the lymphocytes. Dr. Nelson concluded that calfhood vaccination with strain 19 vaccine as practiced in the United States results in a relatively long (five years or more) protection for cattle. The degree of protection appears to be related to the exposure dose of virulent bacteria but, in general, the vaccine protects approximately 70 percent of the vaccinated animals. Dr. Cunningham in explaining the use of strain 45/20 in Ireland presented evidence that, like strain 19, the number of abortions are reduced but vaccination alone cannot be expected to eradicate brucellosis. Strain 45/20 in Ireland is used in adult animals and the entire herd that needs to be protected is injected with two doses of vaccine at approximately six week intervals with boosters at 12 to 18 month intervals. The degree of protection from strain 45/20 bacterin approximated that received from calfhood vaccination with strain 19.

Dr. Plommet, in presenting the evidence that *Brucella* naturally gain entry through the membranes of the eye and upper air passages, indicated that vaccination using strain 19 dropped into the eye produces more efficient resistance to field challenge than does subcutaneous injection. Dr. Plommet explains this statement primarily on stimulation of the IgA antibodies in tears and localized cell-mediated immunity in the adjacent lymph nodes. Dr. Nicoletti reported the encouraging preliminary results of the use of strain 19 vaccine administered to adult cattle via the eye in large dairy herds in Florida.

Dr. William Slatter from Brunette Downs, Northern Territory, Australia, described a procedure that he has used to eliminate brucellosis from a herd of approximately 5000 cattle maintained on vast range areas. Dr. Slatter said, "The control and eradication of brucellosis is very much a joint effort between the producer, the veterinarian, and the laboratory.

Without cooperation between all parties, the scheme is most unlikely to succeed".

R. P. Crawford

R. J. Hidalgo

SYMPOSIUM COMMITTEE

Neville Clarke, Chairman
Charles Boyd
Richard Crawford
Archie Flowers
Richard Hall
Richard Hidalgo
Warren Kilpatrick

Acknowledgements

The editors are deeply indebted to the Symposium participants who graciously accepted the invitation and contributed unselfishly to this comprehensive document on bovine brucellosis. A special thanks is directed to the Symposium Committee and the many unnamed individuals who worked so hard before and during the symposium. We are appreciative of the session moderators, who not only chaired the sessions, but after the symposium edited the tapes and assembled the discussion section. The sponsorship of the Texas Agricultural Experiment Station, College of Veterinary Medicine and the Vice-President for Academic Affairs is acknowledged. In addition, a grant from the King Ranch, Inc. which helped to defray travel expenses of the speakers is truly appreciated.

The editors also wish to acknowledge the invaluable assistance of Mr. John D. Zettelmoyer, Special Assistant to the editors, whose ability, perseverance and extreme dedication made assembly of these proceedings possible. The guidance and counsel of Dr. Neville P. Clarke, Symposium Committee Chairman, and Associate Dean for Research, College of Veterinary Medicine, is also gratefully acknowledged.

We are indebted to the staffs of the Texas A & M University Press and the Biomedical Learning Resources Center of the College of Veterinary Medicine for technical assistance. We also wish to thank the personnel of Executive Services, College

Station, Texas, and the secretaries of the College of Veterinary Medicine, especially Mrs. Diana Berkefelt and Mrs. Jacquelyn Strong for typing the proceedings through its many revisions.

This symposium was the original idea of Dr. Jarvis E. Miller, Director of the Texas Agricultural Experiment Station. Dr. Miller supported the symposium from its initiation to this document. We are grateful for his foresight and influence.

Richard P. Crawford
Richard J. Hidalgo

BOVINE BRUCELLOSIS
An International Symposium

Introduction

The general objectives of the International Symposium on Bovine Brucellosis were to provide a forum for discussion and to produce a reference document containing the current thinking of the international scientific community about brucellosis. The symposium was organized around a series of questions designed to address the current issues of significance to the cattle industry of Texas, other parts of the United States and the world. The intent was to summarize current knowledge about the key issues facing the cattle industry so that: 1. short range decisions about changes in regulatory programs could be made based on having developed the best possible consensus of thinking of the scientific community; and 2. to provide a current review of knowledge as a point of departure for the research project on brucellosis in the Texas Agricultural Experiment Station.

The series of questions formed the basis for the organization of the symposium into five major sessions. Speakers were asked to participate in the symposium from key federal, state and university groups in the United States and from eight foreign countries. Speakers were assigned specific questions to address in their presentations and written papers. The session moderator had the job of summarizing briefly the answers to the questions addressed by the speakers in his session. There followed an active discussion by speakers of the key issues centered in the questions and an attempt was made to secure a consensus from the speakers on the answer to the questions. In the course of discussion, questions from speakers in other sessions as well as from other participants were addressed. The round table discussion was recorded and subsequently edited by the session moderator. The edited discussion is included at the end of the printed papers for each session of these proceedings.

After the symposium was completed, the editors of the proceedings prepared a brief summary of the meeting for interim use pending publication of these proceedings. It is included in the preceeding section of this document to provide the reader an overview of the entire symposium and to place the specific sessions in a total context.

The questions addressed during the symposium are listed below by session:

DIAGNOSIS

1. What is the standard of reference for defining an animal infected with Brucella?

2. Which serologic test or tests used today most accurately designate animals infected with pathogenic B. abortus?

3. Buffered brucella antigen (BBA) test (card test or rose bengal test):

    a. What is the percentage of false positive reactions or overkill observed when the BBA test is used to test cattle for brucellosis?
    b. What is the percentage of false negative reactions observed when the BBA test is used to test cattle for brucellosis?
    c. Is a supplemental test needed to support the results of the BBA test to detect infection, and if so, what test or tests are recommended?
    d. Excluding residual antibody activity from calfhood vaccination, what factors cause false positive or false negative reactions to the BBA test?

4. Is a better test needed for diagnosis of brucellosis in cattle?

5. Are there laboratory procedures that can be utilized to differentiate between bovine antibody responses associated with non-brucella antigens, vaccination, and brucellosis?

6. Brucella ring test (BRT):

   a. What is the established sensitivity of using BRT on bulk milk samples to detect brucellosis in dairy herds?
   b. Is a more accurate or sensitive method or test available?
   c. How often should the test be conducted to monitor brucellosis in dairy herds?
   d. How applicable is the BRT for use on samples of milk from individual cows to detect infection?

7. When using strain 45/20 as a diagnostic reagent in infected herds to detect latently infected animals, which serologic tests are recommended to identify the animals that should be removed from the herd? How severe is the over-condemnation?

8. How effective is strain 45/20 as a diagnostic reagent in infected herds that have been calfhood vaccinated with strain 19?

EPIDEMIOLOGY

1. What percentage of term calves born to infected dams show evidence of infection at birth; at puberty; at first parturition?

2. What environmental factors have been identified that affect the survival of Brucella abortus outside the bovine host?

3. What conditions have been documented that would allow the survival or multiplication of Brucella outside the animal host in sufficient numbers to result in transmission to susceptible cattle?

4. Have there been any documented instances in which bovine brucellosis was acquired by any method other than direct contact with an infected bovine or its secretions, excretions, etc? What danger to cattle is the horse with fitulous withers or poll evil?

5. A number of non-bovine hosts have been reported to be experimentally susceptible to Brucella abortus. Which animal species are likely to be naturally infected and a reservoir of brucellosis for cattle? Which of these species are found in the southern United States and what is the

prevalence of Brucella infection in these non-bovine species?

6. Are there any documented instances of a breed, sex or age susceptibility to brucellosis?

7. In view of the emergence or detection of new Brucella species in recent years, what is the probability that a new species could emerge in cattle after eliminations of Brucella abortus?

8. There is evidence that the portal of entry of Brucella is either ingestion or through the conjunctiva of the eye - which route appears more probable in range cattle? In cattle in confinement?

9. What significance can be associated with the various insects (flies, ticks, lice, etc.) as regards their role in the transmission of Brucella?

IMMUNIZATION

1. What is the definition of a bovine that has been successfully immunized by vaccination? Is the titer of any of the antibody test correlated with the degree of immunity?

2. Brucella abortus strain 19 calfhood vaccination:

    a. Summarizing the data on the effectiveness of strain 19 in immunizing calves - how effective is the procedure?
    b. What are the advantages and disadvantages of strain 19 calfhood vaccination?
    c. How common are persistent strain 19 infections in calfhood vaccinates?
    d. What is the prevalence rate of BBA (card test) reactors in adult cattle that were calfhood vaccinated - those vaccinated at an early age and those vaccinated at a later age?
    e. Is strain 19 transmitted from calfhood vaccinates to other animals in the herd?

3. Brucella abortus strain 19 adult vaccination:

    a. Summarizing the data on effectiveness of strain 19 in immunizing adult cattle - how effective is the procedure?
    b. What are the advantages and disadvantages of strain 19 adult vaccination?
    c. How effective is strain 19 when placed into the conjunctiva of the eye, as opposed to parenteral administration?

4. Brucella abortus strain 45/20 adult vaccination:
   a. Summarizing the data on effectiveness of strain 45/20 in immunizing adult cattle - how effective is the procedure?
   b. What are the advantages and disadvantages of strain 45/20 adult vaccination?
   c. Does 45/20 bacterin interfere with tests to diagnose infection?
5. Can strain 45/20 bacterin be used to increase the immunity in adults that have been calfhood vaccinated with strain 19 vaccine?
6. How effective are the vaccines or bacterins other than strain 19 and 45/20?
7. Is a better immunizing agent needed, and if so, what are the chances of producing one?
8. Can brucellosis be eliminated from a herd by vaccination alone? If not, what is the lowest estimated prevalence that could be achieved?

MANAGEMENT

1. In cattle that have been calfhood vaccinated with strain 19 vaccine:
   a. What is the earliest age recommended for blood testing replacement heifers?
   b. Which test would you use in this situation to detect infection in heifers?
2. At what age should replacement bull calves be blood tested for brucellosis?
3. What precautions are necessary for an individual buying replacement breeding stock to prevent the introduction of brucellosis?
4. Should vaccination be stopped after elimination of brucellosis from a herd? From the county? From the State? If not, when?
5. Is it necessary to have all animals vaccinated to bring brucellosis under control by vaccination? What is the lower limit of percentage of vaccinates needed to influence the spread of the disease in a herd? How should this level of vaccinates be attained - compulsory vaccination?
6. What management principles have been documented to reduce

the transmission of Brucella from infected animals to susceptibles - both intraherd and interherd?

7. What management principles can be employed on herds maintained on range conditions to hasten the elimination of brucellosis infections?

8. Is treatment sufficiently reliable to permit its use, instead of slaughter, in valuable breeding cattle? If so, what drugs are recommended?

9. Is quarantine and the limitation of movement of cattle mandatory in preventing brucellosis?

10. How important is controlled breeding versus year-round calving in eliminating brucellosis from an infected herd?

11. Are there instances or circumstances in which "reactor" animals may remain in the herd or on the premises and still not endanger the remaining non-reactor breeding cattle in the herd?

12. What effect do cortico-steroid drugs have on the animal exposed to or infected with Brucella abortus?

NATIONAL PROGRAMS

1. What is the current program?

2. What changes have been made in the program and what progress in disease reduction can be reported to date?

3. What factors have influenced this success or failure?

4. Is a national system of animal identification essential to a successful brucellosis program?

5. What are the strengths and weaknesses of the slaughter cattle test program as a surveillance tool that is currently being used in the United States?

DIAGNOSIS

Moderator: Neville P. Clarke

A Difficult Disease Called Brucellosis

Brendan Cunningham

When I was invited to open this symposium it seemed appropriate that the opening paper should be entitled "Brucellosis." I got down to the task and found that I was transcribing excerpts from many reputable textbooks on the subject and it eventually dawned on me that I was going to end up trying to write a "half-hour textbook" on the subject, which apart from being impossible, was not going to be very helpful. Most of you know a good deal about brucellosis, and in any case you are as well able to study text books as I am.

So, I scrapped that effort - mainly because brucellosis is a fairly straightforward disease from a textbook. It is only when one becomes involved in working with the disease in the field that one realizes it is anything but a simple disease. For this reason I will go on to deal with some aspects of the disease which to my mind are very important, yet not often discussed in published texts. One of my aims is to make the point from the outset that what we are all going to talk about is "A Difficult Disease Called Brucellosis."

Natural Course of the Disease

> "When a herd first becomes infected the disease spreads rapidly and the number of abortions is usually high, but in succeeding years, although extensive infection is present in the herd, abortions become fewer and fewer provided no

> new animals are introduced.
>
> Abortion is not a constant symptom of this disease. Possibly 20% of infected animals never abort. Eighty per cent of cows which abort do so only once, some twice in successive pregnancies but rarely more than twice.
>
> When new and susceptible animals are introduced into an infected herd these become infected and may abort. Sometimes without the introduction of new stock the disease flares up again" (Gaiger and Davies 1947).

The above brief description of brucellosis was written thirty years ago, and is still a true account. In the meantime we have had the opportunity to become a little more enlightened as to why the disease presents itself in such erratic ways. We have made technical progress in diagnostic tests; in the production and use of vaccines; in the husbandry and management of cattle; as well as in other related areas. I sometimes wonder, have we made the best use of such progress in the control and eradication of the disease, and if not, where and why are we failing?

Whether parturition is premature or full term the foetal tissues and fluids are grossly infected and enormous numbers of organisms are shed in them. The placenta may or may not be retained. Retention would appear to be more related to prematurity of parturition rather than to infection of the uterus and is not a constant feature of the disease. When the placenta is shed involution of the uterus proceeds and the uterus is rapidly cleared of infection so that even four to five days later cultures of vaginal mucous usually reveal very low counts of brucellae or even negative results.

For many years bovine brucellosis was aptly referred to as "Contagious Abortion." This was a very good name as about the only two things one can say about the disease with any reasonable degree of certainty are: 1. It is very contagious, and 2. the only frequent clinical sign or symptom in cattle is abortion.

The disease would be readily manageable if exposure to infection led to: 1. Prompt abortion within a few days, or even a few weeks of challenge; 2. The regular and early development of blood titres; or 3. A positive reaction to some other type of test such as a delayed hypersensitivity test. Unfortunately none of these things happen with any great degree of regularity, so that diagnosis at all times is problematical, and sometimes extremely difficult.

Route of Entry

Although cattle have been infected experimentally by parenteral injection, by the conjunctival, vaginal and intramammary routes, and even through scarified skin, the only route of any real and practical importance in the field is the oral route. Thus most cattle acquire infection by eating, licking or drinking infected or contaminated materials.

Pathogenesis

> "Following invasion and bacteraemic spread the main predilection sites are the pregnant uterus, udder, testicle, accessory male sex glands, lymph nodes, joint capsules and bursae. In calves, infection may persist in the lymph nodes for a short while but is not usually permanent as localization does not occur in the immature udder and uterus. In the adult non-pregnant cow localization occurs in the udder, and the uterus, if it becomes gravid, is infected from periodic bacteraemic phases originating in the udder." (Blood and Henderson 1974).

Erythritol, a carbohydrate substance produced by the foetus and capable of stimulating the growth of virulent strains of B. abortus (Williams, Keppie and Smith 1964) occurs naturally in greatest concentration in the placenta and foetal fluids and is probably responsible for the localization of the infection in these tissues (Keppie et al. 1965). When the invasion of the gravid uterus occurs, the initial lesion is in the wall of the uterus but spread to the lumen of the uterus soon follows; leading to a severe ulcerative endometritis of the intercotyledonary spaces. The allantochorion, foetal fluids, and placental cotyledons are next invaded and the villi destroyed. Abortion occurs principally in the last three months of pregnancy; the incubation period being inversely proportional to the stage of development of the foetus at the time of infection (Thomsen 1950).

Diagnosis

The definitive diagnosis of brucellosis requires the recovery of the causal organism and its positive identification. However, it is not always possible to recover the organism from the live infected animal so that most diagnoses are based on the results of serological tests.

Brucella cells carry antigenic components. Smooth strains of the organism cause the production of at least three kinds of antibodies recognized by different laboratory tests.

1. Agglutinins - Bivalent antibodies which cross-link the cells causing clumping or agglutination.
2. Complement-Fixing Antibodies - Antigen-antibody complexes are formed which require the activation of a complement system that attaches to the Fc end of the antibody.
3. Incomplete Antibodies - Antibodies so named because they do not cause direct agglutination. Their presence can be demonstrated only by the Antiglobulin test (Coombs 1945).

Examination of large numbers of cattle sera suggests that reactions in these laboratory tests are not different expressions of a single population of immunoglobulin (antibody) molecules. Incomplete antibodies do not cause agglutination or complement fixation, complement-fixing antibodies do not cause agglutination, or vice versa. I expect some of the papers to follow will delve more deeply into the structures and properties of immunoglobulins, so I will confine my remarks to some problematic aspects of the disease.

Exposure of Non-Immunized Pregnant Females to B. Abortus

The exposure of non-immunized pregnant heifers or cows almost certainly leads to abortion. A challenge dose of 15×10^6 B. abortus strain 544 given via the conjunctival sac at mid-pregnancy (four to five months gestation) results in abortion in over 90 percent of the animals; the earliest recorded abortion occurred about 37 days after challenge (McEwen et al. 1939).

A dose of 1500 organisms given subcutaneously at 123 to 129 days gestation caused infected parturitions to occur at 266 and 282 days in two of three heifers (Cunningham unpublished). These results endorse Thomsen's observation that challenge early in pregnancy may cause late abortion, but also suggest that cattle might be unusually sensitive to exposure during early pregnancy, particularly so if one considers the subcutaneous route to be less effective than the conjunctival route (McEwen 1940).

Serum Antibody-Titres

Serum antibody-titres (standard tests - SAT, CFT, ABGT) following the challenge to heifers during pregnancy, vary so widely that they cannot be relied upon to give an accurate indication of infection. Many infected heifers abort before serum titres rise and some will even calve (full term) with negative titres. Enormous numbers of Brucella organisms may be in the infected membranes and antibody titres usually become positive within 19 days after parturition. The possibilities underline the importance of completely segregating pregnant females from any possible sources of exposure. The commonest source of exposure is an aborting female and under the conditions of intensive management in Ireland, close daily inspection of pregnant stock is essential. Any stock showing signs of impending parturition should be isolated for the event.

Exposure of Non-Pregnant Heifers to Challenge with B. Abortus

It has long been recorded that non-pregnant immature animals are not very susceptible to infection. Experiments at the Veterinary Research Laboratory, Abbotstown, Dublin would endorse this statement and have produced the following data:

1. Eighteen yearling heifers were exposed to conjunctival challenge with 15 X 10^6 B. abortus strain 544. Serological responses were of a low order and transient - only two animals exhibited transient low positive titres to the Serum Agglutination Test (SAT) and three to the Complement-Fixation Test (CFT). Four months after challenge all animals were negative to standard test interpretations except for one inconclusive CFT (Cunningham 1967).
2. Twenty-four yearling heifers were exposed to conjunctival challenge with 15 X 10^7 B. abortus strain 544. On post-challenge day 11 only two animals exhibited low titres. On day 30, 23 animals had developed high positive titres to SAT and CFT (SAT for 23 animals from

67 to 424 i.u. - mean value 134 i.u.). By day 185 only one animal retained a positive titre (134 i.u.) and two others inconclusive titres (46.5 and 53 i.u.); 21 being negative (< 26.5 i.u.) (Cunningham unpublished).

3. Five pairs of calves (6 to 10 months). Each pair was exposed to a graded dose of 15 X 10^9 down to 15 X 10^5 *B. abortus* strain 544. Seven months later only one animal of the ten exposed to 15 X 10^9 organisms retained a positive SAT titre (80 i.u.). The other nine were negative to both the SAT and CFT (Cunningham unpublished).
4. Six brucellosis-free calves (7 to 45 days of age) were injected with *B. abortus* strain 19 vaccine. Three (7 to 21 days of age) exhibited low serological responses. The other three (29 to 45 days of age) developed high positive titres which did not diminish over a period of 13 months (Cunningham unpublished). This result was rather unexpected. Does it indicate that strain 19 may cause permanent infection in some young calves?

Calves Born of Infected Dams

During gestation in an infected womb the foetus is grossly exposed to *B. abortus*. In the aborted foetus, the stomach contents and lungs are excellent material for bacteriological culturing by the laboratory. The presence of *Brucella* does not appear to be simply due to aspiration of amniotic fluids at the time of parturition as the brain, plus other organs, often yields pure cultures of *B. abortus*. It therefore appears that a *Brucella* bacteraemia may occur in foetuses.

The viable calf born of an infected dam suckles and, in addition to receiving colostral antibodies against B. abortus, ingests large numbers of organisms in the milk (nine out of ten infected cows are infected in the udder and shed Brucella at least intermittently). Thus one might reasonably expect all such calves to become permanently infected - which is in fact very far from the truth.

It is known that in the adult, antibodies are not protective. In colostrum, antibodies are not bactericidal and the high titred colostrum of an infected cow is an excellent material to culture for Brucella. However, in the young calf colostral antibodies appear to be highly protective as they can completely neutralize an injection of strain 19 vaccine anytime up to about four and one-half months of age.

Why should antibodies be protective in the young calf and not in the adult? I don't know that this question can be answered. But we do know that the new-born calf is almost immunologically incompetent. Competence develops quite markedly in the first three months of life but does not reach its optimum until about the age of puberty. When calves born from infected uteri have been suckled on their dams for three months or more and then subjected to an anamnestic test for brucellosis at about 12 months of age - only about 50 percent have given positive reactions of sensitization. This is also quite intriguing - and I doubt very much if it can be ascribed to so called "Immunological Tolerance".

Latency

Another feature of the disease possibly less well-known is latent infection. It is less well known because it becomes a recognizable problem only when the prevalence of brucellosis is low and the area is under very close serological surveillance.

In Holland, Van der Boorn and Vervoorn (1965) reported that "Calves which are born of recently infected mothers and remain alive often infect the herd they join at a later stage." In Ireland about 1968 we recognized it in the field as what appeared to be a "two-year breakdown syndrome".

Briefly, latency is described by that small percentage of heifer calves that acquire infection in early life, pass all official blood tests (usually from 6 months of age onwards) and yet abort during the first pregnancy. They may or may not be daughters of infected dams, but were present in the herd when the last spread of infection occurred. Behaving in this way these heifers can cause serious breakdowns in the final stages of eradication in herds which have been "free of infection" for two years or more.

Non-Specific Antibodies

In a small number of cases we have found animals in known brucellosis-free herds that were classified as reactors; usually only one animal per herd. On investigation of some of these cases we noticed that these animals exhibited positive SAT titres - sometimes 300 i.u.. On the CFT they surprisingly tested negative. Furthermore their titre to the ABGT was the same as their titre to the SAT. As a further check, these animals proved negative to an anamnestic test. It was quite exciting for a while as I thought we had stumbled on to something new. We then found that Andersen of Denmark had already described apparently the same condition in 1961. Although the cause of these reactions has not yet been discovered, other organisms capable of causing cross reactions have been described e.g. Yersinia enterocolitica type IX.

National Program

So much for some aspects of the disease which may cause problems. When one commences to eradicate on a national basis, one formulates a programme. To run the programme we engage staff who along with the stock owners become participants. And to help everyone along we approve a vaccine. All three are highly desirable, even necessary - but in their train they create more problems, some of which we shall no doubt hear about in due course.

References

Andersen, F. M. 1961. Nordisk Vet. Med. 13:289-332.

Blood and Henderson, 1974. Veterinary Medicine. 4th ed., Baltimore: Williams and Wilkins, p. 374.

Coombs 1945. Lancet. 2:15-16.

Cunningham, B. 1967. Proc. B.V.A. Congress, 1967. Vet. Rec. 82:7-11.

Gaiger and Davies. 1946. Veterinary Pathology and Bacteriology. 3rd ed., London: Bailliere Tindall and Cox, p. 249.

Keppie, J.; Williams, A. E.; Witt, K.; and Smith, H. 1965. Br. J. Exp. Path. 46:104-108.

McEwen, A. D. 1940. Vet. Rec. 52:97-106.

McEwen, A. D.; Priestly, F. W.; and Paterson, J. D. 1939. J. Comp. Path. 52:116-128.

Thomsen, Axel 1950. Brit. Vet. J. 106:41-54.

Williams, A. E.; Keppie, J.; and Smith, H. 1964. J. Gen. Microbiol. 30:285-292.

The Diagnosis of *Brucella abortus* Infection in Britain

W. J. Brinley Morgan

Brucellosis in cattle is characterized by many factors, all of which have a marked influence on its diagnosis and on the significance and reliability of tests now available. These factors are:

1. Age - There is an increasing degree of susceptibility from calfhood until sexual maturity is reached. This age-related effect also seems to influence the serological response.
2. Incubation Period - This is a long and variable incubation period. Defined as the period between exposure and abortion, it can vary from about six weeks to eight months. It can be even longer in exceptional cases, for example following neonatal infection when abortion may not take place until perhaps 24 months of age. During this incubation period the results of serological tests may be negative or equivocal (Plommet et al. 1973; Lapraik et al. 1975).
3. Clinical Signs - Abortion is the only clinical feature of the disease although it is not the only cause of abortion. Retention of the placenta is common and in the more chronic form enlarged joints may also occur.
4. Carrier State - Most animals only abort once but they may become chronic symptomless carriers and excretors of the organism even after an apparently normal calving. The disease is highly contagious and can be

introduced into a herd by animals that are in the incubation or chronic stages of the disease.

5. Type and Time of Challenge - The size of the inoculum and virulence of the challenge strain and especially the stage of pregnancy at the time of contact with the organism will greatly influence the results of diagnostic tests immediately after abortion has occurred. A repeat serological test may be required some 14 days after abortion to detect infection (such animals should be kept away from contact with known non-infected animals until their status has been clearly established).

6. Vaccination Status - The use of vaccines influences the results of diagnostic tests. The degree of this effect will depend on the vaccine used, on the age of the animal at vaccination and on the test used. In general, interference with interpretation of the results of serological tests is least when animals are vaccinated with strain 19 as calves (3 - 6 months of age) but recent developments on other tests especially the complement-fixation test and supplemental tests such as the mercaptoethanol and rivanol tests have made the differentiation of vaccinal from infective responses more effective.

7. Individual Variation - In any population of cattle vaccinated with any of the *Brucella* vaccines currently available, the response will range from complete protection to no protection. This wide spectrum of responses to vaccination will also be reflected in a range of serological responses to subsequent challenge which can then vary from a nil serological response (i.e. those that completely resist infection) through

to a complete serological response in those that were fully susceptible.

It follows then that the "ideal" diagnostic test should:

1. detect infection early during the long and variable incubation period.
2. not be influenced by the presence of "non-specific" antibodies.
3. detect the chronic carriers.
4. differentiate a response to vaccination from that of field infection.

The multiplicity of tests currently available is witness to the fact that there is no single test that can completely satisfy all the above criteria. Other criteria which tend to be added are the ease, cost and simplicity of doing and interpreting the tests. However, sufficient information is now known about various tests arising partly from experience in their use and partly from recent advances in studies of bovine immunoglobulins and their properties to comment on their usefulness and limitations. But one fact stands out irrespective of what test(s) are used and that is the importance of conducting sequential tests at properly spaced intervals; these should cover an entire gestation period to take into account the factors already discussed. Three herd tests in quick succession, say at monthly intervals, are not as satisfactory overall as spacing the three tests every three to four months. Although under certain circumstances, such as a herd breakdown, testing would be indicated every month until clear test results had been obtained. But such a herd cannot be really cleared until negative tests covering a whole pregnancy have been produced.

The results of all the serological tests must be interpreted against what is recognised as occurring in known infected animals. Ideally these can be defined as animals which have been exposed to *Brucella* organisms, where the organism has invaded and multiplied in certain tissues such as the placenta and lymph nodes producing lesions and also resulting in a specific antibody response. There is no doubt that *the* definitive test for identifying an animal as "infected with *Brucella*" is the recovery and identification of the organism. There are limitations to this identification partly because of the need for specialized culture media to isolate the organism from a contaminated source (placenta, fetus, vaginal discharge, milk), partly because excretion may be intermittent or may cease although the animal may still be a carrier of the organism, and partly because numerous attempts are needed to have any degree of certainty that the animal is not infected. Cultural techniques do not readily lend themselves to large scale testing but they do have a very essential part to play in diagnosis. No in-depth investigation can be complete without some degree of cultural examinations.

Consequently greater reliance has been placed on the results of various serological tests in defining infected animals. As with the cultural examinations there are certain pitfalls here in relying solely on serological tests. These include:

1. the long and variable incubation period.
2. use of vaccines.
3. variations in individual response.
4. presence of "non-specific" antibodies.
5. response in relation to the stage of pregnancy at time of exposure.
6. response in relation to the degree of immunity.
7. which test(s) to be used and how often.
8. how the test is performed and interpreted.
9. the need for standard or reference preparations to ensure that results are uniform within a country and

can be related to results in other countries.
These factors tend to be influenced also by other factors such as the "traditional" methods used and the differing standards needed for eradication compared with those for the international movement of animals.

The serum tube agglutination (SAT) test is a time-honoured test and, as long as the antigen is properly standardized (against the International Standard anti-*Brucella abortus* serum, Stableforth 1936; Report of FAO/WHO Expert Committee on Brucellosis 1971), it has a useful part to play in diagnosis. But it has shortcomings as a definitive test on the infective status of an animal for many reasons including the following:

1. The test detects "non-specific antibodies" as well as specific antibodies arising from *Brucella* infection and *Brucella* vaccination.
2. In the incubation stage of the disease, the test is often the last to reach diagnostically significant levels.
3. Similarly, after abortion it is often the last to reach diagnostically significant levels.
4. In the chronic stage of the disease, it tends to wane, often becoming negative when the results of some other tests may be positive.

Because, on the one hand, even cattle that have never been exposed to *Brucella* or to *Brucella* vaccines can still have low levels of agglutinins detected by the agglutination test and, on the other hand, some degree of tolerance has to be given for animals vaccinated with strain 19 vaccine, it has been difficult to get complete agreement on SAT antibody levels that can be taken as being negative and positive. In the European Economic Community (EEC) countries, serum agglutinating antibody levels less than 30 i.u. have been accepted as being negative for brucellosis; for animals of a certain age and vaccinated at prescribed ages with strain 19 vaccine, levels of 80 i.u. or over are classed as positive reactions and levels between 30 and 80 as negative as long as the complement-fixation test is negative. In the United States antibody levels of less than 50 i.u. for non-vaccinates and less than 100 i.u. for official vaccinates are accepted as negative so that a greater degree of tolerance has been allowed for official (strain 19) vaccinates. This then is given as indication of the need not to establish positive diagnostic levels too low (too many false positives) or too high (too many false negatives). Our own experience (summarized by Morgan and Richards 1974; MacKinnon 1976) has shown that the use of the SAT alone would over-condemn to the extent of around five percent of the animals and would also miss animals classified as reactors on the basis of the results of all the tests used (13 persent).

The complement-fixation (CF) test has been in use since the early part of this century but its full potential and usefulness was not realized until it was found that the test was useful in differentiating response to calfhood vaccination from that due to infection (Blagoveschtschenskaya 1954). Subsequently, it has been found that the test rarely exhibits non-specific reactions. Unlike the SAT the CF titres do not wane as the disease becomes chronic and very often the CF test reaches diagnostic levels sooner than the SAT after infection (Hill 1963; MacKinnon 1963; Jones et al. 1963; Alton et al. 1975). In addition to these factors, recent technical advances in allowing for much greater speed and accuracy in doing the more labour-intensive test and the availability and recognition of an agreed International Standard for the test (Morgan et al. 1973), have made the CF test the nearest approach to a definitive test for infection.

The rose bengal plate (RBP) or buffered *Brucella* antigen or card test is the latest test to be introduced and was originally developed in the United States by Dr. Pietz and his colleagues following the observations of Rose and Roepke (1957) that the antibody activity of "non-specific" agglutinins was destroyed at a low pH (3.6) whilst that of the "specific" antibody remained unaffected. Since then, the test has been widely evaluated in various countries and results of the test were recently extensively reviewed by Morgan and Richards (1974); MacKinnon (1976); Pilet et al. (1972); O'Reilly and Cunningham (1971) and Alton et al. (1975).

The RBP test was introduced in Britain as an official screening test in 1970 both for the Brucellosis Incentives Scheme and for the Compulsory Area Eradication testing. In Britain all sera are screened using the RBP test; those that are negative are not normally tested further; those that are positive to the RBP are then subjected to the SAT and the CFT and the results interpreted depending on the strain 19 vaccination status of the animal. Table 1 presents the results of testing 10,929 sera from animals in 158 herds with no reactors as judged by the combined use of the RBP, SAT/CFT and where no Brucella abortions had been recorded. One hundred and thirty sera (1.18 percent) were RBP positive and none was positive to either SAT or CFT but 10 showed inconclusive reactions to the CFT. The remaining 98.8 percent of the sera were negative to the RBP and 98.64 percent were also negative to the CFT with 18 (0.16 percent) showing inconclusive reactions to CFT.

Results of the comparison of the RBP, SAT and CF tests conducted on 14,749 animals in 169 herds in which reactors were found are shown in Table 2. The number (and percentage) of RBP reactors rose to 1,627 (11.03 percent); of these, 1,003 (61.6 percent) were positive to the CFT and 433 (26.6 percent were negative to the CFT. Of the 13,122 RBP negative sera, 119 (0.9 percent) were positive to the CFT.

Table 1

Comparison of the Rose Bengal Plate, Serum Tube Agglutination and Complement Fixation Tests Conducted on 10,929 Sera from 158 Herds with no Reactors

Result of SAT(1)	RBP Positive (1.18%) Result of CFT(2)			RBP Negative (98.77%) Result of CFT(2)		
	+	"0"	-	+	"0"	-
+	0	0	0	0	0	9 (0.08%)
0	0	4 (0.03%)	23 (0.21%)	0	3 (0.027%)	103 (0.94%)
-	0	6 (0.055%)	97 (0.88%)	0	15 (0.13%)	10,669 (97.6%)
Total	0	10 (0.09%)	120 (1,09%)	0	18 (0,16%)	10,781 (98,64%)

	Vaccinated	Non-Vaccinated
(1) SAT		
+	≥100 IU	≥100 IU
"0"	>50, <100 IU	>30, <100 IU
-	≤50 IU	≤30 IU
(2) CFT		
+	≥2+ at 1/10	≥2+ at 1/4
"0"	2/4 to 1/10	2/2 to 1/4
-	≤1/4	≤1/2

Table 2

Comparison of the Rose Bengal Plate, Serum Tube Agglutination and Complement Fixation Tests Conducted on 14,749 Sera from 169 Herds with Reactors

Result of SAT(1)	RBT Positive (11.03%) Result of CFT(2)			RBP Negative (88.9%) Result of CFT(2)		
	+	"0"	-	+	"0"	-
+	528 (3.6%)	4 (0.02%)	19 (0.12%)	4 (0.02%)	2 (0.01%)	5 (0.03%)
0	197 (1.3%)	32 (0.2%)	113 (0.76%)	25 (0.16%)	33 (0.22%)	210 (1.4%)
-	278 (1.88%)	155 (1.05%)	301 (2.04%)	90 (0.6%)	227 (1.5%)	12,526 (84.9%)
Total	1003 (6.8%)	191 (1.3%)	433 (2.9%)	119 (0.8%)	262 (1.77%)	12,741 (86.4%)

	Vaccinated	Non-Vaccinated
(1) SAT		
+	≥100 IU	≥100 IU
"0"	>50, <100 IU	>30, <100 IU
-	≤50 IU	≤30 IU
(2) CFT		
+	≥2+ at 1/10	≥2+ at 1/4
"0"	2/4 to 1/10	2/2 to 1/4
-	≤1/4	≤1/2

The combined totals for Tables 1 and 2 are given in Table 3. In Table 4 the results have been analysed for herds without reactors on the basis of:

1. reactors to the RBP test only.
2. reactors to the SAT only (i.e. those with ≥ 30 i.u. or vaccinates under 20 months of age with 30 to 80 i.u. in the SAT but negative to the CFT.
3. reactors on basis of the combined use of the RBP, SAT and CFT as interpreted in our brucellosis schemes.

From Table 4 it can be seen that the use of the RBP test alone is over sensitive even in herds where we believe no infection existed. These herds include a proportion of vaccinated as well as unvaccinated animals. In herds with reactors, 11 percent of the sera gave reactions to the RBP whereas 7 percent of the cattle were subsequently classified as reactors.

Under conditions as they exist in Britain the RBP test on its own is too sensitive but it can be used as an efficient and cheap screening test. The use of the SAT alone, on the criteria advised by the EEC for movement of animals, is far too sensitive in over condemning animals that can be safely retained as *Brucella*-free whilst, on the other hand, it misses a number of animals that are classed as reactors when the CFT is included.

In Table 5 are the serological results in 302 cases of abortion which were confirmed bacteriologically for *B. abortus*. The important features are that:

1. 91.4 percent were positive to RBP.
2. 88.05 percent were positive to CFT at British standard interpretation.
3. 92.68 percent were positive to CFT at EEC interpretation.
4. 66.88 percent were positive to SAT at British standard interpretation.

Table 3

Comparison of the Rose Bengal Plate, Serum Tube Agglutination and Complement Fixation Tests on a Cumulative Total of 25,678 Sera from 327 Herds (Tables 1 and 2)

Result of SAT(1)	RBT Positive (6.8%) Result of CFT (2)			RBP Negative (93.2%) Result of CFT (2)		
	+	"0"	-	+	"0"	-
+	528 (2.05%)	4 (0.01%)	19 (0.07%)	4 (0.01%)	2 (0.008%)	14 (0.05%)
0	197 (0.76%)	36 (0.14%)	136 (0.53%)	25 (0.09%)	36 (0.14%)	313 (1.2%)
-	278 (1.08%)	161 (0.63%)	398 (1.55%)	90 (0.35%)	242 (0.94%)	23,195 (90.3%)
Total	1003 (3.9%)	201 (0.78%)	553 (2.15%)	119 (0.46%)	280 (1.09%)	23,522 (91.6%)

	Vaccinated	Non-Vaccinated
(1) SAT		
+	≥100 IU	≥100 IU
"0"	>50, <100 IU	>30, <100 IU
-	≤50 IU	≤30 IU
(2) CFT		
+	≥2+ at 1/10	≥2+ at 1/4
"0"	2/4 to 1/10	2/2 to 1/4
-	≤1/4	≤1/2

Table 4

Numbers of Reactors on the Basis of Different Tests Conducted on Infected and Non-Infected Herds

Category	Number of Reactors to		
	RBP Test	SAT (1)	Combined RBP, SAT and CFT
10,929 Sera (158 herds with no reactors)	130 (1.19%)	9 (0.08%)	0 0
14,749 Sera (169 herds with reactors)	1627 (11.03%)	562 (3.8%)	1026 (6.96%)
25,678 Sera	1757 (6.8%)	571 (2.2%)	1026 (40%)

(1) SAT titres ≥ i.u. or vaccinates under 20 months - 30 to 80 i.u. SAT, neg. CFT.

Table 5

Serological Results in 302 Cases of Abortion That were Culturally Positive for *B. Abortus*

Results of SAT (1)	RBP Positive (91.4%) Result of CFT (2)			RBP Negative (8.6%) Result of CFT (2)			Total
	+	0	-	+	0	-	
+	196 (64.9%)	5 (1.6%)	0 (0.0%)	1 (1.3%)	0 (0.0%)	0 (0.0%)	202
0	53 (17.5%)	3 (0.99%)	1 (0.3%)	2 (0.66%)	0 (0.0%)	2 (0.66%)	61
-	12 (3.97%)	4 (1.3%)	2 (0.66%)	2 (0.66%)	2 (0.66%)	17 (5.6%)	39
Total	261 (86.4%)	12 (3.97%)	3 (0.99%)	5 (1.65%)	2 (0.66%)	19 (6.3%)	302

(1) and (2) See Table 1 for explanation of footnotes.

5. 87.1 percent were positive to SAT at EEC interpretation.

These figures are virtually identical for a number of surveys which have been made in a number of investigations at our laboratory.

The following are the main factors that can give rise to false reactions to the RBP test:

1. false positive reactions -
   a. vaccination with strain 19 vaccine in calfhood.
   b. vaccination with 45/20 adjuvant vaccine.
   c. maternally derived antibody.
   d. infection with _Yersinia_ _enterocolitica_ type IX (Corbel and Cullen 1970).
   e. infection with salmonella of Kauffman-White group N (Corbel 1975).
   f. human error.
2. false negative reactions -
   a. early incubative stage of the disease.
   b. immediately after abortion.
   c. variations in the rate at which tests reach positive levels.
   d. human error.

It has been observed that in the vast majority of cases following vaccination or following ingestion of maternally derived antibodies the various tests reach negative levels in the same sequence: SAT before RBP before CFT. Under certain circumstances, therefore, an animal may react only to the CF test and be negative to both the RBP and SAT. This can arise in both non-infected (vaccinated) animals as well as in, for example, early infection. Davies (1971), in an analysis of sera tested at Weybridge, estimated that the sensitivity of the RBP (i.e. its ability to recognize true positives on basis of SAT and CFT) was 96.2 percent and its specificity (i.e. its ability to give few false positive reactions) was 97.1 percent. It could be that one explanation for this is that the SAT and RBP tests are mediated by immunoglobulins against surface antigens whilst the CF test also detects subsurface and soluble antigens (Corbel 1972). In particular, after the use of 45/20 adjuvant vaccine, the agglutinated particles are often very small and tightly granular and, therefore, more difficult to detect and read. More recently Plackett and Alton (1975) reported that IgG_2 can inhibit fixation of complement by IgG_1 and IgM thus giving rise to sera reacting to the RBP (and SAT) tests but negative to the CF test. There are also cases where the tests, especially the RBP and CFT, do not always coincide in the time of appearance of positive results. Occasionally the RBP test has not become positive until days after the CFT, and occasionally the reverse takes place.

Human error is always the most difficult to measure and assess since few people will admit to having made an error. Errors can occur at the sampling, identifying, and testing stages: when decanting serum, entering and interpreting results. In spite of in-built quality controls at these stages, errors can creep in and it is for this reason that we addressed ourselves to the question of reducing the chances of errors at the laboratory stage due to fatigue and boredom when very large numbers of samples are tested daily over long periods.

We are currently in Britain testing around five million sera a year by the RBP test of which some two to five percent need further testing by the SAT and CFT. The preliminary screening is done at Veterinary Investigation Centres throughout the country and sera reacting to the RBP test are sent either to the Central Veterinary Laboratories (CVL) at Weybridge or the Laboratory at Lasswade in Scotland for SAT and CF tests. A great deal of research and development effort has been spent in conjunction with a commercial company (Vickers Medical Research organism and/or a positive specific serological response.

2. There is no single test which is guaranteed to identify all infected animals but undoubtedly the CF test is the best which is currently available.
3. A range of tests is now available for diagnosis; they should be used periodically (say every three to four months) to cover a whole pregnancy in order for animals in herds to qualify as brucellosis-free.
4. Because of technical difficulties in subjecting very large numbers of sera to the CFT it is necessary to have a reliable screening test. The RBP (BBA or card test) satisfies the criteria of being an accurate screening test, but is too sensitive to use on its own. The SAT has also a place in routine diagnosis and, alongside the CF test, it should be used as a confirmatory test for sera reacting to the screening RBP test.
5. The rose-bengal plate test is a sensitive and accurate test which lends itself easily to large scale screening of sera. If it is used as the only (or definitive) test, it is too sensitive; the degree of false positive reactions depends on herd history e.g. extent of the use of vaccines. In herds with no history of brucellosis and no reactors disclosed by our standard tests, just over one percent or 10,929 animals reacted to the RBP test. In herds with reactors, 11 percent of 14,749 animals reacted to the RBP test and approximately seven percent reacted to the CF test. Overall, we expect between two and three percent of sera to react to the RBP and to be negative on the SAT/CF confirmatory test.

The percentage of negative reactions in relation to the CF test depends on a number of factors. Generally speaking, the tests become negative in sequence: the SAT before the RBP before the CFT. In herds with reactors (Table 2) 0.8 percent of animals were RBP negative but positive to the CFT. False negative reactions to the RBP are most frequent in calves which have had colostral antibody, in the so-called "problem heifer" reactor and after vaccination with strain 45/20. True false negative reactions arise in the early incubation stage and as variations in the rate of response to the various tests in individual animals. Positive reactions to the RBP test must be supported by confirmatory tests and these should be the combined SAT and CFT. The CFT is accepted as the best definitive test available at present. Recent advances in testing techniques have enabled large numbers of sera to be tested mechanically by the RBP and SAT thus reducing chances of human error.

References

Alton, G. G.; Maw, J.; Rogerson, B. A.; and McPherson, G. G. 1975. Aust. Vet. J. 51:57.

Annonymous. 1971. 5th Report of the Joint FAO/WHO Expert Committee on Brucellosis. Wld. Hlth. Org. Tech. Rep. Ser. 1971, No. 464.

Blagoveschtschenskaya, M. K. 1954. Veterinariya Moscow 31:18.

Corbel, M. J. 1972. Vet. Rec. 90:484.

Corbel, M. J. 1975. J. Hyg. (Camb.) 75:151.

Corbel, M. J., and Cullen, G. A. 1970. J. Hyg. (Camb.) 68:519.

Davies, G. 1971. Vet. Rec. 88:447.

Gower, S. G. m.; Wright, E. C.; Davies, G.; Morgan, W. J. B.; Hopkinson, W. I.; and Gibbs, D. F. 1974. Vet. Rec. 95:544.

Hill, W. K. W. 1963. Bull. Off. Int. Epiz. 60:401.

Jones, L. M.; Hendricks, J. B.; and Berman, D. T. 1963. Am. J. Vet. Res. 24:1143.

Lapraik, R. D.; Brown, D. D.; Mann, H.; and Brand, T. 1975. Vet. Rec. 97:52.

MacKinnon, D. J. 1963. Bull. Off. Int. Epiz. 69:383.

MacKinnon, D. J. 1976. In preparation.

Morgan, W. J. B.; Davidson, I.; and Hebert, C. N. 1973. J. Biol. Stand. 1:43

Morgan, W. J. B., and Richards, R. A. 1974. Vet. Rec. 94:510.

O'Reilly, D. J., and Cunningham, B. 1971. Vet. Rec. 88:590.

Pilet, C.; Toma, B.; and André, G. 1972. Cah. Méd. Vét. 1:1.

Plackett, P., and Alton, G. G. 1975. Aust. Vet. J. 51:374.

Plommet, M.; Fensterbank, R.; Renoux, G.; Gestin, J.; and Phillipon, A. 1973. Ann. Rech. Vet. 4:419.

Rose, J. E., and Roepke, M. H. 1957. Am. J. Vet. Res. 18:530.

Stableforth, A. W. 1936. Bull. Off. Int. Epiz. 12:107.

Brucella Antigens and Serologic Test Results

Lois M. Jones

Although a number of tests are employed in the serological diagnosis of bovine brucellosis, we are still looking for the perfect test, a simple rapid test which will detect an infected animal early in the incubation period as well as at all subsequent stages of the disease. Furthermore, this test should not react with serum from vaccinated animals as it is now evident that vaccination of cattle will have to continue and increase in certain heavily infected areas. Until such a ideal test is devised, we will have to make the best possible use of those presently available.

I plan to talk briefly about what we presently know regarding the antigens and immunoglobulins which are interacting in these tests. Dr. Pietz will talk about the performance of the tests in the field and the recommended test or tests for various situations.

The research workers in Minnesota in conjunction with the USDA laboratories at Beltsville and Ames were examining the immunoglobulins for bovine brucellosis in the late 1950's and early 1960's just when rapid advances were being made in the field of immunology (Amerault et al. 1962; Rose et al. 1964; Rose and Roepke 1964). Christine Rice and her group at Hull, Canada (Rice and Boyles 1971; Rice et al. 1966) also made major contributions to our early knowledge. Certain characteristics of bovine immunoglobulins, such as large molecular weight, heat lability and sensitivity to mercaptoethanol were associated with the immunoglobulin class termed IgM. The other important immunoglobulin class found in serum was of lower molecular weight, was stable to heat and to mercaptoethanol. Two subclasses of bovine IgG were recognized: IgG_1, normally the most abundant in the serum and lacteal secretions, and IgG_2, usually present in low concentrations but can be higher under certain conditions. It was found that antibody of the IgM class was the first to appear in an immune response to infection. IgG appeared shortly thereafter, soon became the predominant class and usually persisted as long as the infection remained. In strain 19 vaccinated animals, IgM appeared first, followed as early as ten days by IgG, the IgG class decreased with time and the occasional persistent agglutinins were attributed to the IgM classes...although this has never been rigorously proved. The antibody is present in such low titer at this time that it is difficult to separate and identify. Low-titer non-specific agglutinins present in some sera from brucella-free cattle were also attributed to the IgM class...but it was never proven that they were antibodies.

Gradually the dogma emerged that the presence of serum antibody of the IgG class was indicative of infection, and IgM antibody was associated with a history of vaccination or was due to non-specific reactions. It appeared advantageous to employ tests which would detect IgG exclusively. Efforts were made to minimize the effect of IgM in the tests. This simplistic approach has been predominant for several years. But it now appears to be in error in several ways. First of all, the so-called "IgG" tests may, in fact, react with immunoglobulins other than IgG. There is now general agreement that IgM does fix complement (Levieux 1974; Rice et al. 1966). It was originally thought that IgM was not reacting in the card test but it has now been shown by several research groups to be active in this test (Allen et al. 1976; Patterson et al. 1976).

Another error was to dismiss the early IgM following infection as unimportant.

The tests which are currently in use in the United States are listed in Table 1.

Table 1

Serologic Tests for Bovine Brucellosis

Tube Agglutination
Plate Agglutination
Mercaptoethanol
Rivanol
Buffered Antigen Tests:
Card (Rose Bengal)
Rapid Screening
Buffered Plate
Complement Fixation
Cold Fixation
Warm Fixation
Anti-Globulin (Coombs)

The same particulate antigen, the whole smooth cell of *B. abortus* strain 1119-3 is employed with all the tests. All of the antigens are prepared and standardized at the Diagnostic Reagents Laboratory, Veterinary Services Laboratories, Ames (Alton et al. 1975). The cell density of the various antigens differ according to the desired sensitivity of the test. The sensitivity of each successive batch of antigen is rigidly controlled by cell density and by testing the new preparation and a standard antigen preparation in parallel with a battery of reference sera (Rose and Roepke 1964). The buffering capacity of the buffered antigens is also checked. In this way, uniform antigens are issued year after year for use throughout the United States. The methods for performing the standard and supplemental agglutination tests are also uniform.

In Europe where each country has its own antigens and methods within a smaller trading area the need for a system to compare diagnostic titers resulted in the establishment of the International Standard for anti-B. abortus serum for the tube agglutination test. Although not routinely used in the preparation of the U. S. antigen, this standard serum (1,000 i.u./ml) gives a titer of 1:1000 with our test, so a titer of 1:100 represents about 100 i.u.

IgM is a very efficient agglutinin and will be detected by the tube and plate agglutination test. The addition of 2-mercaptoethanol (ME) to the tube agglutination test will cause the cleavage of disulfide bonds of IgM and a loss in agglutinin activity. Theoretically only the IgG is detected in the ME test, but this is probably quantitative tather than qualitative. Similarly the rivanol test is supposed to reveal only IgG but results with ME and rivanol are not always identical.

The two IgG subclasses differ in their agglutinin activity. IgG_1 agglutinates poorly except in acid pH or in presence of five percent sodium chloride solution, whereas IgG_2 agglutinates in normal saline but is inhibited by acid or five percent saline (Diaz et al. 1972).

The complement-fixation test (CF) is used in several laboratories in this country, and more widely in other countries. The whole cell tube agglutination test antigen is used for the CF test. The method of performing CF tests vary greatly from lab to lab, not only in temperature or fixation, but in all steps of the procedure. Although comparison of results from lab to lab may be misleading, a given laboratory usually has great confidence in their own procedures and finds the CF test very helpful or even indispensible.

The anti-globulin test has only been used in a few special studies in the U. S. in connection with 45/20 vaccination. Dr.

Nicoletti found that the CF test was as effective as the antiglobulin test in revealing reactors following vaccination in infected herds.

To return to the buffered antigen tests--as you know the card test has been employed as the definitive test under some conditions. In other countries the buffered antigen has been adapted to a plate agglutination test or to automated systems (Miller 1971), and is used as a screening test only. A confirmatory test such as the CF test is run on all positive sera. In the U. S. alternative rapid screening tests have recently been introduced in order to reduce the number of card tests performed annually.

Some labs used the standard plate test at the first dilution only as a screening test (Table 2). It is preferable, however, to use a plate antigen which has been buffered to pH 3.65. 0.03 ml of this blue antigen is mixed with 0.08 ml of serum on the glass plate and read after eight min. in the same way as the standard plate test. The rose bengal stained antigen employed in the card test has been used with Cooke microtiter equipment. A 50 microliter drop of serum and a 25 microliter drop of antigen is placed in the well of the microtiter plate. The plate is put on the vibrator for four min. and allowed to stand at room temperature for an additional four min. before reading. The final concentration of antigen in this test is 2.7 percent which ensures a more sensitive test than the card test. In this way no potentially card test positive sera are missed with the rapid screening test. Sera positive to any of the first three tests are then tested with the card test. It would be preferable if the card test positive sera were confirmed by an additional test such as the CF test or rivanol test. But this is only done in a few places in the U. S. to date.

Although the cell density, the color of the dye and the pH of the diluent varies with each test, the same whole cell,

Table 2

Rapid Screening Tests for Bovine Brucellosis

Test	Cell Density	pH	Quantity of Serum	Quantity of Antigen	Final Conc. of Antigen
Standard Plate	11%	6.4-7	0.08 ml	0.03 ml	3.3%
Buffered Plate	11%	3.65	0.08 ml	0.03 ml	3.3%
Rapid Screening (Microtiter plate)	8%	3.65	0.05 ml	0.025 ml	2.7%
Card	8%	3.65	0.03 ml	0.03 ml	4.0%

smooth *B. abortus* strain 1119-3, is used for all the tests. The antigenic component responsible for the agglutination and CF reactions is part of the lipopolysaccharide-protein complex which can be extracted from the outer membrane of smooth *B. abortus* (Jones and Berman 1976). This complex may be analogous in some ways to the somatic antigens and endotoxins of the Enterobacteriaceae in which repeating units of polysaccharide, and the lipid component which is responsible for the endotoxic properties is also attached to core polysaccharide through KDO.

Rough *B. ovis* lacks the specific smooth somatic antigen but an R-specific antigen can be extracted which cross-reacts with *B. canis* and rough strains such as 45/20. This R-specific antigen can be employed in Ouchterlong gel precipitation or in complement fixation tests in the diagnosis of ram epididymitis (Jones et al. 1975), and has also been employed in gel precipitation with sera from cattle vaccinated with 45/20 (Diaz and Jones 1973). Recently, Miller at al. (1976) have used the R antigen in parallel with the S antigen in CF tests with sera from 45/20 vaccinated cattle. They consider this antigen a useful additional diagnostic test in connection with adult vaccination programs in infected herds or areas.

In the last five years new groups of research workers in France, England, Australia and the United States have been looking at the immunoglobulin classes in *Brucella* antisera and how they function in the serological tests (Allen et al. 1976; Beh 1973, 1974; Corbel 1972; Levieux 1974; Patterson et al. 1976). There has been some disagreement in the results because of the widely different methods chosen for analysis and because sera vary so greatly in their Ig content. As new techniques become available and as more highly trained immunochemists are employed in *Brucella* research, we will acquire a better understanding of the *Brucella* antigens and antibodies than we have today.

References

Allen, G. S.; Chappel, R. J.; Williamson, P.; and McNaught, D. J. 1976. A quantitative comparison of the sensitivity of serological tests for bovine brucellosis to different antibody classes. J. Hyg. Camb. 76:287-298.

Alton, G. G.; Jones, Lois M.; and Pietz, D. E. 1975. Laboratory techniques in brucellosis. World Health Organization Monograph Series No. 55.

Amerault, T. E.; Lambert, G.; Manthei, C. A. 1962. The heat stability of Brucella agglutinins in bovine serum. Am. J. Vet. Res. 23:1023-1026.

Beh, K. J. 1973. Distribution of Brucella antibody among immunoglobulin classes and a low molecular weight antibody fraction in serum and whey of cattle. Res. Vet. Sci. 14:381-384.

Beh, K. J. 1974. Quantitative distribution of Brucella antibody amongst immunoglobulin classes in vaccinated and infected cattle. Res. Vet. Sci. 17:1-4.

Corbel, M. J. 1972. Identification of the immunoglobulin class active in the Rose Bengal plate test for bovine brucellosis. J. Hyg. Camb. 70:779-794.

Diaz, Ramon, and Levieux, Didier. 1972. Role respectif en serologie de la brucellose bovine des antigenes et des immunoglobulines G_1 et G_2 dans les tests d'agglutination, de Coombs et au Rose Bengale ainsi que dans le phenomene de zone. C. R. Acad. Sc. Paris 274:1593-1596.

Diaz, Ramon, and Jones, Lois M. 1973. The immuno-diffusion method for the identification of cattle vaccinated with Brucella abortus strain 45/20. Vet. Rec. 93:300-302.

Jones, Lois M., and Berman, D. T. 1976. Studies of Brucella lipopolysaccharide. Int. Symposium on Brucellosis II, Rabat. Develop. Biol. Standard 31:62-67.

Jones, Lois M.; Dubray, G.; and Marly, J. 1975. Comparison of methods of diagnosis of Brucella ovis infection of rams. Ann. Rech. Veter. 6:11-22.

Levieux, D. 1974. Immunoglobulines bovines et brucellose: I, Purification des immunoglobulines et préparation de leurs antisérums spécifiques. Ann. Rech. Veter. 5:329-342.

Levieux, D. 1974. Immunoglobulines bovines et brucellose: II, Activité des IgG_1, IgG_2, et IgM du sérum dans les réactions d'agglutination, de Coombs, de fixation du complément et dans le test au Rose Bengale. Ann. Rec. Veter. 5:343-353.

Miller, J. K. 1971. Preliminary evaluation of an automated *Brucella* antibody screening system. Res. Vet. Sci. 12:199-202.

Miller, J. K.; Kelly, J. I.; and Roerink, J. H. G. 1976. A complement fixation method for quantitative differentiation of reactions to 45/20 vaccine and *Brucella* infection. Vet. Rec. 98:210-215.

Patterson, J. M.; Deyoe, B. L.; and Stone, S. S. 1976. Identification of immunoglobulins associated with complement fixation, agglutination, and low pH buffered antigen tests for brucellosis. Am. J. Vet. Res. 37:319-324.

Rice, C. E., and Boyes, B. 1971. Serum immunoglobulins in bovine brucellosis. New Zealand Vet. J. 19:146-154.

Rice, C. E.; Tailyour, J.; and Cochrane, D. 1966. Ultracentrifugal studies of sera from cattle vaccinated or naturally infected with *Brucella abortus*. Can. J. of Comp. Med. and Vet. Sci. 30:270-278.

Rose, J. E.; Lambert, G.; and Roepke, M. H. 1964. Ultracentrifugation and heat inactivation studies on seroagglutinins of pregnant heifers artificially infected with virulent *Brucella abortus*. Am. J. Vet. Res. 25:329-332.

Rose, J. E., and Roepke, M. 1957. An acidified antigen for detection of non-specific reactions in the plate-agglutination test for bovine brucellosis. Am. J. Vet. Res. 18:550-555.

Rose, J. E., and Roepke, M. H. 1964. Physichochemical studies on postvaccinal *Brucella* agglutinins in bovine serum. Am. J. Vet. Res. 25:325-328.

Rose, J. E.; Roepke, M. H.; and Briggs, D. R. 1964. Physicochemical properties of nonspecific bovine seroagglutinins for *Brucella abortus*. Am. J. Vet. Res. 25:118-121.

Brucella Antigens and Serologic Test Results

Donald Pietz

The standard agglutination (tube and plate) tests have been used for the detection and diagnosis of brucellosis of cattle since the national eradication program began in 1934. Those conducting research in brucellosis prior to and at that time recognized the deficiencies of agglutination test procedures for the diagnosis of brucellosis. After extensive research on correlating udder infection with agglutination titers, Cotton and Buck (1930) reported in 1939 that low titers (1:100 or less) rarely indicated infection; whereas, over 80 percent of the animals with titers of 1:200 or more were infected.

In 1931 the Committee on Bang's Disease of the U. S. Livestock Sanitary Association (Malcolm 1931) recommended that a uniform procedure for conducting the agglutination test be adopted, using dilutions of 1:50, 1:100 and 1:200. The committee also recommended that animals which were negative at the 1:50 dilution, be considered negative; those with titers of incomplete at 1:50 through incomplete at 1:100 be considered suspicious; and those with titers of complete at 1:100 or greater, be considered positive. However, the committee recommended that agglutination test titers be supplemented with history and clinical aspects of the disease before making a diagnosis, especially in suspicious cases. The committee also stated that interpretation of agglutination titers and subsequent diagnosis should be entrusted only to persons familiar with all aspects of Bang's Disease.

Problems in diagnosing brucellosis using the agglutination test did not deter the authorities from establishing an eradication program. That the program was successful using the standard agglutination tests, is indicated by the fact that the percent of reactors found in herds tested in the eradication program was reduced from 11.5 percent in 1935 to 0.66 percent in 1957 (USDA 1958).

Dr. Lois Jones pointed out that the standard agglutination tests detect all classes of immunoglobulins commonly found in serum; whereas, most of the other serologic tests, often referred to as supplemental tests, differ in their capacity of detecting the various classes of antibody. The acidified plate antigen (APA) test (Roepke et al. 1956) was the first supplemental test to be used for brucellosis. Originally, it was recommended that the test be used to assist in clarifying the status of animals with low agglutination test titers in non-vaccinated herds with no history or other evidence of brucellosis. In 1962 Anderson et al. reported on using the APA, 65°C. heat inactivation, rivanol and serial dilution milk ring tests, along with epidemiology and culturing, to assist in eliminating infection from brucellosis "problem" herds.

Since then other tests have been developed and many studies have been conducted to evaluate the efficacy of these tests for the diagnosis of brucellosis.

The use of supplemental tests as an aid in the diagnosis of brucellosis makes it necessary to have an even greater knowledge and understanding of all aspects of brucellosis than when only the standard agglutination tests were used. When properly used and interpreted, a more accurate diagnosis can be achieved by using supplemental tests. As an example, Nicoletti (1967) found that the efficiency of the BBA (card) test differed in herds on the basis of their history of infection. *Brucella* was isolated from 164/354 (46.3%) card test positive animals in infected herds and 20/253 (7.9%) card test positive animals in herds not known to be infected. In addition, he reported that 22 percent of the tube test negatives--card test positive and 53 percent of the tube test suspect-card test positive animals from known infected herds were culturally positive. Thus the elimination of animals, based on the card test reduced the exposure potential in known infected herds.

In experimentally infected animals, it took an average of 62 days after exposure for the tube test to detect infected animals while it only took 43 days for the BBA (card) test to detect the same animals (Author unpublished).

This evidence indicated the card test should be an effective diagnostic test for detecting early infection and thus achieve eradication more rapidly in areas where high levels of brucellosis existed. Field data (Schilf 1967) from states with a high prevalence of infection revealed 2.84 percent card test reactors during the first six months of 1967 as compared to 2.07 percent plate or tube test reactors during the first six months of 1966. However, fewer tests were required to achieve negative status with the card test. One state reported 1.6 card tests were required as compared to 3.3 plate tests and another state reported 2.18 card tests were required compared to 3.46 plate tests. Another state reported 76.1 percent of the herds negative on first retest using card test compared to 55.2 percent using plate test.

The percentage of false positive reactions or "overkill" when the BBA (card) test is used varies, depending on the conditions existing in the herd or area. In my estimation, the effectiveness of a test must be based on the end results, that is the total number of animals removed in the process of eliminating infection. Experience in the field has shown me that field personnel who removed standard agglutination test suspect animals, which certainly was over condemnation, cleaned up infected herds faster and had fewer chronically infected problem herds than those that did not (Author unpublished).

The number of false positive reactions to the BBA (card) test in areas with low levels of infection will vary, depending on the amount of vaccination and the age of vaccination with strain 19 vaccine. However, the test should not be used in a diagnostic test in these areas--only as a screening test or, when standard or buffered antigen screening tests with greater sensitivity are used, it should be used as a supplemental test. A battery of serologic tests supplemented by epidemiology and culturing, are recommended procedures in herds with evidence of brucellosis in areas with low levels of infection.

It is difficult for me to determine the percentage of false negative reactions observed when the BBA (card) test is used to test cattle for brucellosis. Since the average interval required to detect infection is shorter than with the tube test, and since the test is usually more sensitive than the other supplemental tests, false negative reactions should be rare.

Supplemental tests are recommended to support the results of the BBA test, or any other test, used to detect infection in areas with low levels of brucellosis. In this country the mercaptoethanol and rivanol tests are most commonly used because they are easier to conduct than the CF test. More than one supplemental test should be used because patterns of results differ in herds with infection from herds with "cross" reactions. Under field conditions, various biologic products, such as shipping fever, leptospirosis and mastitis bacterins have been incriminated, but workers have not been able to duplicate the results by inoculating the same products into animals under experimental conditions. By using more than one supplemental serologic test and the serial dilution milk ring test (BRT), these reactions can usually be differentiated from reactions due to brucellosis.

It is difficult to say what factors, other than vaccination with strain 19 vaccine, may cause false positive reactions to the card test. Pasteurella (Mallman 1930; Berman 1956; King 1961; Morse et al. 1953), Vibrio (Kiggens et al. 1955; Morse et al. 1953), Salmonella (Morse et al. 1953), and Yersinia (Hurvell and Lindberg 1973; Fribourg-Blanc 1971) organisms have been reported to cross react with *Brucella*. However, I know of no work that has been done to elucidate the problem these agents might cause in using the card test for the diagnosis of brucellosis.

I know of no specific factor that may cause false negative reactions to the BBA tests, except that there are animals that have excessively long incubation periods and others that abort prior to developing a serologic response. However, to my knowledge, these animals will not be detected by any of the serologic tests presently being used.

The supplemental tests can be utilized to differentiate between bovine antibody responses associated with non-*Brucella* antigens, vaccination and brucellosis; however, I want to emphasize that the tests themselves do not make that differentiation. The individual must conduct an epidemiologic investigation, perform a battery of serologic tests, conduct the serial dilution BRT and culture milk and/or tissues, and use the "pattern of results" together with the epidemiologic and culturing information to make a diagnosis.

In answering the question as to which serologic test or tests used today most accurately designate animals infected with pathogenic *B. abortus*, I again must give the answer--it depends on the conditions that exist in the herd or area. In an area with a low incidence of infection, as I stated earlier, a combination of tests is most accurate. My personal preference is to use the card, mercaptoethanol, rivanol, tube, and serial dilution milk ring tests because they are quite easy to do and

I have had experience in evaluating the results. When we have used the CF test, it usually has been in conjunction with previously mentioned tests. Rarely has it provided additional information.

In infected herds or areas with a high prevalence of infection, in my opinion, the BBA (card) test most accurately designates animals infected with B. abortus. Serologic tests are usually evaluated by comparison with the ability to isolate Brucella from the milk. This is not the most accurate method of determining the status of an animal since studies have shown that Brucella was isolated from the milk of only 45 percent of the animals from which Brucella was isolated (Nelson et al. 1966). There is considerable lag time between exposure and the development of udder infection; therefore, the less sensitive the test, the better the correlation will be with udder infection.

A more effective method of evaluating a test is to slaughter each animal at the time of the test, culture multiple tissues and compare the results with the results of each serologic test. My hypothesis is that the BBA (card) test would correlate best with the isolation results.

The brucella ring test (BRT) was first used and evaluated in the U. S. in 1958 (Roepke et al. 1950). The test was conducted on a sample obtained from two to three cans of milk of each herd. It was reported that 68 percent of the herds considered infected on the basis of serologic results, were positive to the BRT. Investigation revealed that the BRT was positive on 88 percent of the herds in which the reactor animal(s) were in production at the time of the test.

Most milk is now being stored in bulk tanks and we sometimes question what effect this has on the sensitivity of the test.

Roepke and Stiles (1970) have estimated the probability of the BRT detecting one reactor cow in different sized herds (Table 1).

Table 1

Probability of Detecting Milk from One Reactor Cow in Different Sized Herds Using Milk Ring Test

No. Cows in Production	Estimated Probability	Lower 95% Confidence Limit
1	0.993	0.975
2	0.984	0.965
4	0.967	0.950
8	0.931	0.907
12	0.871	0.825
25	0.818	0.770
50	0.696	0.653
100	0.521	0.474
200	0.389	0.343
400	0.248	0.207

Roepke and Stiles, Am. J. Vet. Res. (1970).

The effectiveness of the BRT in states with relatively small herds is demonstrated by the BRT results for Minnesota in 1975 (Table 2) (Thomas).

Table 2

BRT Data, 1975

	Minnesota	California
No. BRT Sucp. Herds	77	62
% BRT Susp. Herds	>0.1%	0.2%
No. BRT Susp. Herds Infected	6	27
% BRT Susp. Herds Infected	7.8%	44%
No. Cattle in Infected Herds	250	9461
Average No. Cattle/Infected Herd	42	350
No. Reactors Initial Test	9	118
Average No. Reactors/Infected Herd	1.5	4.4

As a result of studies by Vanderwagen, Nelson and Kimberling (unpublished), the state of California has varied the sensitivity of the BRT according to the size of the herd. The BRT is conducted on one, two or three ml of milk, or on samples collected from segments of the herd (Table 3).

Table 3

Adjustment of BRT by Herd Size

No. Animals (2 years of age or over)	BRT Sample Size
5-200	1 ml
201-500	2 ml
501-900	3 ml
901 or more	segment, each representing less than 120 lactating cows

Even by increasing the sensitivity in large herds, the BRT is not as effective in detecting infection as it is in small herds (Table 2) (Vanderwagen). However, the BRT is more effective than market cattle identification (MCI) in California (BRT - 4.4 reactors per herd; MCI - 7.7 reactors per herd). In addition, the BRT with increased sensitivity is more effective than the standard one ml test that was being used (Table 4)(Vanderwagen 1965).

Since only a small quantity of antigen (0.03 ml) is required for such a large test sample (1 to 3 ml), the BRT is a very sensitive test procedure. I know of no other test that could compare with the BRT in sensitivity and accuracy when properly used. The BRT should be conducted at least three times, and preferably four times, per year. When conducted two times per year, some cows will be lactating only during one of the tests. Therefore, only one complete herd test is

Table 4

Comparison of Herd Size to BRT Suspicious Rate and Infection Rate, California, 1965

Herd Size		BRT Suspect Rate		Infection Rate of BRT Suspect Herds	
Range	Average	Range	Average	Range	Average
41-90	63	4.1-3.7%	3.9%	24-43%	36%
130-160	145	2.3-2.1%	2.2%	41-52%	47%
180-245	220	1.5-1.3%	1.4%	60-85%	77%

obtained. When four BRT tests are done per year, it is likely that an individual cow will be missed only on one test and, therefore, three complete herd tests are obtained.

The BRT should be used only as a supplemental test on individual animals. Udder infection normally follows systemic infection and there usually is not a significant level of antibodies in the milk until after the udder is infected. Therefore, it is almost impossible to get ahead of the spread of infection by using the BRT on individual animals. California did a considerable amount of work using the whey plate test for the detection of infected animals, but the procedure proved not to be successful in eliminating brucellosis from herds (Vanderwagen).

Summary

1. There is no single best test for detecting all animals infected with virulent Brucella. Each test has deficiencies which are most evident under a particular set of circumstances. By using a battery of tests rather than relying on a single test, one can hopefully minimize the deficiencies.

2. In a total eradication effort, false negative animals to any test should be of major concern. For this reason, the margin of error should be in favor of "overkill". The likelihood of false negatives to the card test is very remote. It probably occurs only in recently infected animals which have not had time to develop a detectable serologic response and in those infected pregnant animals which develop a response only after calving.
3. It requires a considerable amount of information and work to be able to consider a card reaction as a false positive with confidence. In areas or herds where there is a high incidence of infection, card positive animals should be considered and treated as being infected until proven otherwise. In areas where the incidence of infection is low or in herds otherwise negative, card positive animals should be isolated and their status determined using a battery of tests, culturing, herd history and other information as available in making a determination on the proper disposition of an animal.
4. There is no finite procedure for determining whether or not a reaction to a test is stimulated from prior vaccination, exposure to a heterologous organism or infection. The results of a battery of tests, culturing, epidemiology and any other information available must be used in making a determination. Most importantly to coming up with the right answer is experience in properly weighing all information available. Only by using knowledge gained through training and experience can the probability of making the right decision be elevated to an acceptable level.
5. The BRT is a highly sensitive test for detecting brucellosis in an infected herd. Ways of increasing the sensitivity in large herds has been discussed. The major deficiency in the test is a failure to properly apply the

test and the principles involved. If sampling intervals are optimized, if attention is paid to details such as the type of samples collected, the way the test is conducted and if there is immediate follow-up and testing of suspicious herds, the efficiency of the test would probably approach the limit anyone could expect from a serologic procedure.

References

Anderson, R. K.; Pietz, D. E.; Nelson, C. J.; Kimberling, C. V.; and Werring, D. F. 1962. Epidemiologic studies of bovine Brucella in problem herds in Minnesota. Proc. 66th Ann. Mtg. U. S. Livestock San. Ass'n., pp. 109-118.

Berman, D. T. 1956. The effect of bacterins containing Pasteurella multicida on agglutinins for Brucella in cattle. Proc. 60th Ann. Mtg. U. S. Livestock San. Ass'n., pp. 97-103.

Cotton, W. E., and Buck, J. M. 1930. Bureau of animal industry researcher on infectious abortion. Proc. 34th Ann. Mtg. U.S. Livestock San. Ass'n., pp. 306-325.

Fribourg-Blanc, A. 1971. Immunofluorescence study of antigenic relationships between Brucella and some strains of Yersinia enterocolitica. Ann. N. Y. Acad. Sci. 177:37-38.

Hurvell, B., and Lindberg, A. A. 1973. Serological cross-reactions between different Brucella species and Yersinia enterocolitica. Acta. Path. Microbiol. 81:113-119.

Kiggens, E. M.; Plastridge, W. N.; Williams, L. F.; and Easterbrooks, H. L. 1955. Cross agglutination between Vibrio fetus and Brucella abortus. Am. J. Vet. Res. 16:291-294.

King, N. B. 1961. Effect of three shipping fever bacterins on Brucella titers in cattle. J.A.V.M.A. 139:678-680.

Malcolm, P. 1931. Reports on the committee on Bang's Disease. Proc. 35th Ann. Mtg. U.S. Livestock San. Ass'n., pp. 323-332.

Mallman, W. L. 1930. The interagglutinability of members of the Brucella and Pasteurella genera. J.A.V.M.A. 77:636-638.

Morse, E. V.; Restic, M.; Robertstad, G. W.; and Schnieder, D. W. 1953. Cross agglutination reactions among Brucella, Vibrio, and other microorganisms. Am. J. Vet. Res. 14:324-327.

Nelson, C. J.; Anderson, R. K.; Kimberling, C. V.; and Pietz, D. E. 1966. Epizootiologic factors of bovine brucellosis: Comparative bacteriologic studies of infected herds. Am. J. Vet. Res. 27:1515-1520.

Nicoletti, Paul. 1967. Utilization of the card test in brucellosis eradication. J.A.V.M.A. 151:1778-1783.

Roepke, M. H.; Paterson, K.; Driver, F. C.; Clausen, L. B.; Olson, L.; and Wentworth, J. E. 1950. The Brucella abortus ring test. Am. J. Vet. Res. 11:199-205.

Roepke, M. H.; White, T. G.; Stiles, F. C.; and Driver, F. C. 1956. Studies on a differential test for nonspecific Brucella agglutination reactions in bovine serum. Proc. 60th Ann. Mtg. U.S. Livestock San. Ass'n., pp. 109-118.

Roepke, M. H., and Stiles, F. C. 1970. Potential efficiency of the milk ring test for detection of brucellosis. Am. J. Vet. Res. 31:2145-2149.

Schilf, E. A. 1967. Brucellosis card test. Proc. 71st Ann. Mtg. U.S. Livestock San. Ass'n., pp. 93-94.

Thomas, J. E. Personal communication.

Unpublished data. Donald Pietz.

USDA, ARS, Animal Disease Eradication Division. FY 1957. Statistical tables showing progress of the eradication of brucellosis and tuberculosis in livestock in the U.S. and territories.

Vanderwagen, L. C. Personal communication.

Vanderwagen, L. C. 1965. Report written to E. F. Chastain entitled "Evaluation of BRT program."

Development and Evaluation of Serological Tests

Godfrey Alton

I have been asked to "talk to" two specific questions and would like to try to dispose of these first.

Question No. 1 is: Do we need a better test for bovine brucellosis? A number of countries have succeeded in eradicating bovine brucellosis using tests presently available. On the other hand, the epidemiological model for brucellosis eradication developed by the Veterinary Epidemiology and Preventive Medicine Unit at the University of Melbourne predicts that a slight improvement in diagnostic efficiency would pay large dividends in an eradication campaign. Particularly in the later stages of a campaign, greater specificity is required especially in distinguishing vaccinal antibodies from those resulting from infection.

The second question is whether laboratory procedures can distinguish nonspecific antibodies and those produced by vaccination, on the one hand, from those resulting from infection, on the other.

As regards nonspecific antibodies; Feinberg and Wright (1951) demonstrated that people recovered from tularaemia and people vaccinated against cholera had high serum agglutination titres against brucella antigen when the tests were incubated at 37°C whereas, these titres disappeared when the tests were incubated at 60°C. Titres in people suffering from brucellosis were very little affected by these differences in temperature. We would assume that nonspecific antibodies in cattle would behave in the same way. Assuming that the antibody destroyed by heat was IgM, then it is likely that the mercaptoethanol and rivanol tests would have given the same result as heat inactivation.

Regarding antibodies that arise following strain 19 vaccination, the development of the vaccinal infection leads to the production of IgM, IgG_1 and IgG_2 antibodies. The infection is fairly short lived and antibody levels soon fall, thus about six months after vaccination IgG_2 has disappeared from the serum but low levels of IgG_1 and IgM persist for some time longer (Beh 1974). The IgG_1 is responsible for the complement fixation reaction but presumably at six months post-inoculation the level is not high enough to give a positive reaction. The IgG_1 is a poor agglutinator so the agglutinating effect of the serum is due to IgM which may be destroyed by heating or mercaptoethanol treatment or precipitated by rivanol. Thus, from about six months after vaccination, the supplementary tests mentioned and the complement-fixation test (CFT) are negative in vaccinated animals, whereas there may be enough of the right kind of antibody present in untreated serum to cause a suspicious or a positive reaction in the buffered brucella antigen or serum agglutination tests. In animals infected with virulent Brucella higher levels of IgG_1 and IgG_2 are generally present and the CFT and the supplemental tests are likely to be positive.

There is some doubt about the part played by IgM in the CFT. Allan et al. (1976) report that IgM is very active in fixing complement but it may be inactivated by heating at 60°C in serum, whereas pure IgM is not inactivated at this temperature. Most of the supplemental tests depend on the elimination of IgM for their effect. I would like to point out, however, that IgM is the first class of immunoglobulins to appear after infection and if an eradication system, to be successful, requires the early detection and elimination of infected cattle, then these tests may suffer a disadvantage.

To summarize on this second question, it is possible to distinguish nonspecific antibodies and those that persist after strain 19 vaccination from the antibody associated with established infection, but the tests that are capable of doing this with the exception of the CFT are likely to suffer some time lag in early infections and this may account for the fact that though there have been supplemental tests available for a good many years now, none of them have really been widely accepted.

So far, we have talked about vaccination with strain 19. There have also been efforts made to distinguish antibodies resulting from vaccination with the rough strain 45/20 vaccine. Comparative tests with rough and smooth antigens have been reported for agglutination by Shimizu and Shibata (1962), for gel diffusion by Diaz and Jones (1973) and for complement fixation by Miller et al. (1976).

For the remainder of my paper I will confine myself to describing some of the test procedures that we investigated while formulating standard procedures for use in Australia.

The Buffered Brucella Antigen Tests

Many different techniques have developed for doing this test and I expect that many variations in sensitivity have arisen. What I am about to say probably does not apply to the card test as carried out in the United States. The Australian state laboratories generally conduct this test, 80 sera at a time, in a WHO haemagglutination tray. Twenty-five μl of serum are measured into each well with a sampler having a disposable tip. When all the sera have been dispensed, 25 μl of antigen is dropped into each well. The plate is rotated by hand on the bench vigorously for a few seconds then placed in a rotary agglutinator as shown. After four minutes, the tests are read over a white light and positive reactions are noted as 1+, 2+, and 3+ according to the degree of the reaction. The test is evaluated very severely since it is a screen test and the sera positive to the rose bengal test are retested by the CFT. The proportion of rose bengal reactors that react to the CFT varies, mostly due to the varying levels of strain 19 vaccination. Over-all, perhaps one CFT positive emerges from every three rose bengal reactors. In the State of Victoria, owing to compulsory strain 19 vaccination, currently about 12 percent of cattle tested are reacting to the rose bengal test and 2.5 percent to the CFT. We believe that the rose bengal test misses very few infected cattle.

The Serum Agglutination Test

This test has been the sole diagnostic procedure used in successful eradication campaigns from Norway to Tasmania. There has, however, been a good deal of evidence presented indicating that this test is by no means the most effective for the diagnosis of brucellosis in individual cattle. Nicoletti and Muraschi (1966) reported that the agglutination test failed to classify 39 percent of culture-positive cattle as reactors. In a later article, Nicoletti (1969) reported that the agglutination test failed to classify correctly 48 percent of another group of culture-positive cattle. The results of our own investigations in Australia (Alton et al. 1975) using the European rather than the USDA technique for the test supported those of Dr. Nicoletti. We found that 11 percent of culture-positive cattle had less than 100 i.u. of antibody per ml of serum and four percent had less than 30 i.u. The work of Renoux et al. (1971) also supports these findings and the same authors also observed that the agglutination test was rather late in becoming positive following infection. The CFT generally becomes positive sooner, a fact also observed by Morgan (1974). The work quoted also demonstrates what I think has been acknowledged for a long time, that the agglutination test gives many more indeterminate reactions than does, for example, the CFT or some of the so-called supplemental tests, especially in areas where strain 19 vaccination is practiced. It is also an established fact that the agglutination test stays positive longer in strain 19 vaccinated animals than some of the other diagnostic tests e.g. the CFT and most of the supplemental tests.

The agglutination test is much less affected by previous vaccination with 45/20 adjuvant vaccines than is the CFT. Also, if used alongside the CFT, as is done in Britain, the agglutination test must have value since the weakness of the complement fixation test, at least with the techniques using warm fixation is the occurrence of prozones and, as will be described later, these prozoning sera, by their very nature, are good agglutinating sera. We feel that apart from these two situations the use of the agglutination test is difficult to justify especially in an area where strain 19 vaccination is being practiced.

The Complement-Fixation Test

The CFT is a complicated procedure and perhaps in the early days of brucellosis eradication was considered too difficult for the mass testing of cattle in eradication campaigns. Information accumulated over the years (Burki 1963; MacKinnon 1963; Nicoletti and Muraschi 1966; Nicoletti 1969; Morgan 1974; Alton et al. 1975) has indicated that this test is more specific than the agglutination test and is especially useful in cattle that have been vaccinated with strain 19 vaccine. Improvements in the technique of the test and especially the development of automated micro-methods have increased enormously the reproducibility of the test and the number of sera that can be handled by each worker.

There are a number of different techniques available for the CFT and for anyone starting to use this test I would recommend the United States Department of Health, Education, and Welfare's Public Health Monograph No. 74, first printed in 1965, as essential reading. The test can be done in tubes in any desired volume; a total volume of one ml is convenient. The test may be done in this volume in WHO haemaglutination plates. The development of the microtiter system, however, allows a variety of mechanical aids to be applied to the system and also minimise the quantities of reagents used. Titrations are usually done in tubes in total volumes of one milliliter even when the microtiter system is used in the diagnostic test.

The first part of the test, the reaction involving serum, antigen and complement, may be done either at 37°C for one hour or in the refrigerator overnight. When there are only a few samples to be tested, there is little doubt that fixation in the cold is preferable, it gives higher titres and is much less liable to give prozones. However, laboratories using complement-fixation on a large scale in eradication programmes invariably use warm fixation. It is more convenient, if only because there are only four overnights in a five-day working week.

One of the drawbacks of the CFT is its dependence on the use of an accurately titrated quantity of complement and, unfortunately, complement is the most fragile reagent involved. The serologist, in deciding on a method for titrating complement, has the choice between using a chosen number of units based on the amount of complement required to lyse 100 percent of the erythrocytes in the system or a number of units based on the amount of complement required to lyse 50 percent of the erythrocytes present. We believe that the 50 percent unit is the more accurately definable quantity of complement and this is what we use.

The Australian veterinary laboratories have agreed on a standard complement-fixation procedure. Let me describe briefly how this is done; details are about to be published in the Australian Veterinary Journal. The test is done in micro-titer plates and the total volume is 0.1 ml (25 μl of each reagent: serum, antigen, complement and haemolytic system); the various reagents used are titrated in tubes in one ml volumes. Successive samples of serum are placed in successive first wells in the microtiter plate, 12 sera per plate. The serum does not need to be measured but must be at least 50 μl to allow the mechanical diluter to pick up efficiently. The row of first wells containing serum is taped with a strip of cellotape and placed in a hot-air oven for 30 minutes at 58°C; the oven should be fitted with a fan. After inactivation, diluent is added to all wells except those containing serum and the serum is diluted mechanically right across the plate. The second well of each row contains a 1:2 dilution of serum; it acts as an anti-complementary control and receives diluent instead of antigen, and, of course, complement. The test proper begins at the third well in which the serum dilution is 1:4 and extends to the eight and last well (serum dilution 1:128). Antigen and complement (five, 50 percent haemolytic units) are added to all wells from the third in each row to the end. The plates are placed in a bacteriological incubator at 37°C for 30 minutes after which the haemolytic system is added. The plates are then incubated for a further 30 minutes at 37°C this time on a shaker. Except during the inactivation of the serum the plates are not taped. The results are read after centrifuging the plates or allowing them to stand in the refrigerator for at least two hours. They may be read from above over a white light or from below using a magnifying mirror. A reaction at 1:4 may be considered as positive or negative at the discretion of the attending veterinarian; normally when definite reactors are present in the herd a reaction at 1:4 would be considered positive. A reaction at 1:8 is always considered to be positive.

Prozones in the Complement-Fixation Test

A prozone is a series of reactions in which some of the lower dilutions (more concentrated serum) are negative and one or more higher dilutions is positive. We believe (Plackett and Alton 1975) that in bovine serum this is usually due to non-complement fixing antibody of the immunoglobulin sub-class IgG_2 interfering with the activity of the complement-fixing sub-class IgG_1 In fact, if there is enough IgG_2 present in the serum of a Brucella-infected animal then the complement-fixing activity of the IgG_1 may be suppressed and the CF test is negative. The prozone phenomenon is more evident when warm fixation is used. It is, however, very rare for the reaction to be totally suppressed.

The effect of mixing fractions containing complement-fixing antibody (IgG_1) with various quantities of non-complement-fixing antibody (IgG_2) can be expressed in agglutinating units since IgG_2 is invariably a good agglutinating antibody. This data shows prozones are more easily produced with warm fixation but not entirely absent with cold fixation.

Increasing the concentration of the antigen in the CF test reduces the extent of the prozone, but this is not a practical solution since the sensitivity of the test is thereby reduced to an unacceptable degree. The prozone problem is greatly reduced by adopting the cold, overnight fixation method in routine testing, but I have never found any laboratory handling large numbers of bovine sera that was prepared to change from warm to cold fixation. What several diagnostic laboratories in Australia are prepared to do is to separate those sera that give a 3+ reaction to the rose bengal test and are negative on the warm CF test and to retest them with the cold fixation technique. Consideration of how the problem of prozones could be overcome led to the development of a new and simpler haemolytic test which I shall now describe.

The Indirect Haemolysis Test for Bovine Brucellosis (IHLT) (Plackett et al. 1976)

This test depends on the fact that a brucella lipopolysaccharide antigen will attach itself to an erythrocyte. If this coated erythrocyte comes in contact with a complement-fixing specific anti-brucella antibody in the presence of excess complement it will lyse. In the absence of specific antibody it will not lyse. All the reagents can be added at the same time and prozones do not occur; an additional advantage is that the sensitivity of the test does not depend on the presence of an accurately titrated amount of complement as does the CFT. Bovine erythrocytes from an animal lacking the J factor are normally used for testing bovine sera in the IHLT. Larger quantities of complement are used than in the CF test and this requires a microtiter system; however, the test is conveniently done in this system. The necessity for coating erythrocytes daily is a drawback. The IHLT has the advantage that it is very little affected by vaccination by strain 19. Figures given in the original publication suggest that cattle vaccinated by strain 19 will be completely negative by eight weeks, at most, after vaccination. In animals vaccinated with 45/20 adjuvant vaccines, on the other hand, the IHLT remains positive longer than the agglutination test or the CFT. This test needs more evaluation but all the work that we have done since the original publication suggests that it may eventually prove to be a better diagnostic test than we mentioned at the beginning.

Evaluation of Serological Methods

There seem to be three main ways of going about evaluation of serologic methods. The first is to compare a new method with an established method using large numbers of serum samples, some from known free herds and others from infected herds, without the infection status of each individual animal being known. This method suffers from the obvious defect that where the tests give different results on individual animals it is generally not known which test is giving the right result. However, meaningful conclusions have been arrived at.

The second method is to try to establish bacteriologically the infection status of the animal whose serum is being used. There are certain problems associated with this method. When animals are found to be negative at autopsy there is always a doubt about the effectiveness of the culture methods, and even with those animals from which a few brucellae are isolated, one doesn't know whether or not they would ever be capable of infecting other contact cattle.

The third method is but an idea; I don't know if anyone has tried it. Surely if you wish to determine which of two methods is best at doing a specific job, the logical way would be to try them both under identical conditions. That is, carry out a test and slaughter campaign on a certain number of herds using one method and an equal number of similar herds using the other. If all other things could be made equal except the tests, significant differences in performance should be detectable.

References

Allan, G. S.; Chappel, R. J.; Williamson, P.; McNaught, D. J. 1976. J. Hyg. Camb. 76:287-298.

Alton, G. G.; Maw, J.; Rogerson, B. A.; and McPherson, G. G. 1975. Aust. Vet. J. 51:57-63.

Anonymous. 1965. HEW Public Health Monograph No. 74.

Beh, K. J. 1974. Res. Vet. Sci. 17:1-4.

Büki, F. 1963. Bull. Off. Int. Epiz. 60:419-432.

Feinberg, R. J., Wright, G. G. 1951. J. Immunol. 67:115-122.

MacKinnon, D. J. 1963. Bull. Off. Int. Epiz. 60:383-400.

Miller, J. K.; Kelly, J. I.; Roerink, J. H. G. 1976. Vet. Rec. 98:210-215.

Morgan, J. W. B. 1974. Vet. Rec. 74:510-517.

Nicoletti, P., Muraschi, T. F. 1966. Am. J. Vet. Res. 27: 689-694.

Nicoletti, P. 1969. Am. J. Vet. Res. 30:1811-1816.

Plackett, P., Alton, G. G. 1975. Aust. Vet. J. 51:374.

Plackett, P.; Cottew, G. S.; and Best, S. J. 1976. Aust. Vet. J. 52:136-140.

Renoux, G.; Plommet, M.; Philipon, A. 1971. Ann. Rech. Vétér. 2:159-171.

Shimizu, T, Shibata, S. 1962. Nat. Inst. Anim. Hlth, Quart. 2(1):15-20.

Use of 45/20 Bacterin to Detect Latent Infection in Brucellosis

Paul Nicoletti

The variable incubation period of brucellosis has been recognized for decades. Cows may be infected early in pregnancy and exhibit no serologic or clinical evidences until abortion in late gestation or after a normal but infected parturition. Young heifers may have similar syndromes. A practical method to detect latent carriers of Brucella infections would be a most valuable asset in the elimination of the disease.

Tacken in 1964 suggested that inoculation of strain 19 vaccine or a killed adjuvant vaccine would produce a stronger and more lasting reaction on the complement fixation test in infected heifers. He concluded that the procedure salvaged 519 of 554 young cattle on 70 farms which would have been slaughtered when depopulating infected herds.

In a series of papers, Cunningham (1968; 1970) and Cunningham and O'Connor (1971) reported on studies using the anamnestic system on artificially or naturally exposed cattle and strain 19 vaccinates. The experiments were based upon the following principle. Exposure to smooth strains of Brucella results in a serologic priming (Figure 1). These cattle under field conditions would be in one or more of the following categories:

1. Strain 19 vaccinates.
2. Exposed to field strains with subsequent infection.
3. Exposed to field strains with resistance to infection.

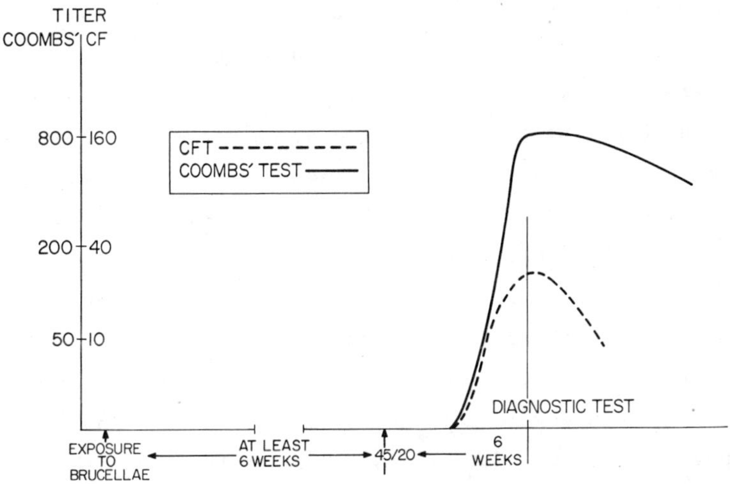

Figure 1. The Anamnestic Test

After a suggested period of at least six weeks for priming or sensitization to develop (Cunningham 1968), an injection of 45/20 vaccine results in a secondary type serologic response with maximum titers at approximately six weeks post-inoculation. The Coombs or complement fixation (CF) tests are performed. Complete agglutinins are usually not present or are in low titers on conventional tests.

The effect of 45/20 vaccination was studied by Cunningham (1968) on 18 heifers which had been exposed to an infective dose of virulent strain 544. The heifers were divided into three groups and inoculated with 45/20 three to eight months after exposure. Seventeen of the 18 heifers had positive Coombs test titers and 15 were CF test positive. He concluded that the level of Coombs titer following a single injection of 45/20 adjuvant vaccine may be used as a highly accurate diagnostic test in previously unvaccinated cattle. Following a second injection of 45/20, the CF and Coombs tests would have little practical diagnostic value.

In an expansion of earlier studies, Cunningham (1970) inoculated three groups of heifers with 45/20 vaccine. Group A was heifers which had been vaccinated as calves with strain 19, group B was eight heifers vaccinated as calves with strain 19 and challenged with virulent strain 544. Group C was 14 previously unvaccinated heifers which were also exposed to virulent strain 544. All cattle were inoculated with two doses of 45/20 vaccine. In Group A all 12 strain 19 vaccinated heifers developed high Coombs and CF titers after one injection of 45/20. Similar results were obtained with Group B. In Group C, all 14 heifers developed high Coombs test titers and 12 developed positive CF test titers. None of these cattle were apparently infected.

We recently examined the sensitivity of the anamnestic procedures under field conditions on strain 19 vaccinates (Nicoletti, in publication). A total of 79 strain 19 vaccinated cattle in three herds were given 45/20 vaccine and 16 (20 percent) were CF test positive and 20 (25 percent) were Coombs test positive by the criteria used for classification. The variations between controlled and field conditions, such as differences in exposure and calf vaccination methods, could explain the wide range of percentages of strain 19 vaccinates responding to anamnestic tests.

The use of 45/20 bacterin as a diagnostic aid in large herds was reported by Reid and Harvey. Three large herds were studied. In a herd of 522, 67 or 13 percent were slaughtered after they were positive to anamnestic tests. In another herd, a subgroup of 354 cattle was inoculated and approximately ten percent were reactors. The third herd was divided and in 125 cattle, 56 positive CF reactors were slaughtered. The unmated heifers were also inoculated and 143 of 1443 (10 percent) were reactors on the first or second CF test after inoculation. Twenty-nine heifers were eventually slaughtered when the CF titers persisted. The authors concluded that the anamnestic procedure was very useful in eliminating infection in all the herds studied. The procedure was later expanded to examinations of imported cattle to hopefully detect latent infections.

A large number of problem herds were studied by Cunningham and O'Connor (1971). The 53 herds contained a total of 879 cattle which were subjected to the anamnestic test. Of these, 226 (26 percent) were judged to be reactors on the Coombs test. An additional 78 cattle (9 percent) were considered suspicious and 43 of those were eventually slaughtered. A total of 275 of 879 (31 percent) of the cattle were removed on the results of the anamnestic and further tests. Although some problems arose in a few herds, the procedure was considered highly successful in eliminating infection.

None of the reported studies using 45/20 vaccine as a diagnostic aid included bacteriologic studies on slaughtered cattle to examine the sensitivity and specificity of the procedure or to compare the Coombs and CF tests. In an attempt to resolve some of these questions, we studied four infected herds (Nicoletti). Cattle were tested using conventional tests and reactors to the rivanol test were removed. The remaining cattle were inoculated with 45/20. An anamnestic test was performed six to seven weeks post-inoculation and cows with positive titers on CF and/or Coombs tests were purchased for further serologic and bacteriologic studies. A total of 319 cows in these herds received 45/20 bacterin and 64 (20 percent) were Coombs test positive. Fifty of the 64 or 16 percent of the total were CF test positive. In addition, in one herd, five bulls were inoculated and three had positive Coombs but no CF test titers.

Isolation facilities for individual cattle did not exist for cows purchased from two of the four herds and it was possible that transmission occurred among cattle after purchase from one herd. Twelve cows were culture positive within three to four weeks after purchase. An additional six cows were culture positive at various intervals of up to six months after the cattle were purchased. All 12 culture positive cows which were sold within one month after purchase were positive on both CF and Coombs test at the time of purchase. Therefore, 12 of 50 (24 percent) of the CF positive and 12 of 64 (19 percent) of the Coombs test positive cattle were considered infected when purchased. No conclusions can be made about the other six culture positive cows.

Several serologic tests were performed at intervals on all purchased cows. These included the plate, tube, card, mercaptoethanol, rivanol, CF, and Coombs tests. The rivanol test proved to be the best indicator of culture findings.

Five herds in Mississippi and Texas have been studied using 45/20 vaccine in an anamnestic system. Epidemiologic and serologic details will be published elsewhere. Some of the effects of the procedures may be summarized.

Herd No.	Herd Size*	No. Reactors*	No. Cows Inoculated	Anamnestic Test Reactors	No. Additional Reactors**	Remarks
1	154	21	121	33	16	- Abortion immediately prior to anamnestic test.
2	48	2	46	7	0	- Herd apparently free at time of anamnestic test.
3	57	2	54	13	4	- Reactor calved within 2 weeks of 45/20 inoculation.

Herd No.	Herd Size*	No. Reactors*	No. Cows Inoculated	Anamnestic Test Reactors	No. Additional Reactors**	Remarks
4	100	2	98	11	5	Reactor calved between inoculation and anamnestic test.
5	82	2	80	12	4	Reactor with young calf at time of inoculation.

* At time of 45/20 inoculation ** On subsequent herd tests.

Herd 1 was sold for slaughter approximately one year after the anamnestic test. One reactor was found on a herd test immediately before sale of the herd.

Exposure prior to the inoculation of 45/20 and before the anamnestic test is the probable explanation for additional reactors in herds 1, 3, 4, and 5. The last reactors were removed from herds 3, 4, and 5 after six, four, six months, respectively. Cattle in all herds were given a second injection of 45/20 bacterin at seven weeks (herds 3, 4, and 5) or 12 weeks (herds 1 and 2) after the first inoculation. The effects upon the elimination of brucellosis from herds 3, 4, and 5 are unknown.

The timing of the diagnostic procedure using 45/20 vaccine is based on an assumption that it may take up to six weeks for an animal to be sensitized, or primed, by field exposure to *Brucella abortus* (Cunningham and O'Connor 1971). The added six weeks from the time of inoculation of 45/20 until serologic tests are performed permits a period for infected cattle to possibly expose other cattle. An alteration of the anamnestic system, such as a specific skin allergen, could prove very useful.

It is obvious that controlled breeding is necessary for the

principle of anamnesis in diagnosis to have maximal effects. Unfortunately, most dairy and beef herds do not follow this practice.

Perhaps research will provide a more practical method of diagnosis of latent Brucella infections and also solve additional problems in brucellosis control.

References

Cunningham, Brendan. 1968. Serological response in cattle following vaccination with S. 19 and killed Brucella 45/20 adjuvant vaccine. Vet. Rec. 82:3-7.

Cunningham, Brendan. 1970. Vaccination of cattle with killed 45/20 adjuvant vaccine: Effects on serological and milk ring tests when used in cattle previously exposed to infection or vaccinated with S. 19. Vet. Rec. 86:2-7.

Cunningham, Brendan, and O'Connor, Michael. 1971. The use of killed 45/20 adjuvant vaccine as a diagnostic agent in the final stages of the eradication of brucellosis: The clearance of brucellosis from problem herds by interpretation of anamnestic serological responses. Vet. Rec. 89:680-686.

Nicoletti, Paul. A bacteriologic and serologic study of cows responding to Brucella strain 45/20 vaccine in an anamnestic system. Submitted for publication.

Reid, M. A., and Harvey, P. R. 1972. The use of Brucella abortus 45/20 adjuvant vaccine as a diagnostic aid in the brucellosis eradication campaign in Papua, New Guinea. Aust. Vet. J. 48:495-499.

Tacken, P. H. W. Vaccination of young calves as an aid to detect infection with Brucella abortus Bang during youth. T. Diergeneesk. 89:1703-1708. Abs. 2883 in Vet. Bull. 35 (1965).

Diagnosis Discussion

DR. NEVILLE CLARKE (Texas A&M): To initiate our discussion, I will try to briefly summarize the papers in this session in the context of the key questions which were posed to the speakers. As regards a standard of reference for defining an animal infected with brucellosis, the unassailable method is to culture the organism, although failure to do so is not definitive proof of lack of infection. There are batteries of serological tests used in different countries that are more or less recognized as standard without there really being recognized international standards. All speakers agree that multiple tests increase the confidence in the diagnosis, and that sequential tests over time also provide better insight than single tests. All speakers agree that supplemental serological tests are needed to accurately designate animals as being infected with *B. abortus* by serology. There is agreement as to the utility of screening tests such as the rose-bengal or card test provided supplemental tests are used. The complement-fixation test is the supplemental procedure of choice in most countries other than the United States, where the rivanol and mercaptoethanol supplemental tests are preferred for most uses. Some of the differences in opinion result from variations in procedure and interpretation; there is some evidence the complement-fixation test may become negative sooner than other tests after adult vaccination. The rivanol and mercaptoethanol tests are simpler to conduct.

EDITORS NOTE: As was pointed in later discussion, there continues to arise confusion over terminology in speaking of evaluation of diagnostic tests. The following simple chart and example are inserted here to clarify communications:

		Disease Status	
		Infected	Non-Infected
Test Result	positive	true positive	false positive
	negative	false negative	true negative

$$\text{Sensitivity} = \frac{\text{true positive}}{\text{true positive + false negative}} \text{ X } 100$$

$$\text{Specificity} = \frac{\text{true negative}}{\text{true negative + false positive}} \text{ X } 100$$

$$\text{Overkill} = \frac{\text{false positive}}{\text{true negative + false positive}} \text{ X } 100$$

Overkill is not, as is sometimes stated, the percent of test positives that are demonstrated to be false positives.

For Example: If 100 cattle were tested and ten positive sera were identified; and if subsequently, seven of the ten were confirmed as being positive with supplemental tests and all test negatives were true negatives, then the following would be the results:

Sensitivity = 7/7+0 X 100 = 100%

Specificity = 90/90+3 X 100 = 97%

Overkill = 3/90+3 X 100 = 3%

The buffered brucella antigen (BBA) test is used in one form or another by most countries as an initial screening tool. "Overkill" using the card or rose-bengal test was estimated to vary between one and three percent, depending on the level of infection and vaccination history in the herd. False negative reactions were estimated to be of the order of one to two percent. All speakers agree that supplemental tests are needed to support results of the BBA test. Dr. Morgan specifically addressed the question of factors causing false positive and negative reactions to diagnostic tests. Other than residual antibody activity from vaccination, false positive reactions are observed in association with ingestion of colostrum from infected dams, cross reaction with certain bacteria and human error. False negative reactions are observed during early incubation of the disease, immediately after abortion, as a result of variations in rate to achieve detectable positive level of antibody and human error. There was uniform agreement among the speakers that a better test is needed for diagnosis of brucellosis, particularly for detecting the latently infected animal or the infected animal soon after abortion. A more specific test is needed to avoid overkill and there is need for doing a better job of separating the infected animal from the vaccinate. Although better diagnostic methods are advocated, most speakers believe that experienced use of the battery of available tests will allow differentiation between infected and vaccinated animals and that these methods are sufficient to justify proceeding with national eradication programs. Dr. Pietz covered the brucella ring test (BRT), citing data to show its sensitivity as a function of sample size, including samples from individual cows. Dr. Nicoletti stated that strain 45/20 vaccine has use under carefully controlled conditions as a diagnostic tool. The anamnestic response to this vaccine may be used to improve detection of the latently infected animal, although intercurrent use of strain 19 vaccine tends to confound results.

This is obviously a very superficial set of generalizations to a very detailed and comprehensive group of presentations. Its main purpose, other than to summarize, is to focus discussion into the more controversial, and, therefore, more interesting areas. To this end, I would like the speakers to come back again to the issue of choice of serologic supplemental tests. Specifically, could you address the comparison between the complement fixation test and the other supplemental tests such as the rivanol and mercaptoethanol procedures?

DR. LOIS JONES (University of Wisconsin): We have some data on the complement fixation test, comparing its performance with bacteriological examinations of milk. It is an unpublished collection of data made some years ago which Dr. Berman is prepared to give.

DR. DAVID BERMAN (University of Wisconsin): May I first compliment the moderator on the summary. I think it was admirably done. What I would like to emphasize, as has been previously done, is that we tend to get bogged down in details of procedures on diagnostic tests and neglect, to some degree, the necessity of understanding the circumstances under which they are to be applied. If we are dealing with areas in which there is a high prevalence of infection with vaccination, then we have to look at the results of our tests in one way; if we are dealing in areas in which there is a low prevalence of infection with vaccination, we have to look at the results of our tests in another fashion. When we talk about the complement fixation (CF) test, as came out in an earlier discussion, we are really talking about data from a series of CF tests. No two of us conduct the test exactly alike even though sometimes we say we do. And this is not all bad. It is not all bad simply because when a laboratory has worked out, with adequate cultural backstopping, the limits and characteristics of its CF test, then the test can be usefully employed. (Editor's note: The following material was provided by Dr. Berman after the symposium for inclusion below.)

Published data on the relative efficiency of the standard tube agglutination test (SAT) and the complement fixation (CF) test in identifying infected cows are relatively scarce. I want to present some unpublished data accumulated from 1960-65 by Drs. Joe Hendricks, Brian Espe, Lois Jones, and myself. This was a time when Wisconsin was moving from modified-certified status to certified-free status (achieved in 1965) and during which intensive problem herd work was in progress. The CF test is the one described by us (Jones, Hendricks and Berman 1963). The relationship of SAT titers and isolation of B. abortus from milk only, from 623 cows, vaccinated as calves with strain 19 is shown in Table 1.

Table 1

Relationship of SAT Titers and Isolation of B. Abortus from Milk of Vaccinated Cows in Infected Herds

Titer	Number	Brucella +	Brucella -
0-I 50	78	2	76
50-I 100	121	14	107
100-I 200	154	24	130
≥ 200	270	95	175
Total	623	135	488

It can be seen that approximately 12 percent of the cultures (16 of 135 isolations) were isolated from cows with titers of incomplete 100 or less. The CF test results are shown in Table 2 for the same 623 cows. It is clear that bacteriologically proved infection was found in only one animal with a CF less than 2+ at 1:40.

Table 2

Relationship of CF Test Reactions and Isolation of *B. Abortus* from Milk of Vaccinated Cows in Infected Herds

Titer	Attempts	Isolations
0 -1(20)[1]	238	0
2(20) -1(40)	82	1
$\geqq$ 2(40)	303	134
	623	135

[1]Figures represent degree of fixation (at dilution of serum).

It should be emphasized that this represents only a single attempt at isolation and from milk only, and it is to be anticipated that more intensive bacteriological investigation would disclose somewhat higher infection rates in these animals. However, the distribution of rates of infection among CF titer groups is not likely to be greatly influenced, as shown in Table 3 which contains data from animals, in infected herds,

Table 3

Relationship of CF Test Reactions and Isolation of *B. Abortus* from Milk and Tissues of Vaccinated and Unvaccinated Cows in Infected Herds

Titer	Attempts	Isolations
0 - 1(20)	55	2
2(20) - 1(40)	30	7
$\geqq$ 2(40)	293	224
	378	233

whose tissues were also cultured if *Brucella* had not been isolated from the milk. These animals were all selected on the basis of positive or suspicious reactions of any of the serological tests.

Several salient points may be derived from these data, as well as the experience in Wisconsin and elsewhere in applying them to decisions in classifying animals in the eradication program. First, the CF test identifies infected animals more efficiently than the SAT; secondly, it is possible to set a CF titer tolerance for officially vaccinated animals in infected herds with a low probability that they will prove to be infected with virulent organisms. The operational decision as to what titer is used will depend on many factors such as: extent of infection in the herd, number and frequency of previous tests, traffic of animals into and out of the herd, etc.

DR. CLARKE: Thank you very much. Dr. Morgan, would you speak to this question too, please, sir?

DR. BRINLEY MORGAN (Weybridge, England): Thank you very much. I would like to reiterate what the last speaker has said. I have found in my experience over the last twenty-five years working with *Brucella* that you are invariably wearing at least two hats. One is where you are in a very clean environment where you can take an awful lot of chances and the other hat is where you are working in an infected environment where you cannot afford to take any chances at all. There is also, I think, a marked difference as to whether you are in effect in the process of actively eradicating the disease or you are in the fortunate position where you have eradicated the disease and are only concerned with the movement of animals. You can afford to have different criteria for the two things: one for the interstate movement of animals; and another for the actual eradication of the disease. On the question of difference in use of diagnostic tests, I think the difference is partly in the way we do the test. I think there are two types of complement people. There are the cold fixers and there are the hot fixers.

We did an international exercise some years ago at my laboratory comparing the tests against the standard reference serum and I think at the end of the day it showed there was not any real basic difference as to whether you were a cold fixer or a hot fixer, but I am quite sure that part of the difference between Dr. Jones and myself is based in effect on a different diagnostic level of tests. We classify as infected animals those which are non-vaccinated with CF titers of more than 1:4. And our evidence is based on the correlation between this and actual infection. Dr. Jones mentioned using as the diagnostic criterion a positive reaction at 1:40 and I think this gives us the level of difference that we are finding. Similarly, this explains the apparent difference as to which of the tests become negative first, second, last and so on. I think the apparent difference again between us is basically due to the fact that although we are talking about the CF test, this can give the impression that we are talking about the same test. We are talking about a range of tests of varying degrees of sensitivities and so on. And I am quite sure that this is the basic difference between us. Now, I think it is essential for us to resolve it. Certainly in Europe where we have within the European Economic Community (EEC) regulations defining animals as positive and negative and so on, we have really very quickly had to come to grips to sort out the differences between ourselves. Nobody likes to change their minds, their method of interpretation or the way they have traditionally been used to doing tests. There comes a time when somebody has got to change. I would like to make a plea that in all our interpretations of these tests that as much use as possible be made of the International Standard Anti-*Brucella abortus* Serum. It is widely accepted for the agglutination test. It is also widely available and suitable for correlating and interpretating the results of the CF test. I would make a plea that this must be done.

DR. CLARKE: I wonder if I could ask Dr. Pietz to comment on the comparison between the mercaptoethanol and rivanol tests and the complement fixation (CF) test. As all of you know, we in the United States are using the former two routinely now. They are easily applied in laboratories that are not terribly sophisticated.

DR. DONALD PIETZ (USDA, Iowa): I do not think there is a tremendous amount of difference between using a battery of supplemental agglutination tests and what you get using CF tests. However, as it has been pointed out before, you need to have the technical capability of doing a CF test and your probability of getting erroneous results using that test is much greater, I think, than using the more simplified test. As Dr. Alton pointed out, there are potential problems with prozone type reactions, which we have noted with warm fixation for years in our laboratories. If you are going to rely only on the CF test and a screening test, I think you are in trouble. This is why we have always used a battery of tests because if you are looking at the results of a battery of tests, you can pretty well determine what is probably going on in that herd and/or animal. As I mentioned in my presentation, the tests themselves do not make the diagnosis, you do. It is necessary to take a lot of things in consideration and I would not have any problems in using the CF test as one of the battery, but I would not use it alone.

DR. MORGAN: But there is no question of using it on its own, and I do not think anybody has said that we only use the CF test. I would really query, too, whether you need the implied degree of sophistication for doing the CF test, especially with the terrific advances now available in getting reproducible complement standard antigens, reference positive and negative sera and so on. And I would see no real difficulty in this becoming widely used as one of the tests that can be done. The prozone thing, I think, needs to be kept in some degree of perspective. We come across them, but as the exception rather than something that we see very frequently. And, we see them because we do not do a single CF test. We do at least four dilutions, but we also do the serum agglutination test along side it and we can easily pick these out because the serum is positive on rose-bengal test with a high agglutination titer and a negative CF test. When this occurs, clearly something has gone wrong. Only sometimes it is the prozone and sometimes it is straight human error. I think we need to be terribly careful in having built in quality controls all along the line. Otherwise, I think we are in danger of trying to find highly detailed sophisticated scientific reasons for just somebody's having transcribed results incorrectly.

DR. CLARKE: Have there been side by side comparisons in recent times of the modern innovation of the complement fixation test with the other tests? Could you address that please, Dr. Nicoletti?

DR. PAUL NICOLETTI (USDA, Florida): We are doing thousands of CF tests and we have four other tests we are comparing to the CF test to check against the possibility of prozones. I can almost categorically state that prozones are simply no problem. We have rarely found prozone. I think Dr. Alton suggested in his paper this morning, and certainly Dr. Jones and I have discussed this many times, that the probable explanation for this is the difference between the warm and cold fixation. I think it has quite well been concluded that with cold fixation there is much less of a probability of having a prozone phenomenon than in the warm fixation. We are not doing a comparison of warm and cold, but I can categorically state prozones are not a problem to us.

DR. CLARKE: What can you say about the utility of the CF test as an incremental capability above the present rivanol and mercaptoethanol type tests? In other words, given that you are in the field currently doing the standard supplemental tests that we do now, what would you gain by doing the CF test in addition to, or in lieu of these tests?

DR. NICOLETTI: Well, I would, of course, quite closely agree with Dr. Pietz in suggesting that the CF test in most cases parallels the results of some of the other supplemental tests. I am particularly talking in terms of rivanol. We see very little difference between those two tests in comparisons with culture positive animals. What we are seeing, and this will perhaps be brought up tomorrow in my paper, is that the CF test is, in fact, going negative more rapidly than any of the other tests, including the rivanol test. So I think this may be one reason to include the CF test in the battery.

DR. PIETZ: Going negative in what situations?

DR. NICOLETTI: This is following strain 19 vaccination in adult cattle. But I think, perhaps, a parallel could be made in younger animals. After the CF test, the rivanol would be the first one which would go negative. But I think there would be instances where the rivanol test reaction may persist and a CF test would be negative.

DR. PIETZ: Yes, that is true. If in the detection of developing titers in animals you use a battery of supplemental tests and the card test, the card test will usually become positive first, followed by the mercaptoethanol and the rivanol. In vaccinated animals then, as the titer recedes, the negative status is achieved in reverse order. The rivanol usually is the first to go, mercaptoethanol second, and the card test last. With the standard agglutination test, the titer may be in the negative or suspect range (used in the diagnostic criteria for lactating animals) and the animal may or may not be negative on the card test. But from the evidence in the field, in the early studies using the card test, in the vicinity of 90% of those animals would be negative to the card test that had agglutination titers from vaccination.

DR. CLARKE: Dr. Morgan, have you had experience comparing these several tests?

DR. MORGAN: Well, yes. We have done quite a lot, especially with the mercaptoethanol and rivanol tests. And in quite marked contrast with what Dr. Nicoletti was saying, we were finding that neither of these two tests, mercaptoethanol or rivanol, were giving us information additional to the CF test. So, at the end of the day we stopped with the CF test, the test we knew most about.

DR. CLARKE: Let me make sure I understood. While they were not giving you additional information, were they giving you approximately the same information?

DR. MORGAN: No, we were finding a number of cases that were negative to the mercaptoethanol and rivanol tests and positive to the CF test. I must stress, of course, we are using a fairly severe CF test (2+ at 1:4-1:10). Whereas, in your country, you are using 1:20 and 1:40 and this may be significant.

DR. CLARKE: One of the things that perhaps we ought to do before our time gets away is to pay a little more attention than we did during the presentations to the new developments that show promise of separating the vaccinal reaction to strain 45/20 from infected animals. Several of the speakers discussed the use of the new methods by Miller for separating the vaccinal reactions with strain 45/20 from reactions of infected animals. They all agreed that additional research is necessary to really validate this procedure. Is this something that shows considerable promise? Can you tell us whether we ought to be looking carefully at that as a way of increasing our chances of being able to use adult vaccine?

DR. MORGAN: I have an impression that this is rapidly becoming a modern bandwagon. I know a lot of people working on exactly this. Is this not so, Dr. Jones?

DR. JONES: I think the problem is going to be with strain 45/20 vaccinated animals from an infected area. You can do parallel CF with the smooth antigen and the rough antigen but what if you get titers with both? Then, where are you? And, there is some low titer to the smooth antigen even in the disease-free strain 45/20 vaccinated animal. So it is a matter of establishing the levels of differentiation. Much must be done with this before we can say, I think. This question was brought up in my paper as well.

DR. MORGAN: I think we need to be fairly careful in this kind of differentiation between strain 45/20, field infection, strain 19 and so on. At the end of the day, certain criteria have to be laid down. I think that the only usefulness of any attempt at differentiating between the strain 45/20 and field infection would be in the infected environment where the vaccine has been used in order for you to make some kind of attempt to so decide which of the animals to get rid of now and which you do not. But, at the end of the day you have to satify your national criteria. You cannot have animals, as I see it, having had strain 45/20 vaccine with CF levels or agglutination levels of any test which is a recognized test, above what you have recognized and laid down as the minimum level. And, we would not allow animals to be retained as official brucella-free with titers of CF antibodies to smooth antigen of 2 in 10, even though we are fairly convinced that they were strain 45/20 vaccinates with titers to the rough antigen of five times or ten times higher. I think this is something we have to recognize.

DR. CLARKE: If I understand what you are saying, in your country you would slaughter the animal positive to a standard CF test, even if she were shown to be also reacting to the strain 45/20.

DR. MORGAN: We might not slaughter the animal in the initial stage of clearing up the herd, but at the end of a day I do not think we would accept it.

DR. CLARKE: I wonder if there are areas that the speakers would like to discuss with each other that we have not specifically teased out here as questions. I would like to make sure that we have a chance to do that before our time slips away.

DR. PIETZ: The question was asked: Is a better test needed for diagnosis? I think the two speakers indicated that there is need for a better test and I encourage research to develop better tests, but at the same time, I do not think we should lose sight of the fact that we can eradicate the disease with what we have, if we use them correctly. We have to use what we have at the present time effectively and, at the same time, encourage research to develop methods that can improve our ability to eradicate the disease.

DR. MORGAN: Can I also, Mr. Chairman, strongly reiterate what Dr. Pietz has just said. I also am quite convinced the range of tests we now have available, which have been well evaluated in various countries, are adequate for eradicating brucellosis in cattle. But, we would like also, human nature being what it is, to have something which is better or easier to do. But I am also quite convinced we have adequate tests.

If I may, Mr. Chairman, mention one area which I think we have touched on and this is what Dr. Nicoletti talked about earlier. This is the latent period or incubation period (call it what you like). I do not know if you can really differentiate between them. All the records from the eradication herds that we have in Britain go into a computer. We have taken a long time to decide exactly what are the right questions to ask the computer and we are beginning to get results back now, in the last six months or thereabouts. And there is, I think, a little problem concerning these heifers born of infected animals. I have no idea of the size of this problem, but it is something which does occur. On the other hand, we did an experiment not too long ago where we took groups of calves and gave some of them strain 19 vaccine and gave another group a virulent challenge strain. At the same time we took another group of adult cows that had not previously been vaccinated and we gave half of them strain 19 vaccine and half of them the virulent challenge strain. Now I must add straightaway that the size of the virulent challenge strain was quite large. It was 80,000 million strain 19 and we gave 80,000 million of the 544 strain, so it was a very hefty challenge. We got a pattern of results which was connected not so much to the virulence of the strain but to the age of the animal. And we found that the calves responded to the virulent challenge strain in the same way they behaved to the strain 19 vaccine; the titers shot up as you would expect them to do when large doses are given subcutaneously and they eventually became negative. The adult animals behaved not quite in this clear cut way but the titers rose and they persisted for very much longer than in the young calves. There was a slight difference between the strain 19 and the virulent 544. Now these are small numbers of animals, half a dozen in each. We followed the young animals straight through. We got them at two years of age or thereabouts and followed them through calving and in no case was there any change in the titer and in no case at subsequent examination of milk, colostrum and so on or at post mortem examination were we able to recover *Brucella* even from those calves that had been given the virulent challenge strain. These are the two extremes of the situations as I see it. These are small numbers of cows where after we put virulent field infection into them, they recovered. Yet, on the other hand, we have perhaps a much larger field of evidence that calves can in effect occasionally retain infection into adult life. LaPracke, who has been working in my laboratory in Scotland, has documented just one or two of these field type of cases.

DR. CLARKE: Dr. Morgan did mention we would be touching on this later in our meeting and I think that is a subject for considerable discussion either this afternoon or tomorrow. I know Dr. Plommet from France has some experience to report to us regarding calfhood infection. We also know that USDA is giving some serious consideration to increasing their research effort in this area so it does remain an area that I think most of the people working in the field now agree is one that has to have additional attention. Are there other comments from the speakers or from speakers who did not speak this morning?

DR. FRANK HAYES (University of Georgia): Repeated reference has been made to cultural procedures. Could someone be a little more exact on that? What tissues should be examined and what media used?

DR. PIETZ: I would say that most of the culturing is done on milk only and the isolation results are compared with the serologic results to evaluate the effectiveness of the serologic procedures. It takes quite a while for the udder to become infected. In most cases, of course, this depends on the resistance of the animal and the amount of exposure, but the udder does not become infected, generally speaking, for quite some time; in fact, we had animals that we purchased from infected herds that were in the reactor range on the standard agglutination test but they did not have antibodies in the ring test. We kept these animals on hand for a six-month period and studied the development of antibodies in the udder. This was about 20 years ago. We could isolate Brucella from the milk of these animals from a few days to a few weeks before they developed high milk titers. In two of these animals that never did develop milk titers, we isolated Brucella from the tissues when we sent them for slaughter, so the organism does tend to localize in the udder but it also may localize in other areas. The types of tissues that are desirable to culture include milk, of course. The supramammary lymph nodes are the tissues of choice. I do not recall the exact percentage but probably in the vicinity of 60 percent of the animals from which you can isolate Brucella, you would be able to culture the organism from the supramammary lymph nodes. We would normally culture: milk, supramammary lymph nodes, iliac lymph nodes, lumbar lymph nodes, the spleen, uterus and retropharyngeal lymph nodes.

DR. CLARKE: Thank you. I will mention one or two more things that were not mentioned this morning, specifically in the area of new diagnostic tests. There are a number of groups, including ourselves here at TAMU, who intend to evaluate some tests that are not commonly used today. I will just mention the automation of the enzyme labeled antibody (ELA) test as it has been developed by the people at the Los Alamos Scientific Laboratories. The general area of cell mediated immunity (CMI) may perhaps offer some opportunities for a look at the latent carrier at an earlier stage before she shows up serologically. I would like to turn now to see if there are questions from the audience that they might like to address to the speakers.

DR. THEODORE KRAMER (Auburn University): I would like to address myself to all the hot-fixers and cold-fixers. I believe there is one aspect in CF testing that we have not considered and which is common to many bacteria and yeast. This is the alternative pathway of complement. My question is: Does Brucella trigger the alternative pathway of complement and if so, would this explain the advantages which I seem to gather of a cold fixation over hot fixation?

DR. JONES: I cannot answer that.

DR. ALTON: I do not know the answer to your question at all. We examined the sera of a number of culture positive animals. The number of serologic positives is the same by cold and warm fixation. The cold fixation, with the same set of materials, gives approximately one to two times higher titer. There is no more to it than that, I think. The results you get are comparable. It is mostly a question of convenience. This slight problem of prozones which occurs both in warm and cold is much more pronounced in the warm fixation.

DR. KRAMER: With regards to the difference in results with prozone attributed to IgG_2, it is also known that immunoglobulin aggregates will trigger the alternative complement pathway and some of the complement fixation results might be artifacts in this respect.

DR. CLARKE: Are there any other questions from the audience?

DR. JAMES WHITTEM (Australian Embassy, Washington, D.C.): Where you are doing large volume testing, can you afford to apply a battery of tests? Can you have a consensus about a single supplementary test which will take 80 or 90 or 95 percent of the work on the first round of testing and then have a special laboratory for the problem herds?

DR. PIETZ: It certainly is not recommended to use a battery of tests when you have a lot of infection. The diagnosis of brucellosis is on a probability basis. You can take a serologic test such as the standard agglutination test that has been used for years and use it to reduce the infection to a low level. Then you can start using supplemental tests. You could supplement it in certain instances or certain herds. The card test in comparison to the standard agglutination test does away with the suspect categories. The card test detects some of those suspects as potentially infected and others as negative or potentially not having the disease. And so, in essence, we are pulling these animals out a little sooner, if we use only the reactor range, than if we use only the standard agglutination test. You have to recognize that at that point in time some of those animals may overcome that exposure. You have a choice.

Do you want to use another test that is less sensitive? This is fine if you can isolate those animals from the negative animals. If you have the facilities to do that, I have no qualms, but if you do not, I think it is better to take those animals out and clean up infection sooner. Then, once you get down to the problem and you have low level infection, then you can start bringing in the supplemental tests, epidemiology, etc. Another thing, in the development of the card test, when the acidified plate antigen was first developed and used, it was run at the 1:25 dilution along with the plate test at 1:25 dilution and many serums that were positive on the plate test at 1:25 were negative on the acidified plate antigen. Others were positive but the agglutination was comparable to the acidified plate antigen. Whereas, there were other serums that were negative or showed weak reactions on the standard plate but they came out and hit you in the eye with acidified plate antigen. These, it turned out in later investigation, were usually chronic carriers. This is the advantage of the card test and one of the reasons why it was developed to be used in these herds that were hard to handle, to get these chronic carriers out. There are reasons for a lot of these things and there is no way or no test that I know of that can tell you which individual animal is not infected or is infected. You have to make a decision one way or the other, i.e. take out a lot of animals with a sensitive test to clean up sooner or putz around and leave infection in there to expose other animals.

DR. CLARKE: In the case of our state, the overall herd infection rate is of the order of two percent or less. Is it not practical to run supplemental tests on the relatively small number of reactors that you would get into in a situation like this?

DR. PIETZ: Yes.

References

Jones, L. M.; Hendricks, J. B.; and Berman, D. T. 1963. The standardization and use of the complement-fixation test for the diagnosis of bovine brucellosis, with a review of the literature. Am. J. Vet. Res. 24:1143-1151.

EPIDEMIOLOGY

Moderator: Leon H. Russell

The Epidemiology of *Brucella abortus*

Winthrop C. Ray

Intensive study on the various aspects of brucellosis occurred during the first 35 years following Bang's report on the isolation and identification of the organism in 1897. The observations and comments of these early workers are remarkable because of their relevancy to today's questions. Much of the basic epidemiology was described by 1930 and remains but to be rediscovered by each succeeding generation. I do not mean to discount the tremendous advances that have occurred in the last 45 years or the excellent work that has been accomplished to expand and refine our knowledge on brucellosis. However, in spite of the available knowledge that has been accumulated, there are some facets of brucellosis that are still unclear and need to be answered more fully. Many of these areas will be topics for discussion here this week.

The epidemiology of a disease is not static. Changes in the agent, the host or the environment affect the complex interrelationships that exist in brucellosis thereby influencing the epidemiology of this disease. Most changes are subtle and not of apparent significance. Other changes have greater visibility and require appropriate adjustments in program procedures.

One of the factors that has altered the epidemiology of bovine brucellosis has been the successful application of control and eradication procedures in a large number of herds. Reduced prevalence of the disease was largely accomplished by removal of those infected animals from the population that responded to the test procedures in a predictable manner. The infected herds subjected to similar procedures which still remain in the population are often referred to as "problem herds" because they do not respond in a predictable and identifiable way. As the proportion of "problem herds" increases among the total infected herds, the apparent epidemiology is altered.

Another factor which influences the epidemiology of the disease is the collective influence of livestock management and livestock industry practices. Modernization of farms and the accelerating trend toward larger and more compact operations increases animal population densities and subjects animals to greater stress. Higher requirements for individual animal production, coupled with the use of mechanized equipment operated by unskilled and often disinterested farm laborers, adversely influences the degree of attention and care that can be focused on individual animals or groups of animals to implement good animal health programs. It is imperative that an awareness be maintained of livestock husbandry and industry practices so that the affect on the disease can be detected if it occurs.

A comprehensive review on the epidemiology of brucellosis is beyond the scope of this discussion. Various facets of the disease will be considered in detail by the other speakers this week, and I want to avoid unnecessary duplication if possible. The areas I will specifically address are: Brucellosis in Calves, Brucellosis in Horses, Growth Requirements, and the Survival of the Organism in the Environment. Also, I will briefly comment on selected epidemiologic factors as observed in the United States.

There are three "classical" *Brucella* organisms, two of which commonly occur in the U.S.A. *B. melitensis* has been detected occasionally in goat herds in the South-Central and Southwestern United States but is presently unknown in the U.S.A. Only *B. abortus*, biotypes I, II, and IV and *B. suis*, biotypes I, III, and IV exist in native animal populations. *B. suis*, biotype IV, affects reindeer and caribou in Alaska and is not found in domestic swine. The infections in cattle caused by the three biotypes of *B. abortus* are epidemiologically indistinguishable as are the infections in swine caused by *B. suis*, biotypes I or III (Nelson 1966). When infections occur in other than the preferred host, for example, *B. suis* in cattle or *B. abortus* in swine, the disease syndrome is altered (Meyer 1964). Udder but not uterine infections are usually observed in cattle with *B. suis* infections. Transmission of *B. suis* from cow to cow or to the progeny occurs rarely, if at all. *B. canis* and *B. neotomae* are not associated with brucellosis in livestock and *B. ovis*, while prevalent in sheep-raising areas, does not interfere with the diagnosis or epidemiology of the classical infections.

The susceptible host range for *B. abortus* and *B. suis* is very broad, and a large number of animals have been reported as affected on the basis of serologic or bacteriologic results. However, there is no evidence, based on limited surveys nor on experience in the eradication program, to support the contention that wildlife in the United States form a natural reservoir of *Brucella* infection. The only recognized exceptions are elk on certain concentrated feedgrounds, bison, caribou and some herds of feral swine.

Dr. Hayes will discuss the role of wildlife in detail, but it is important to stress that even though the list of susceptible animals is impressive, the number of biologic reservoirs other than cattle and swine appears to be quite limited. Circumstantial evidence of this conclusion is provided by the failure to reestablish *Brucella* infection on premises stocked with susceptible animals after herd depopulations. Under depopulation procedures, only the bovines are slaughtered and special precautions are not taken other than to clean and disinfect the buildings and not to restock for 30 days. Other domestic animals remain on the premises and no vector control is instituted to control ticks or flies nor to control rodent or wild carnivore populations. Reinfection of cattle premises, under these circumstances, is rarely reported.

Brucella is a highly invasive organism that can penetrate the host defences through various routes (Berman 1950). Ingestion is believed to be the most common route of invasion in cattle. Cattle frequently lick aborted fetuses, placentas, and external genitalia of infected cows. Other routes of exposure include mucous membranes of the eye, nostril, and reproductive organs. Invasion through the skin has also been reported. Venereal transmission is an important epidemiologic factor in the spread of swine brucellosis but not bovine brucellosis. Artificial insemination of contaminated bovine semen, however, greatly increases the risk of infection (Manthei et al. 1950).

Brucellosis in Calves

The role of calves in perpetuating the disease within a herd is a subject of renewed interest. Several of the early workers in brucellosis investigated Brucella infection in calves and most concluded that calves were highly resistant to the disease even though temporarily harboring the agent. Connaway (1923) noted that occasionally a calf of an "abortion" infected cow becomes permanently infected with Brucella before birth or from the milk of the dam; but as a rule, the calf overcomes the infection.

Hart and Woods (1925) fed calves 75 to 90 billion organisms twice daily for two to six months and examined tissues bacteriologically for Brucella up to 18 months after the last feeding of contaminated milk. In their work, lymph tissue from all 15 calves fed contaminated milk for two days up to five weeks were positive for Brucella. These calves were slaughtered at intervals varying up to four weeks after the last feeding. Another calf fed contaminated milk for 12 weeks was bacteriologically positive seven weeks later. One of the four calves fed contaminated milk for four to six months was bacteriologically positive 11 weeks later. Eleven calves fed contaminated milk for six months and slaughtered after completion of gestation were negative. Carpenter (1924) reported that Brucella could not be recovered from tissues of calves fed contaminated milk (30 billion twice daily) more than 28 days after weaning. Some calves were fed for 63 days with similar results. Barger and Hayes (1924) demonstrated that both naturally contaminated and artificially contaminated milk was infectious for calves. Brucella was detected in the feces of calves throughout the feeding period beginning on the seventh day and terminating on the 28th day. Brucella was recovered from regional lymph nodes up to 19 days after weaning. The usual failure to isolate Brucella from the lymph nodes three to four weeks after the cessation of feeding contaminated milk lead to the conclusion that young calves are highly resistant.

Brucella agglutinins were usually absent in these trials during the time the young calves were fed Brucella contaminated milk. Ranney (1934) purchased ten calves, two to three months of age, and fed them artificially contaminated milk daily for ten weeks. Virulent brucellae were isolated from the feces of each calf during the feeding period. Brucellae were not found in the feces seven days after the last feeding of contaminated milk in this trial. Rettger and White (1918) concluded that calves fed raw milk from infected cows after six months of age could and did develop persistent infection leading to abortion and reactor titers, but there was insufficient evidence in their report to exclude later exposure.

Other workers (Hignett and Nagy 1964) have noted that young calves exposed to Brucella, and later re-exposed when six months of age or older, frequently exhibit a diminished or altered immunologic response compared with control animals. Others have noted that animals exposed as calves that resist infection are susceptible to exposure as adults.

Fitch et al. (1941), established a brucellosis-free herd by isolating calves from infected dams. This study was undertaken because of the continuing controversy concerning the possibility that Brucella could remain dormant and undetected in the lymph nodes of the calf until breeding age. They also were interested in possible modes of transmission from the dam to the daughter either prenatally or postnatally. Brucella was isolated from the placenta of 19 and from the colostrum of 44 of the 46 dams. The neonatal calf was allowed to nurse its dam twice daily for one week. After the first week, the calf was fed milk from negative cows. When the blood titer became negative, the calf was bathed and put in the isolation barn with other progeny of reactor cows. Forty-three cows were followed through at least one parturition without any evidence of Brucella infection. All told, the 43 animals had a total of 95 lactation periods during the six-year investigation with 93 placentas recovered and cultured and 257 milk samples cultured.

In spite of these data and other similar evidence, field reports based on circumstantial evidence occasionally cited the introduction of calves as the most likely source of infection in newly infected herds. Also, occasionally, observations on the cause of recurrence of disease in previously infected herds cited the introduction of natural additions into the adult producing herd. The calves were born to infected dams or reared on contaminated premises without exhibiting evidence of brucellosis until after calving.

Plommet (1973) reported that four out of 22 heifers born of experimentally infected cows, separated at birth, and raised in isolation units were shown to be infected shortly before or after their first parturition. The four animals remained serologically negative until the middle or end of the gestation period.

Because of the importance dormant infections in calves could have in an intensive short term eradication program, we are planning to study this facet of the epidemiology in greater depth. Based on field observations over the years, it is believed that the frequency and persistence of infection in calves lies somewhere between that reported by Fitch and Plommet. Certainly in the long run, this aspect has not prevented the elimination of brucellosis from numerous herds, but it may well have served to delay progress in achieving this goal for some.

Brucellosis in Horses

Equine brucellosis was recently reviewed by Denny (1973). Horses are susceptible to Brucella infection and can be experimentally infected by various routes and methods of exposure. Natural infections are usually, but not always, associated with close contact with infected livestock. Brucellosis in horses probably occurs most commonly as a latent or as a subclinical disease; but under favorable conditions, clinical signs may be manifested as bursitis, stiffness, osteomyletis, osteoarthritis, suppurative bursitis, or abortion. Fechner and Meyer (1961) indicated that two horses developed fistulous withers 14 and 32 months, respectively, after exposure to aborting cattle. Brucellae tend to localize in infected horses in the bursae, tendons, muscles, and joints rather than tissues of the repoductive system or embryonic tissues. Abortions, although infrequent, have been reported (McCaughey 1967). Isolation of Brucella from feces of horses segregated from other animals has been reported by Karlson and Boyd (1940), but the frequency of such shedding is apparently low.

Most workers suggest that horses are infected by contact with infected cattle and not that cattle are infected by contact with horses. B. suis has also been isolated from a few cases following association with infected swine (Portugal 1971). However, any time a horse or any other animal aborts and discharges large numbers of Brucella, there is a possibility of transmission to susceptible animals regardless of species.

Serological surveys in the United States on horses indicate that horses are involved in those areas where the prevalence of bovine brucellosis is relatively high. In fiscal year 1974, 7.2 percent of the horses tested were diagnosed as positive. In fiscal year 1975, this was 11 percent; but most of the horses were tested in States with relatively high bovine infection rates and were selected for test by association with cattle on infected farms or by presence of signs such as fistulous withers. In fiscal year 1976, 2,174 horses were tested in South Carolina, a brucellosis-free state, without any positives found.

Growth Requirements

Brucella, in common with most bacteria, have rather specific growth requirements. McCullough et al. (1947) found that thiamine, niacin, cystine, histidine, tyrosine, phenylalanine, tryptophane, and magnesium salts were necessary for growth. They also reported additional nutrients were needed for maximum growth. Gerhardt (1958) reported that a nitrogen source such as asparagine, glutamic acid, or histidine was essential for maximum growth.

Brucellae have a relatively slow multiplication rate. The initial growth rate may be very slow, especially when only a few brucellae are present. Borts (1946) reported that some cultures required more than 30 days incubation on nutrient medium on initial isolation. Others advise holding all culture plates eight to ten days (Alton et al. 1975) before discarding on initial isolation attempts. Our usual practice is to discard culture plates after seven days of incubation.

Survival of the Organism in the Environment

The survival of viable brucellae has been investigated by several workers under various conditions. These attempts were to determine if, under controlled environmental conditions, Brucella could be recovered after varying intervals. In most instances, a large initial inoculum was used without determining the percentage of cells that remained viable. However, in the investigation by Kuzdas and Morse (1954), a titration of viable organisms was performed after specified intervals. From these results, it was obvious that although the brucella culture survived, a steady reduction in viable cells occurred under the conditions studied with the exception of materials held below freezing.

Long survival times have been reported for Brucella by various authors. Some of these are cited here as examples of the conditions investigated:

Cameron (1932)	4 1/2 hours exposed to direct sunlight
	Less than 4 days dried quickly in soil
	5 days when dried in burlap in laboratory
	30 days when dried in burlap in cellar
	66 days in wet soil in cellar
	72 days when dried in absence of nutrients

	72 days in soil dried quickly in February 121 days when dried in presence of nutrients
Kuzdas and Morse (1954)	12 hours in urine at 37°C and pH 8.5 6 days in urine at 8°C and pH 8.5 1 day in raw milk at 37°C 1 day in raw milk at 25°C 2 days in raw milk 8°C 800 days in raw milk at -40°C 188 days in manure sterilized at 37°C 0 days in manure untreated at 37°C 29 days in manure untreated at 25°C 385 days in manure untreated at 8°C 121 days in manure untreated at -3°C 670 days in manure untreated at -40°C

The decrease in survival at -3°C in the Kuzdas and Morse experiments may be explained by the deleterious effect of the "freeze-thaw" action on bacterial cells. Death at the time of freezing is considered to be mechanical due to formation of extracellular ice. Death after freezing is thought to be due to concentration of solutes in the "intercrystallic film."

Brucella-infected carcasses were also examined for survival of the agent in the spleen by placing the carcasses on the ground surface and by burying the carcasses in two feet of soil. Comparisons between summer and winter seasons were also made in this study. Brucella survived 44 days in carcasses placed on the ground in January and February compared with 29 days when buried in the summer. Brucella were found to survive only one day in guinea pig carcasses when placed on the ground in the summer.

King (1957) found that liquid manure tanks did not support the survival of Brucella more than four hours. The temperature reached 158°F in the winter and 170°F during the summer when the manure pit was approximately one-fourth full.

In summary, the survival of Brucella discharged into the environment is dependent on many factors. Under appropriate conditions, the organism survives for long periods of time. It does not tend to multiply but merely persists. A number of factors combine to make Brucella a poor survivor outside of its host. Brucella has a relatively slow multiplication rate or generation time and because of its relatively slow growth, it is not a good competitor with the saprophytes for the available nutrients. It is easily overgrown by contaminants under ideal optimum growth conditions.

The organism is readily killed by heat-pasteurization (fifteen minutes at 143°F or 15 seconds at 160°F). The organism is relatively susceptible to the common disinfectants and is inactivated by acid conditions below pH 5.5. It does persist exceptionally well under freezing or cold conditions or in cool protected areas away from direct sunlight. Survival of viable Brucella has been demonstrated under appropriate conditions, but it has not been shown by these experiments, nor by field observation, that Brucella persist or multiply in significant numbers to create a significant risk of reinfection of susceptible animals reintroduced to the affected premises. This should not be construed to mean that the existence of favorable environmental conditions should be ignored. Recognition of conditions such as improper disposal of a fetus is an important step in correcting the potential problem.

References

Alton, G. G.; Jones, Lois M.; and Pietz, D. E. 1975. Laboratory techniques in brucellosis. World Health Organization, p. 33.

Barger, E. H., and Hayes, F. M. 1924. The discharge of Bacterium Abortum in the feces of calves fed milk containing the organism. J.A.V.M.A. 19(3):328-336.

Berman, D. T. 1950. The natural course of bovine brucellosis In Third Inter-American Congress on Brucellosis, Washington, D.C., Pan American Sanit. Bur., p. 104.

Borts, I. H.; McNutt, S. H.; and Jordan, C. F. 1946. Brucella melintensis isolated from swine tissues in Iowa J.A.V.M.A. 130:966.

Cameron, Hugh Stuart. 1932. The viability of Brucella abortus Cornell Vet., 22:212-224.

Carpenter, C. M. 1924. Bacterium Abortum invasion of the tissues of calves from the ingestion of infected milk. Cornell Vet. 14(1):16-31.

Connaway, J. W. 1923. Agric. Exp. Station, Univ. of Missouri, Bull. 201, p. 4.

Denny, H. R. 1973. A review of brucellosis in the horse. Equine Veterinary Journal 5(3):121-125.

Fecher, J., and Meyer, W. 1961. Brucellosis in horses. Abst. in Vet. Bull. 31:2844.

Fitch, C. P.; Boyd, W. L.; Kelly, Margaret D.; and Bishop, Lucille M. 1941. An extended study of female offspring of positive Bang's, diseased cattle. J.A.V.M.A. 99:413.

Gerhardt, Phillip. 1958. The nutrition of Brucellae. Bact. Rev. 22:81-98).

Hart, George H., and Woods, Gladys M. 1925. The location and longevity in calves of Bacterium Abortum ingested with milk, and its effect on the agglutination titer of their blood. Hilgardia 1(10):204-226.

Hignett, P. G., and Nagy, L. K. 1964. Effect of exposure of very young calves to virulent Brucella abortus on their serological response to re-infection by the same organism at six months of age. Nature 201(4915):204.

Karlson, A. G., and Boyd, W. L. 1940. Brucellosis in horses: A study of five cases without clinical symptoms. J.A.V.M.A. 97:576-580.

King, N. B. 1957. The survival of Brucella abortus (USDA strain 2308) in manure. J.A.V.M.A. 131(8):349-352.

Kuzdas, C. D., and Morse, E. V. 1954. The survival of *Brucella abortus*, USDA strain 2308, under controlled conditions in nature. Cornell Vet. 44:216-228.

Manthei, C. A.; DeTray, D. E.; and Goode, E. R., Jr. 1950. *Brucella* infection in bulls and the spread of brucellosis in cattle by artificial insemination. Proceedings of the A.V.M.A. Meetings 87:177.

McCaughey, W. J., and Kerr, W. R. 1967. Abortion due to brucellosis in a thoroughbred mare. Vet. Rec. 80(5):186.

McCullough, W. G.; Mills, R. C.; Herbst, E. J.; Roessler, W. G.; and Brewer, C. R. 1947. Studies on the nutritional requirements of *Brucella suis*. J. Bact. 53:5.

Meyer, Margaret E. 1964. The epizootiology of brucellosis and its relationship to the identification of brucella organisms. Amer. J. Vet. Res. 25(105):553-557.

Nelson, Claude J.; Anderson, R. K.; Kimberling, C. V.; and Pietz, D. E. 1966. Epizootiologic factors of bovine brucellosis: Comparative bateriologic studies of infected herds. Vet. Res.--A.V.M.A. 27(121):1515.

Plommet, M.; Fensterbank, R.; Renoux, G.; Gestin, J.; and Philippon, A. 1973. Brucellose bovine experimentale: XII, Persistence to adult age of congenital infection in the heifer. Ann. Rech. Veter. 4(3):419-435.

Portugal, Manuel A. S. C.; Nesti, Albino; Giorgi, Waldyr; Franca, Enio Nogueira; and de Oliveira; e Brasilio S., Jr. 1971. Brucellosis among equine caused by *Brucella suis*. Arq. Inst. Biol. (S. Paulo) 38(3):125-132.

Ranney, Alvert F. 1934. The elimination of *Brucella abortus* from the feces of calves taking infected milk. Cornell Vet. 24:244-253.

Rettger, L. F., and White, G. C. 1918. Storrs. Agric. Exp. Sta. Bull. 93, pp. 217-224.

Studies on Experimental Brucellosis in Cows in France

Michel Plommet

In 1967 we undertook careful studies on experimental infection. During seven experiments, we have inoculated a total of 344 heifers, generally during their first gestation, seldom before their first insemination. According to the purpose of the experiment, heifers were vaccinated or not, or underwent various treatments. The challenge, dispensed by conjunctival route, was constant: 15×10^6 Brucella abortus, strain 544 (Weybridge).

Analyses conducted as shown in Figures 1 and 2 compared:

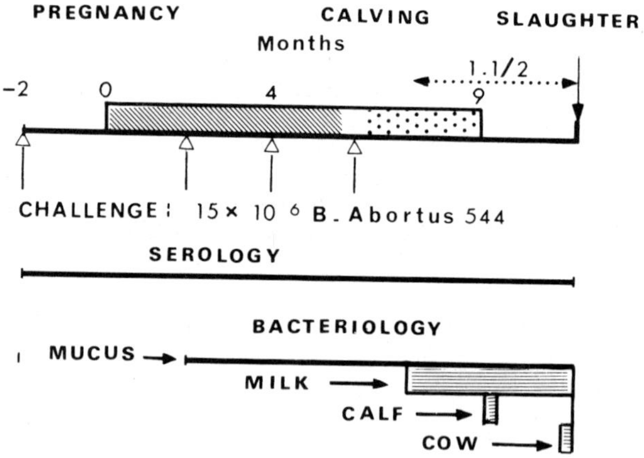

Figure 1

Experimental Design in Experimental Brucellosis Studies in Cattle

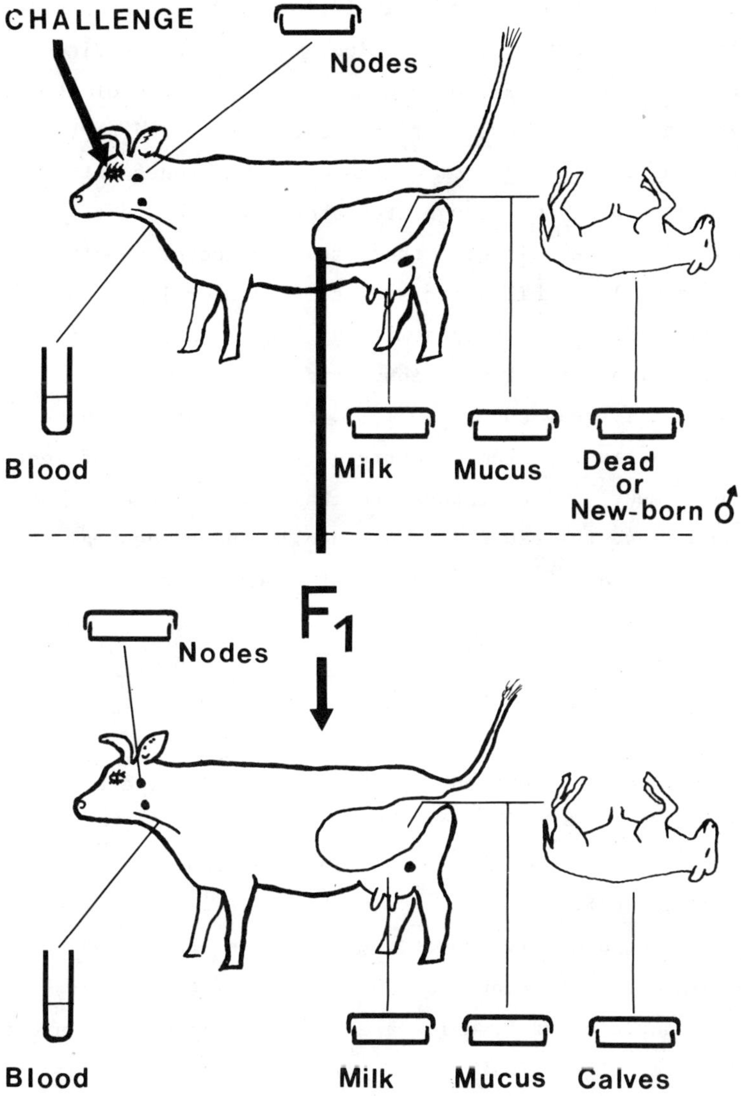

Figure 2

Design: Mother to Daughter Transmission Experiment

(Plommet et al. 1973)

serological response (sero-agglutination [Agg], complement fixation [CF], other tests); isolation of Brucella on selective media from colostrum, milk, vaginal mucus, uterine discharges; isolation of Brucella from organs and lymph nodes of aborted calves and some calves, mostly males, slaughtered at birth; and isolation of Brucella from organs and lymph nodes (at least 20 samples) on all cows slaughtered about six weeks after calving or abortion. We will give the results concerning pathogenicity and epidemiology while stressing some more or less known aspects of brucellosis epidemiology, which should be taken into account for an efficient prophylaxis.

We will study successively: 1. the route of inoculation--the conjunctival portal of entry; 2. the influence of gestation and treatment on the response to challenge; 3. the serological responses; 4. the excretion of Brucella and congenital brucellosis; and 5. the survival of Brucella outside the bovine--liquid manure and wild rodents.

Route of Inoculation - Conjunctival Portal of Entry

In natural infection, four portals of entry are generally recognized:

1. The congenital or transplacental route, which will be studied further.

2. The digestive route, by ingestion of milk or contaminated water. This route has been studied with calves. Very large quantities of Brucella are needed to induce an infection, which does not remain for a very long time in the female calf (Nagy and Hignett 1967). In the male, the infections obtained by such passage would be the origin of the organisms observed in adults (Rankin 1965). Because calves born to infected mothers are often born infected, contamination with milk probably plays a negligible role in practice, except in calves

suckling nurse cows.

3. The udder route, by transfer of bacteria from an excreting udder to a non-infected one through milking and inoculation in the same way as in mastitis. This rarely studied route could be of some importance within milk herds (Kerr and Rankin 1959).

4. Conjunctival and upper air-passages. This route is usually chosen for experimental inoculation because it is probably the most frequent one under natural conditions. Fensterbank (Personal Communication 1976) justifies such a choice by showing that colonization of the lymph nodes of the head draining the face area is about as frequent in natural disease as after artificial conjunctival inoculation (Table 1).

Table 1. Infection of the Lymph Nodes of the Head of Non-vaccinated Cows Inoculated by the Conjuntival Route and Cultured Approximately Six Months Later and of Naturally Infected Cattle Sampled at the Abbattoir (Fensterbank - personal communication 1976)

Source of Infection	Number of Isolations	Total No. of Cattle
Conjunctival Challenge, Strain 544, 15×10^6 organisms	49	66
Naturally Infected (Abattoir)	13	23

$X^2 = 2.48$ P = 0.10

The process of penetration through the mucous membrane and the transport of the bacteria to the lymph nodes of the head are not well known. The bacteria probably adhere to the epithelial cells. Conjunctival vaccination with strain 19 induces the synthesis of specific IgA in tears (Levieux Personal Communication 1974). These IgA antibodies could eliminate adherence and reduce penetration. Colonization of the nodes of the head is made in a preferential way, though not exclusively on the inoculated side, by following a frequency order showing that penetration is more likely at the level of the orbital and upper pharyngeal cavities (Plommet and Plommet 1976, Table 2).

Table 2. Colonization of the Lymph Nodes of the Head of Calves 15-30 Days after Conjunctival Inoculation with 10^9-10^{10} *Brucella abortus* Strain 19 in the Right Eye (Plommet and Plommet 1976)

Lymph Node Colonized	Right	Left
Parotid	34	10
Submaxillary	25	7
Retropharyngeal	10	2
Total Number of Calves	59	

Once in the node, *Brucella* may be stopped or may spread through lymph and blood passages to target organs according to the resistance of the subject and the virulence of the strain (McCullough 1970). Humoral factors, probably antibodies, interfere at this stage allowing blockage in the lymph node (Pardon 1976). The conjunctival vaccination induces a colonization of nodes of the head and stimulates the competent cells which, since they are located along the route of natural infection, will be the first to react in case of further contamination (*Brucella* exposure). In our opinion, this could explain why conjunctival vaccination is more efficient than classical vaccination by the subcutaneous route, and could be even more protective when performed in a bilateral way (Plommet and Fensterbank 1976).

Influence of Gestation and Treatment on the Response to Challenge

We used a challenge dose that would infect about 100% of the cows, based on the works of McEwen, Priestley and Paterson (1939). Our results confirm that choice because nearly 100% of the pregnant cows were infected (Table 3).

Table 3. Infection Determined by Bacteriological Examinations of Treated and Untreated Cows Challenged During and Prior to Pregnancy with 15 x 10^6 Brucella abortus Strain 544 (Fensterbank et al. 1975; Fensterbank - Personal Communication 1975)

Status of Cows	Infected	Total
Untreated		
Pregnant	60	62
Non-pregnant	7	11
Treated*		
Pregnant	9	18
Non-pregnant	2	22

*10g oxytetracycline administered intraperitoneally in a single dose 10 days after challenge.

The influence of gestation is evidenced by the fact that the inoculation performed two months before insemination infected only seven of eleven cows. The influence of a treatment with oxytetracycline (one I/P injection of 10 g.) ten days after inoculation is quite evident as well, and also depends upon the stage of gestation (Fensterbank, Plommet and Pardon 1975).

We explain these facts as follows: the antibiotic limits the colonization in the lymph nodes to a level corresponding to a lower inoculum (Philippon et al. 1971) and gestation speeds up the infection spreading process to the target organs. When circumstances of the colonization lead to a low level node colonization which develops slowly, there is an induction of a sufficiently strong immunity so that some cows, even during gestation, completely recover without noticeable serological reactions. Such an interpretation has suggested to us the process of vaccination by conjunctival route (Plommet and Plommet 1975); moreover, it allows for a better understanding of the evolution of brucellosis within a herd.

Brucellosis can, in fact, break out in a herd either suddenly or in a progressive form. As time goes by, it progresses toward a reduction in the frequency of abortions and in infections, sometimes to the point of complete disappearance, as long as new animals are not introduced into the herd. Although differences of virulence between infecting strains can be documented, it seems more probable to me that the degree and the moment of exposure of the herd are, in reality, the decisive factors of this evolution. Repetition of low-level exposure of non-pregnant animals is, in a way, a natural vaccination, although not without a considerable risk of accident.

Serological Response to Experimental Infection

The rapidity of serological responses to the same inoculum is relative to the stage of gestation (Fensterbank, Plommet and Pardon 1975, Figures 3 and 4). On the average, the agglutination and the complement fixation tests became positive four weeks after the inoculation carried out during the fourth

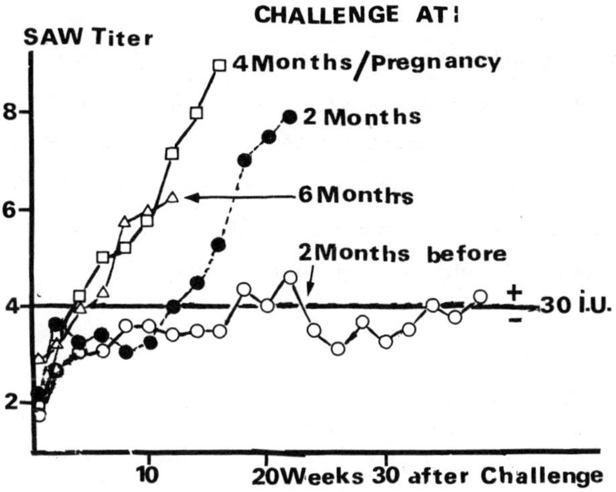

Figure 3

Serologic Response (Agglutination) According to the Time of Pregnancy at Challenge (Fensterbank et al. 1975)

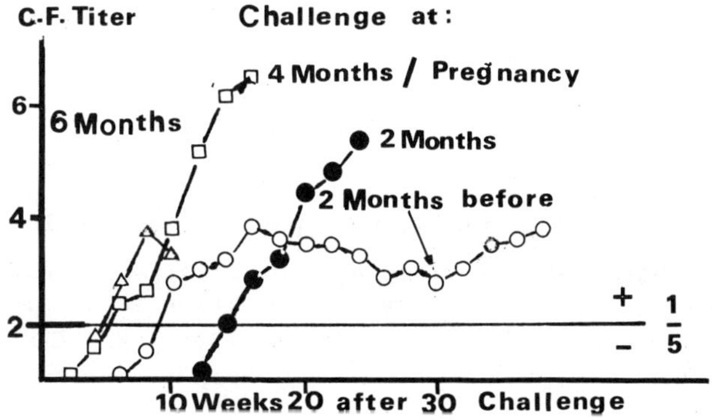

Figure 4

Serologic Response (Complement Fixation) According to the Time of Pregnancy at Challenge (Fensterbank et al. 1975) or sixth month of gestation and about ten weeks after the inoculation made two months before or two months after insemination. However, there are important differences in results from individual animals, to the extent that even after calving, some cows that are actually infected (isolation of Brucella at slaughter) are still negative to all serologic tests. Fensterbank (Personal Communication 1975) has pooled the data showing the time when the tests become positive in relation to calving and the manner in which this takes place (Table 4).

Table 4. Comparison of the Serologic Responses (Agglutination or Complement Fixation) to the Time of Calving in Cows Experimentally Infected Near the Time of Parturition (Fensterbank - (Personal Communication 1975)

Calving Status	Time of Infection in Reference to Calving (Weeks)				
	-5	-3	-1	+1	+3
Abortion	42*/77**	62/80	69/-	78/-	75/75
Premature (Living)	17/19	18/-	18/-	19/-	19/-
Full Term (264 days)	39/67	41/-	50/-	53/66	57/65

* Total number of cows giving a positive serologic response (either agglutination or complement fixation) before calving.
** Total number of cows giving a positive serologic response (either agglutination or complement fixation) after calving.

Three weeks after calving, which is considered the very best time for serological diagnosis, eight cows out of 65 (full term) were still negative, although actually infected; 56 of the 65 had excreted Brucella at calving (four of which had negative serology) and nine did not excrete Brucella and could be considered simply infected carriers.

Excretion of Brucella and Congenital Brucellosis

Excretion by vagina and milk is well known; the results of an experiment are given in Figure 5 (Philippon, Renoux and Plommet 1970 and 1971 a).

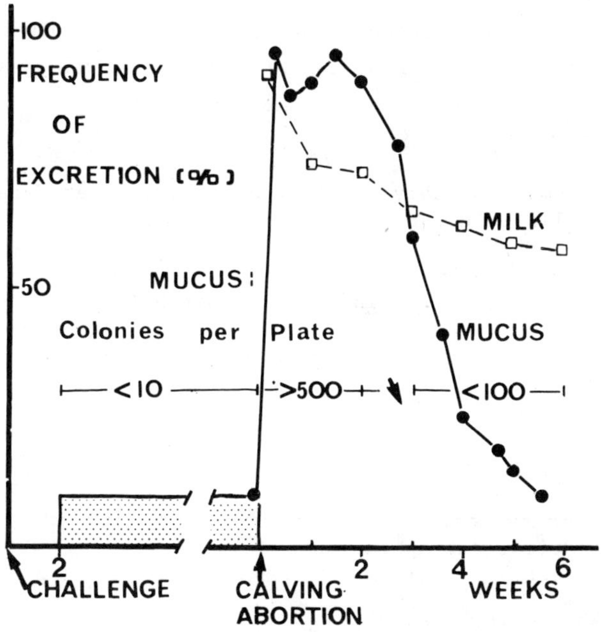

Figure 5

Brucella in Vaginal Mucus or Postpartum Discharges and in Colostrum or Milk (Philippon et al. 1970, 1971a)

Before calving or abortion we found small quantities of *Brucella* in vaginal mucus (less than ten colonies per plate) in 11 percent of the samples (135/1259) from the tenth day after inoculation onward. At calving, whether normal or by abortion, almost all samples contained a large number of *Brucella*. This excretion decreased rapidly and disappeared entirely by the 40th day post-parturition. There was also a very high rate of excretion by way of the udder (91 percent) the first day after calving. It then remained at a moderate rate without any notable reduction during the observation period.

The presence of *Brucella* in the calf, whether stillborn or alive, born to an infected mother is, from an epidemiological point of view, a particular way of excretion. Table 5 (results

Table 5. Number of Calves Infected at Birth That Were Born to *Brucella* Infected Cows (Plommet et al. 1973)

Sex of Calf	Infected at Birth/Total		
	Aborted	Premature	Term (264 Days)
Male		6/7	4/10
	24/25		
Female		X*/11	X*/11
*X (Hypothetical-extrapolation of male data)		9	3
Still Infected as Pregnant cows		1	3

of two experiments) shows that calves born before term are nearly always infected, whether stillborn (aborted) or alive (premature). Male calves born at term to infected cows (that are nearly always excreting Brucella from genital passages) are, on the other hand, not always infected at birth (Phillipon, Renoux and Plommet 1971 b).

In these two experiments (Table 5), live female calves were separated from their infected mothers immediately after birth, raised in conditions of strict isolation until puberty, inseminated, and then submitted to the system of analysis as outlined in Figure 2. Four of these F_1 females were found to be infected by isolation of B. abortus strain 544. Strain 544 had been inoculated into their mothers three years beforehand. Serological tests carried out from the age of a few months until slaughter gave slightly positive transitory reactions in two of the infected heifers and entirely negative results until the end of gestation for the other two heifers (Figure 6, Plommet et al. 1973).

The facts shown by these experiments are very important because they contradict the accepted general opinion that calves, infected at birth, recover by themselves in the first months of life. They also showed that serological tests used in this experiment were more or less pointless on heifers. These facts have since been confirmed in England (Lapraik et al. 1975). We cannot gauge with precision the frequency of this means of transmission and conservation of brucellosis under natural conditions. However, we can be sure that:

1. Our conditions of isolation exclude all possibility of outside contamination.

2. The four infected heifers were born to vaccinated cows; the three born at the normal time were probably only slightly infected at the time of birth. It appears that calves born prematurely, and thus more highly infected at birth, recover more frequently than those born at term (Table 5).

3. The facts were established by two successive experiments performed at one year's interval. Three more recent

Figure 6

Serologic Tests in Four Female Calves Born from Infected Cows. The tests were performed from eight months of age to the end of the first pregnancy. Bacteriological test results from vaginal mucus, colostrum and milk (Lait) are shown below each graph. I = insemination Avort. = abortion Abat = slaughter (Plommet et al. 1973)

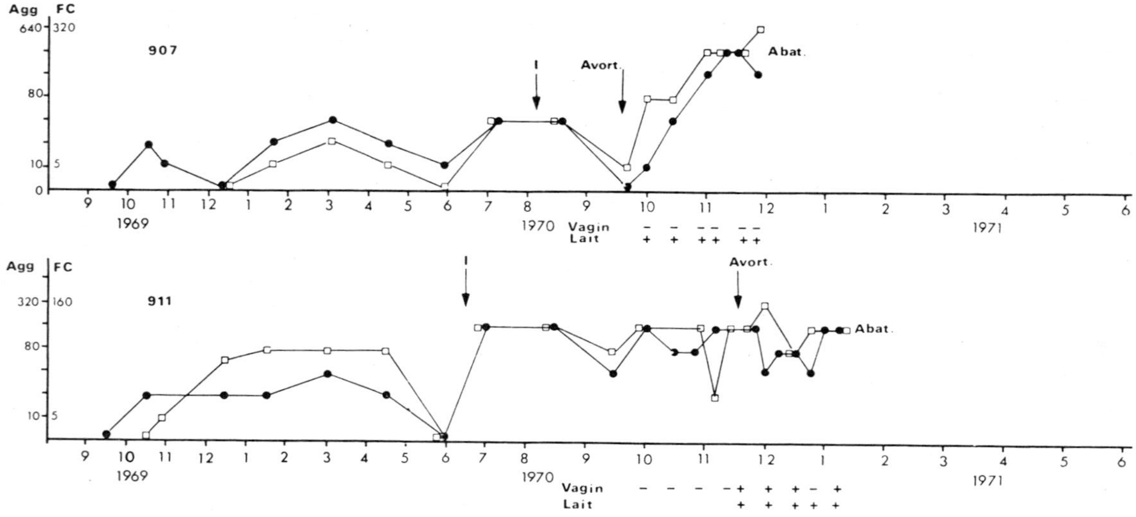

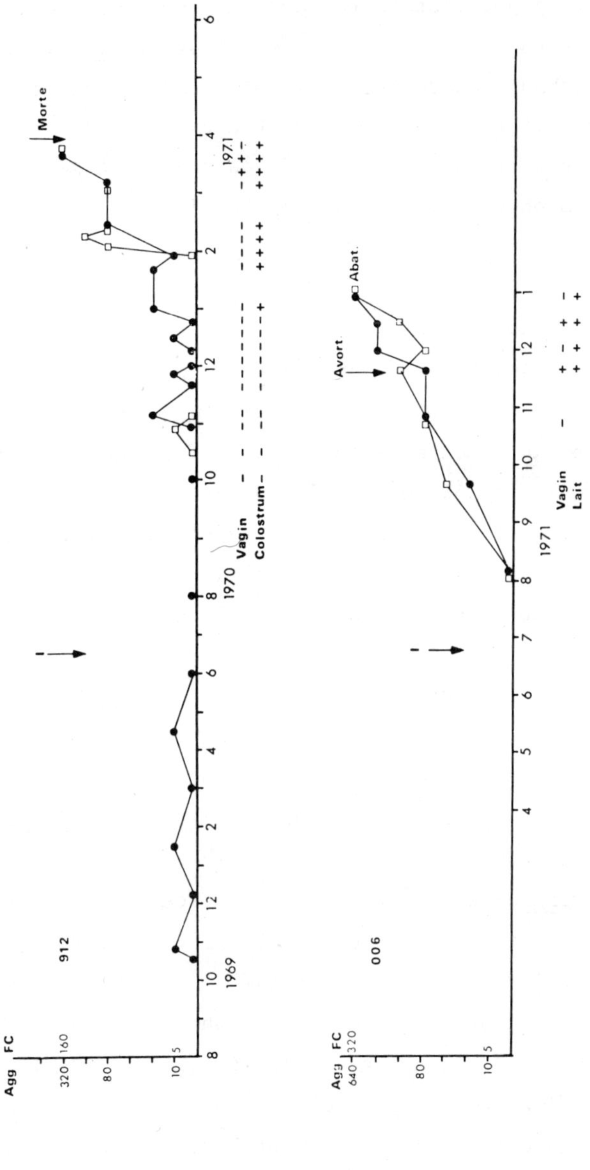

Figure 6 Continued

experiments on 21 heifers have not shown congenital transmission. Therefore, the frequency observed is a total of 4/43 (9 percent).

4. All experiments were carried out on cows of the same breed (Friesian) and with one strain (544) of B. abortus.

5. Although congenital transmission had not been established before on an experimental basis, control programs in certain countries (Denmark and Nederlands) take it into account from observations made in the field (Plommet et al. 1973).

Survival of Brucella Outside the Bovine - Liquid Manure and Wild Rodents

In the experimental stable of the Station (experimental isolation unit for 50 cows), liquid manure is stored in eight separate tanks of 50 m^3 which permits conservation for three months. In designing this equipment we did not think that the Brucella in the manure would survive longer than this.

We noted that following two abortions (the placentas having been collected and destroyed) the number of Brucella in one tank reached 3×10^4 per ml of liquid manure. After a series of abortions this number can reach 1×10^5 per ml. This corresponds to an excretion of at least 8×10^{11} Brucella per cow. Enumerations made approximatively every second month have shown that Brucella survive without noticeable decrease for at least eight months. A method of simple disinfection by adding xylene (1/1000) has been perfected (Plommet 1972). We have not studied the role of liquid manure in the dissemination of brucellosis in open-grazing cattle, but it is very likely that manure spraying or pollution of running water with manure are of considerable importance in inter-herd communicability. In France, observations made in the field show that certain epidemics of brucellosis follow the streams and rivers in the same way as salmonellosis.

The role of wild rodents as a reservoir of infection has been studied at the laboratory in three different circumstances. Verger (1970) made a survey in the southern part of France where ovine and caprine brucellosis (*B. melitensis*) is frequent. He was unable to isolate *Brucella* from any of the 941 samples collected, principally from *Apodemus sylvaticus* and *Microtus agrestis*. Not knowing what to do with the liquid manure from our experimental unit before disinfection was perfected, we used to spread it out in an isolated wood lot near the Centre. No *Brucella* was found in 167 small wild mammals trapped in this wood (Verger Personal Communication 1971). Finally, on a farm in the west of France where a brucellosis outbreak with abortions was occurring, 252 wild mammals were caught and analyzed. The strain of *B. abortus* isolated in cattle, which had a particular epidemiological character, was found in three field mice (*Apodemus sylvaticus*) caught in a hedge where two cows had aborted two months previously. None of the 129 wild rodents captured two months later in the same place were found to be infected (Verger and Dufresnoy 1972). Consequently we think that if contamination of certain wild rodents is possible, the role of these animals as a reservoir of infection is negligible.

Conclusions

The work carried out in our laboratory in the last ten years has revealed the following new factors concerning the epidemiology of bovine brucellosis: congenital transmission occurs from mother to daughter at a rate difficult to predict; the infection evolves unnoticed in the heifer until the time of her first gestation; the first manifestation of infection can be an excretion of *Brucella* by mammary secretions *prepartum* or an abortion; the very long period of survival of Brucella in liquid manure; and the not-very-frequent and slight but nevertheless positive vaginal excretion of Brucella during gestation and before parturition. Other facts have also been confirmed or specified: the absence of a measurable serological reaction after calving in certain cows carrying infection and the influence of the degree of exposure and the time it takes place in the development of infection.

These facts have the following immediate implications on prophylaxis: careful control of heifers born to infected mothers; dangers of liquid manure; control of contagion at the moment of calving, but also before and after; and the restrictive interpretation of individual serological diagnosis. They also suggest the following new points for research: how to avoid congenital transmission; how to recognize latent infection in heifers; and how far can vaccination help to control contagion in or between herds?

References

Fensterbank, R.; Plommet, M.; and Pardon, P. 1975. Traitement de la brucellose bovine par l'oxytetracycline. Ann. Rech. Vet. 6:43-66.

Kerr, W. R. and Rankin, J. E. F. 1959. The spread of brucellosis within herds: the milk problem. Vet. Rec. 71-224.

Lapraik, R. D.; Brown, D. D.; Mann, H.; and Brand, T. 1975. Brucellosis: A study of five calves from reactor dams. Vet. Rec. 97:52-54.

McCullough, N. B. 1970. Microbial and host factors in the pathogenesis of brucellosis in Mudds, Infectious agents and host reactions, Philadelphia: Saunders Co.

McEwen, A. D.; Priestley, F. W.; and Paterson, J. D. 1939. An estimate of suitable infective dose of B. abortus for immunization tests on cattle. J. Comp. Pathol. 52:116-128.

Nagy, L. K. and Hignett, P. G. 1967. The long-term effects of *Brucella* infection of newly born calves. Res. Vet. Sci. 8:247-255.

Pardon, P. 1976. Colonisation ganglionnaire, splenique et hepatique par *Brucella abortus* chez des souris, immunisees ou non, inoculees par voie sous cutanee plantaire (To be published).

Philippon, A.; Renoux, G.; and Plommet, M. 1970. Brucellose bovine experimentale: III, Excretion de *Brucella abortus* avant et apres la mise-bas. Ann. Rech. Vet. 1:215-224.

Philippon, A.; Renoux, G.; and Plommet, M. 1971a. Brucellose bovine experimentale: IV, Excretion de *Brucella abortus* par le colostrum et le lait. Ann. Rech. Vet. 2:59-67.

Philippon, A.; Renoux, G.; and Plommet, M. 1971b. Brucellose bovine experimentale: VI, Infection par *Brucella abortus* des veaux a la naissance. Ann. Rech. Vet. 2:69-76.

Philippon, A.; Plommet, M.; Renoux, G.; Gestin, J.; and Fensterbank, R. 1971. Brucellose bovine experimentale: VII, Influence sur l'evolution de l'infection d'une faible concentration d'oxytetracycline dans l'organisme au moment de l'inoculation. Ann. Rech. Vet. 2:147-157.

Plommet, M. 1972. Survie de *Brucella abortus* dans le lisier de bovins: Desinfection par le xylene. Ann. Rech. Vet. 3:621-632.

Plommet, M.; Fensterbank, R.; Renoux, G.; Gestin, J.; and Philippon, A. 1973. Brucellose bovine experimentale: XII, Persistance a l'age adulte de l'infection congenitale de la genisse. Ann. Rech. Vet. 4:419-435.

Plommet, M. and Plommet, A. M. 1975. Vaccination against bovine brucellosis with a low dose of strain 19 administered by the conjunctival route: I, Protection demonstrated in guinea pigs. Ann. Rech. Vet. 6:345-356.

Plommet, M. and Plommet, A. M. 1976. Vaccination against bovine brucellosis with a low dose of strain 19 administered by the conjunctival route: II, Determination of the minimum dose leading to colonization of the regional lymph nodes of cattle. Ann. Rech. Vet. 7:In Press.

Plommet, M. and Fensterbank, R. 1976. Vaccination against bovine brucellosis with a low dose of strain 19 administered by the conjunctival route: III, Serological response and immunity in the pregnant cow. Ann Rech. Vet. 7:In Press.

Rankin, J. E. F. 1965. Brucella abortus in bulls: A study of twelve naturally infected cases. Vet. Rec. 77:132-135.

Verger, J. M. 1970. Enquete sur la presence eventuelle de Brucella chez certaines especes sauvages de France, de l'ordre des rongeurs, des insectivores et des carnivores. Ann. Rech. Vet. 1:141-147.

Verger, J. M. and Dufrenoy, J. 1972. Isolement de Brucella abortus biotype 1 chez le mulot (Apodemus sylvaticus). Ouest Medical 25:989-991.

Epidemiological Odds and Ends

Margaret E. Meyer

Non-Bovine Reservoirs of Brucella Abortus

The non-bovine species of domesticated livestock that are susceptible to Brucella abortus are sheep and goats, swine, and horses. However, it is unlikely that these animal species are infected.

In comparison to cattle, sheep and goats are relatively resistant to infection with Brucella abortus. Infections have been established experimentally, but natural infections have occurred very infrequently and abortions are rare (Meyer 1964). In the reported instances of B. abortus infections in sheep in the United States (Luchsinger and Anderson 1967; Stoenner 1951) and elsewhere (Alsup 1969; Young 1953; Bannantyne 1960) this species of animal became infected by having been exposed to aborting cattle. However, B. abortus infection is not self-perpetuating in sheep or goats and these animals cannot seriously be considered as a natural reservoir of infection for cattle.

Swine also are relatively resistant to infection with B. abortus. This organism has been recovered from tissues of swine that were in contact with infected cattle (McCullough et al. 1949), and swine fed milk that contained the organism, but there has been no documented or reported occurrence of abortion in swine from infection with B. abortus. Clearly, this species of animal is not a reservoir of infection for cattle.

There are numerous reports in the literature of *B. abortus* having been recovered from the lesions of fistulous withers and poll evil in horses (Meyer 1974). This is not of widespread occurrence in horses, but rather is sporadic and usually confined to individual or "singleton" animals. If the lesions are draining, it is possible that an infected horse could transmit the disease by direct contact to cattle. However, horses have never been viewed as a measurable threat in serving as a reservoir of *B. abortus* infection.

Even though none of these kinds of livestock are a clear and present danger to cattle, they should not be completely discounted as potential reservoirs of infection. When epidemiological investigations fail to reveal a conventional and obvious source of infection, these animals could conceivably be exotic, obscure and infrequent sources of infection.

It also behooves epidemiologists to remember that sheep and goats can transmit *B. melitensis* and swine can transmit *B. suis* to cattle. While abortion in cattle from *B. melitensis* is rare, and has not been known to occur as a result of *B. suis* infection, nonetheless, infected cattle can shed both these species of organisms in their milk and will show positive serological reactions.

In addition to the domesticated species of livestock that are susceptible to infection with *B. abortus*, many species of wild animals also are susceptible to infection with this organism. Some, but certainly not all, of these kinds of animals can be found in Texas. Wild animals that are known to be susceptible to *B. abortus* and that are found in Texas include various species of rodents, jack rabbits, several species of deer (White tail and Desert mule deer, Axis, Sika, Red and Fallow deer), elk, bison, sheep (Desert Bighorn, Oudad, Mouflan, and Barbados), and foxes (Grey, Swift, Kit, and Red). Details on wildlife as reservoirs of infection will be presented by another participant.

Insects and Their Transmission of Brucella

The idea that insects might transmit Brucella organisms first occurred to Horrocks and Kennedy (1906) after they isolated B. melitensis from four mosquitoes caught in a hospital ward housing patients with undulant fever. Other members of the Mediterranean Fever Commission, in carefully designed feeding experiments, later examined several kinds of blood sucking and biting insects for their potential ability to transmit brucellosis. Several species of Culex and Anopheles mosquitoes were allowed to feed on specially infected guinea pigs (intracerebrally inoculated to produce an acute bacteremia in five to six hours) and later the mosquitoes were allowed to bite healthy guinea pigs or monkeys. While it was possible to recover up to 5,000 B. melitensis organisms from mosquitoes that had fed on infected guinea pigs and even though the organisms survived in the mosquitoes up to four days, transmission from one animal to another animal did not occur as a result of mosquito bites. In similar experiments, it was found that up to 50,000 B. melitensis organisms could be recovered from the stomach and intestines of biting flies (Stomxys calcitrans), and that the organisms could persist in the fly up to five days. However, no transmission occurred between infected guinea pigs and healthy monkeys, guinea pigs, or young goats as a result of bites with these flies. Dog fleas (Pulex serraticeps) and rat fleas (Pulex sciurorum) fed on their respective experimentally infected hosts failed to transmit the disease to other dogs or rats.

Various Soviet investigators have recovered Brucella from the several kinds of ticks, including Haemophysalis concinna and H. punctata (Galuzo 1946-1956), Ixodid ticks

(Arshaktuni 1955), Dermacentor marginatus (Kusov and Rementsova 1957), Hyalomma marginatum (Pritulin 1957), and Ornithodorus lahorensis (Rementsova and Kusov 1950). As with flies and mosquitoes, Brucella organisms can be recovered from ticks that have fed on animals with a bacteremia, but no evidence has yet been forthcoming that establishes ticks as vectors of Brucella infections.

Brucella neotomae was recovered from fleas (Orchopeus sexdentatus) taken from a wood rat and the suggestion was made that fleas and other arthropods may have a role in transmitting brucellosis among wild life (Thorpe et al. 1965).

The most recent suggestion concerning insect transmission of brucellosis was made by Vaskevich, after he found that 11 to 44 percent of the first stage larvae of the reindeer warble fly (Oedemangena tarandi) collected from naturally infected reindeer yielded cultures of B. suis, type 4. Also 37-60 percent of the first stage larvae collected from experimentally infected deer were positive for Brucella.

However, actual transmission of brucellosis from one infected herd to a "clean" herd has not been shown with warble flies, fleas, ticks or mosquitoes. There is, however, the possibility that flies congregating *en masse* on infective material such as a fetus could mechanically transmit organisms to animals nearby in the herd.

Age, Sex and Breed Susceptibility

Cattle are less susceptible to infection prior to sexual maturity than after maturity. Any observed differences in breed susceptibility among dairy animals is probably more apparent than real. The smaller breeds, such as the Jersey, mature earlier and, thus, the increase in susceptibility occurs at an earlier age. However, there is no evidence to indicate that the total number of Jerseys that become infected is either more or less than any other dairy breed.

For rather obvious reasons, there is considerably less information on brucellosis in males than in females. In one of the more recent studies on infection in bulls, Cedro (1967) collected blood samples and also genital organs for culture from 211 bulls at a slaughterhouse in Buenos Aires. He found that all but 69 of the bulls had a blood agglutination titer of 1:12.5 or higher and he recovered B. abortus from 24 or 11.3 percent of the animals (six of the isolates were from bulls without a titer). The titers and the isolates were approximately equally distributed among all the breeds included in the sample--Dutch Argentine, Hereford, Aberdeen Angus, Shorthorn, and Charolais. He concluded that breed was not associated with susceptibility to infection with B. abortus.

Emergence of New Species

During the last two decades, three new species of Brucella have been recovered in "nature"--Brucella neotomae from woodrats; Brucella ovis from rams; and Brucella canis from dogs.

Recently, an organism essentially indistinguishable in vitro from B. ovis was derived in the laboratory (Meyer 1976). The basic mechanism responsible for its derivation was incomplete reversion of L-forms to their original parental characteristics. More precisely, a number of strains of B. abortus, type 2 were exposed to a physiological concentration of progesterone. This steroid hormone triggers B. abortus to grow in the cell wall defective and cell wall deficient (L) form. When the L-forms were grown back on media without the inducing agent, they did not completely revert to the parental characteristics either morphologically or biochemically. After having returned to conventional growth in the cell wall intact form, the L-forms had incompletely reverted and now had mucoid colonial morphology and the metabolic pattern of B. ovis. The evolution of B. ovis in nature probably occurs by this same mechanism.

The probability that a new species could emerge in cattle after the elimination of Brucella abortus is remote, because:

1. Not all strains of B. abortus can be induced to form L-type organisms.
2. When a strain is inducible, the normal course of events is for it to completely revert to the parental form; incomplete reversion is rare.
3. In the event a strain incapable of complete reversion encounters the inducing agent in vivo and forms a "new" species, it then has to be transmitted to another host. Since B. neotomae, B. canis and B. ovis all have narrow host ranges, presumably another "new" species derived by the same mechanism would also characteristically have a narrow host range. An incomplete revertant is not infectious for the same host as is the parent form from which it is derived, so to be transmitted, just the right new host would have to be in the right place, at the right moment. What we are really talking about then is, could a strain of B. suis go through this process and then be infectious for cattle? Possible, but only remotely probable.

References

Alsup, T. N. 1969. Abortion in sheep associated with Brucella abortus infection. Vet. Rec. 84:104-108.

Arshaktuni, G. A. 1955. The role of ixodid ticks in the transmission of brucellosis infection in sheep and goats. Tr. Arm. Vet. 8:39-44.

Bannantyne, C. C. 1960. *Brucella abortus* infection in a black face ewe. Vet. Rec. 72:660-661.

Cedro, V. C. F.; Cisale, H. O.; and Farti de Meraldo, L. R. A. 1967. Brucellosis in bulls: Agglutination titres and bacteriological diagnosis. World Health Organization WHO/Bruc/67.302.

Collier, J. R., and Molello, J. A. 1964. Comparative distribution of *Brucella abortus*, *Brucella melitensis*, and *Brucella ovis* in experimentally infected pregnant sheep. Am. J. Vet. Res. 25:930-934.

Eyre, J. W. H.; McNaught, J. G.; Kennedy, J. C.; and Zammet, T. 1906. Report upon the bacteriological and experimental investigations during the summer of 1906. *In* Report of the Commission to Investigate Mediterranean Fever, part VI London: Harrisons, pp. 73-99.

Galuzo, I. G. 1946-1956. Blood sucking ticks of kazakhstan, parts 1, 2, 3, 4. Alma Ata: Acad. Sci. Kaz. SSR Press.

Horrocks, W. H., and Kennedy, J. C. 1906. Mosquitoes as a means of dissemination of mediterranean fever. *In* Report of the Commission to Investigate Mediterranean Fever, part IV London: Harisons, pp. 70-91.

Kusov, V. N., and Rementsova, M. M. 1957. On the natural infection of ticks *D. marginatus* with brucellosis and leptospirosis. Alma Ata: Acad. Sci. Kaz. SSR Press, pp. 92-94.

Luchsinger, D. W., and Anderson, R. K. 1967. Epizootiology of brucellosis in a flock of sheep. J.A.V.M.A. 150:1017-1021.

McCullough, N. B.; Eisele, C. W.; and Pavelcheck, E. 1949. Isolation of *Brucella abortus* from hogs. USPHS Rep. 64:537-538.

Meyer, Margaret E. 1964. The epizootiology of brucellosis and its relationship to the identification of *Brucella* organisms. Am. J. Vet. Res. 25:553-557.

Meyer, Margaret E. 1974. Advances in research on brucellosis, 1957-1972. Advances in Veterinary Science and Comparative Medicine 18:231-250.

Meyer, Margaret E. 1976. Evolution and taxonomy in the genus *Brucella*: Concepts on the origins of the contemporary species. Am. J. Vet. Res. 37:199-202.

Meyer, Margaret E. 1976. Evolution and taxonomy in the genus Brucella: Contemporary evolutionary status of the species Brucella abortus. Am. J. Vet. Res. 37:203-205.

Meyer, Margaret E. 1976. Evolution and taxonomy in the genus Brucella: Steroid hormone induction of filterable forms with altered characteristics after reversion. Am. J. Vet. Res. 37:207-210.

Meyer, Margaret E. 1976. Evolution and taxonomy in the genus Brucella: Progesterone induction of filterable forms of Brucella abortus, type 2, with revertant characteristics essentially indistinguishable in vitro from those of Brucella ovis. Am. J. Vet. Res. 37:211-214.

Pritulin, P. I. 1957. On the transmission of brucellosis by pasture ticks Dermacentor nuttalli and Hyalomma marginatum. Vet. Med. 7:31-33.

Rementsova, M. M., and Kusov, V. N. 1950. On the question of the role of the tick Ornithodorus lahorensis in the dissemination of brucellosis. News Acad. Sci. Kaz. SSR, Series on Parasitology, 8:128-125.

Støenner, H. G. 1951. Isolation of Brucella abortus from sheep. J.A.V.M.A. 118:101-102.

Thorpe, B. D.; Sidwell, R. W.; Bushman, J. B.; Smart, K. L.; and Moyes, R. 1965. Brucellosis in wildlife and livestock of west central Utah. J.A.V.M.A. 146:225-232.

Vaskevitch, R. B. 1972. The reindeer warble fly, Oedemangena tarandi, as a carrier of brucellosis. Veterinariya (Moscow) 49:46.

Young, S. 1953. Preliminary report on a Brucella infection in a ewe. Vet. Rec. 65:247-248.

Epidemiology Discussion

DR. LEON RUSSELL (Texas A&M): I'll try to summarize these three fine papers and ask for discussion of the points on which there appears to be lack of complete agreement. Looking at the questions concerning epidemiology - Question number (1): What percentage of term calves born to infected dams show evidence of infection at birth; at puberty; and first parturition? Apparently in Ireland, as Dr. Cunningham mentioned this morning, it is the practice to separate the newly born calves from the dam and put them in a different environment. This apparently is designed to stop the transmission of *Brucella* infections. In your experiment, Dr. Plommet, you demonstrated that one could isolate the organism from the fetus before parturition. Would you like to discuss this congenital or vertical transmission?

DR. MICHEL PLOMMET (Nouzilly, France): Dr. Ray has given a review of the literature which indicated that vertical transmission *in utero* is unlikely, but more likely to occur in the newborn calves fed milk for several days. If you take the calf *in utero* before birth and the calf is infected, the infection occurs *in utero*, not afterwards. And if infection occurs *in utero*, infection which may occur afterwards has no importance at all. We took about 15 calves *in utero*, one week or two weeks before normal time of parturition, and some of these were already infected. We isolated the organism from lymph nodes and the stomach, also frequently and early from the lungs. So infection is acquired mostly *in utero*.

DR. WINN RAY (USDA, Maryland): I'm afraid I may have given the wrong impression. I didn't mean to infer that calves were infected by feeding contaminated milk rather than *in utero*. The study that I was reporting was work done in the twenties and was designed to take newborn calves and feed them contaminated milk, either naturally or artificially; and in those instances and conditions, the organism was not normally detected more than about 30 days after weaning and they were usually weaned at an early age, 15 or 30 days of age. The organism disappeared in another 30 days, but there were some exceptions. The question of when the calves become exposed and which is the most important route, I don't believe has really been answered. I think most people feel that *in utero* exposure is of most importance. We plan to conduct some studies to determine if calves exposed *in utero*, and not through contaminated milk, present the kind of an epidemologic picture that Dr. Plommet has described. We also want to examine calves that are only exposed through contaminated milk and not *in utero*. So we are going to take some animals that are born of infected cows, separate them at birth, and keep them isolated from potential exposure after birth. We are also going to take a similar group of calves that are born of negative dams and feed them contaminated milk from infected cows and determine what the infection rate may be in that group. We also hope to determine how long they are fed this contaminated milk and if this has any bearing on the degree of infection that may be found in each group. So we plan to wean some calves after seven to 30 days of nursing, and another group we will wean at seven to nine months. We also want to look at calves that are born of negative cows, but raised in an infected environment to see if animals that have been neither exposed *in utero* or exposed through contaminated milk may pick up the infection and display this long incubation period.

DR. RUSSELL: Dr. Cunningham, would you like to comment on your program or recommendation for the newborn calves?

DR. BRENDAN CUNNINGHAM (Dublin, Ireland): I think you're misquoting me on the question of separating the calves from the dam and keeping them in a negative environment. The calves I talked about spent three months suckling the dams. When they got to a year old we tried to examine these calves to see how many of them had the infection as indicated by blood titers. Now as far as I recall off the top of my head, there were only about two percent of the calves born of infected dams and suckled on infected dams for three months which had any sort of blood titer at a year of age. So in the rest of them, the 98 percent, we injected 45/20 vaccine to see if we could elicit a positive anamnestic response. And in these, we got a positive anamnestic response only in 50 percent. This is quite interesting, I think, because it means that the calf for at least three months of its life is not sensitizable by the *Brucella* organism. Whether its due to the immaturity of the calf or to colostral protection from the dam, I just don't know. This is still an open question.

DR. DAVE BERMAN (Universitv of Wisconsin): Dr. Russell, I wonder if I could make a comment. I think that Dr. Plommet's observation is a very important one, but I think it's also very important that it be set in context. And I know that Dr. Plommet and I have discussed this and we are in agreement. It seems to me that we have to look at the epidemiological context within which the situation arises. I know, looking retrospectively at some of the problem herds that Dr. Ray investigated when he was in Wisconsin, that our inability to clear the herds was traceable to infection remaining in heifers. Vaccinated heifers which were the offspring of infected dams, and reared in isolation, when we assiduously tested them before they were mixed with the other animals it became quite clear that we were able to clear those herds. And I think, in retrospect, some of those situations represented animals comparable to what Dr. Plommet has seen. These animals were in heavily infected herds in an area that became clean, by and large, by the pursuit of the conventional procedures. And I think we must recognize that while this situation clearly occurs, we don't know its frequency and we have to investigate it when the situation demands it while we continue to learn more about the phenomenon through the kinds of investigations that USDA is now sponsoring.

DR. RICHARD CRAWFORD (Texas A&M): Let me ask Dr. Plommet, if you will, to come back to the latency of the infected calf that was born to an infected dam. You had one set of experiments in which there were four calves that were born to infected cows that did develop the disease at their first parturition. Did I understand you correctly to say you repeated this experiment under the same set of circumstances but the second time you got no infection? Is that a correct translation?

DR. PLOMMET: Not exactly, because we have had a different kind of experiment each year and from the experiment done this year, for example, we will keep the heifers from the infected mothers. But the mothers were sometimes vaccinated, sometimes treated, and sometimes used for other kinds of experiments. So we had four successive experiments done with these heifers; the first year three heifers were positive and the second year one was positive. So the first two experiments gave us four positive heifers. And we have since had two experiments with no infected heifers, but the circumstances of the infection of the mothers were not the same, and it is difficult to assess the exact percentage in field conditions.

DR. R. J. AVERY (Ottawa, Canada): We have been talking about the calf from the positive dam. For a number of years in the eradication program of Canada, we have removed positive dams and left the calf. Lately we have been taking the calf from the positive dam, but not bothering to test the calf. We have made this kind of an *ad hoc* observation just discussed. It seems to be in the calves which were born to positive dams, and the problem is in herds where we had a completely negative test on all mature animals; these calves, which are now mature animals, react during their first parturition. This, of course, created problems because we again had a positive herd. In the last two years, we have not left calves from positive dams in a herd. I know we are talking about eradication programs now, and we are going to talk about management later, but Dr. Ray, would you like to comment? What is your feeling about leaving these calves, not talking too much of scientific evidence, but from the practical application of your eradication program? What have you done about these calves from positive dams in the past and what are you doing at the present time?

DR. RAY: Dr. Berman mentioned that when I was in Wisconsin there was a problem of retention of infection in the young heifers. As they matured and came into production, some of these were found to be infected, and as a consequence of this, and later work duplicating that kind of observation, the testing age of heifers was reduced from 30 months to 20 months of age for dairy and to 24 months for beef. We did not feel that this is really adequate for the known infected herd, and in our recommendations on handling infected herds we state that calves 12 months of age and over, regardless of vaccination history - even if they were only vaccinated a couple of months previously, should be included in testing programs. The calves or heifers at this age, the short yearling heifer on up to the animal that is ready to calve, would not necessarily be interpreted on the basis of the standard interpretation of the test. We want to include these animals in the herd test so that we, at least periodically, can establish baseline titers and baseline reactions. As the animals mature and are bred and approach calving, if there are some shifts in the serologic pattern, we try to remove these animals prior to premature or normal calving with subsequent serological shifts. So, we have been aware of this problem, but we haven't tried to change the rules of the program to routinely remove both the dam and its calf because of the cost. We are not sure it is entirely necessary because the percentage of calves born of infected dams that are later found to be infected at parturition seems to be relatively small.

DR. RUSSELL: Along that line, Dr. Plommet mentioned that the heifers would not show a positive serologic reaction until about three weeks after calving.

DR. RAY: Some don't, but many do. You can identify many of them before calving and before they apparently have a chance to spread brucellosis; but it's not 100 percent by any means.

DR. RUSSELL: I believe that the next two questions are very similar, therefore, we will discuss both questions at the same time.

Question (2): What environmental factors have been identified that affect the survival of Brucella abortus outside the bovine host? And Question (3): What conditions have been documented that will allow the survival and multiplication of Brucella outside the animal host in sufficient numbers to result in transmission? Dr. Ray pointed out the fact that Brucella needs moisture, maybe a little bit of coldness, darkness and probably some nitrogenous substances for the bacteria to persist in the environment. Any deviation from this, i.e. high temperatures and drying, would reduce the viability and probably inactivate the organism. However, Dr. Plommet did point out the very high concentration of Brucella abortus in liquid manure. It was not proven whether this indicates multiplication of Brucella or a great degree of survival; but this was a liquid, moist environment, protected from sunlight and certainly high concentration of nitrogenous substances were present for the organism to use as a source of energy and food.

DR. RAY: I'd like to go back to one point on which there seems to be conflict. Dr. Plommet has mentioned the long term survival of the organism in the manure tank and Dr. King has reported that Brucella only last four hours. I think one of the important things that was said here was when Dr. Plommet reported that the temperature in the manure tank in France reached a temperature of 15 degrees centigrade, which would permit the survival of the agent for a long period of time. In the manure tank that Dr. King was talking about they were getting temperatures of 45 to 50 degrees centigrade or maybe higher. So the temperature differential is probably the key point in the apparent discrepancy between Dr. Plommet's report and what I said. While I was in the state of Washington, liquid manure tanks were becoming popular. One of the first herds that I worked on there had just converted to a liquid manure tank. This question came up at that time because the farmer immediately spread the manure on his pasture where the dairy cows were being pastured. The cows were never fenced off that land, but just avoided the pasture for a few days after it was freshly sprayed with the liquid manure. We took temperatures of that manure tank and, I don't recall precisely what they were, but they were in the range of what Dr. King has reported, 170 to 180 degrees fahrenheit, which made us feel quite confident that we weren't spreading any Brucella on the pasture. In fact, we were able to free the herd of brucellosis quite readily in spite of this situation. So, I think that we aren't really that much in conflict in our stories.

DR. RUSSELL: Question (4): Have there been any documented instances of bovine brucellosis that was acquired by any method other than direct contact with an infected bovine or its secretions, excretions, etc.? What danger to cattle is the horse with fistulous withers or poll evil? Both Dr. Meyer and Dr. Ray answered this and mentioned that the equine animal was probably of less danger to the cow than the cow was to the horse. However, if you have a premise of low prevalence, a horse with a tremendous amount of exudate from the fistulous withers, as in the case mentioned by Dr. Ray, could contaminate the environment and possibly transmit Brucella abortus to susceptible bovine animals. Whether other types of indirect transmission are involved, we should consider Dr. Plommet's information concerning liquid manure where he made the statement that brucellosis outbreaks may follow the contaminated waterways or the rivers in much the same pattern as does salmonellosis of the bovine. So this could be an important type of indirect transmission of brucellosis. Dr. Plommet, would you clarify that?

DR. PLOMMET: These observations were made very often in our country where villages are on hills. There are villages on hills and villages down on the river, and very often when epidemics of brucellosis start near the villages on the hills, the villages below the hill on the river will be infected about one or two months after the outbreak on the hill. But the reverse does not occur. So this is taken by a lot of people in our country as evidence of transmission by the water in the river. I really don't know, but the survival of Brucella in water and in liquid manure is really an important fact. I don't know about the composition of the tank fluid, but in the tank, which was underground, the temperature was less than 15 degrees centigrade and the pH was about neutral. In this condition, the survival of Brucella is absolutely perfect. And even after eight months, you only have to take one drop of this manure to infect a cow--so the spraying manure process I showed you in a picture is something very terrible. I still do not have scientific evidence of transmission by this way, but where observation was made on one experimental area which was about one kilometer from the land where the manure was sprayed, we observed one infection in which Brucella was isolated from the lymph node from the head of one heifer. We observed this transmission by chance, and although it was not the salvage requirement, we did have the chance to determine the biotype of Brucella. It was biotype one, which is the most important one in our part of France. So, this infection may have been transmitted by other ways than by the spraying process even though I feel it was most likely by this way.

DR. RAY: We also have had numerous observations in this country of brucellosis following a stream or river and some people have gone to great lengths to describe these kinds of situations. I think on closer observation of the circumstances of infected herds along streams and the effect on herds downstream from the infected premises, it usually has been concluded that there were also means of transmission other than having the Brucella carried through the water. Rather than water transmission, it has been stray animals moving from pasture to pasture or the animals congregating along the banks of the stream, along a common fenceline, under a shadetree where a lot of the animals may be aborting or freshening, or something of this sort, that provided more direct contact than did water transmission. We have generally adopted the feeling in this country that Brucella in waterways is not a very important epidemological factor in the spread of the disease because of the dilution involved. But if you have a stagnant pool or some kind of a swampland that remains wet and protected from the sun, you may have a situation develop in that kind of an environment which may cause some increase in transmission. But most of the events where streams have been incriminated, on more careful examination of other factors, have incriminated a more direct type of transmission.

MR. HILMAR MOORE (Richmond, Texas): I'm not clear as to the period of transmission from a calf born to an infected mother and to the period of transmission from an infected cow.

DR. PAUL NICOLETTI: I have done no personal studies on this, but if we can go to the textbook references which currently suggest that when the fluids from the parturition disappear, the transmission of the organisms largely disappears. I think we have two other possibilities of transfer: (1) the surface contamination and (2) the possible fecal transmission or emission of the organisms. I think these two different things, from the standpoint of the surface contamination, would be directly related to the aspects discussed in terms of survival of the organisms outside the host. From the standpoint of fecal emission of the organisms, I think the general feeling is that after the first few bowel movements this largely disappears.

DR. RAY: I would like to elaborate a little on Dr. Nicoletti's remarks about the communicable period of a cow. Most cows are going to shed the organism from shortly before parturition until three or four weeks afterwards. There are a number of cases reported in the literature in which the individual animals may continue to shed the organisms in uterine or vaginal discharges continuously for as long as 101 weeks. Most animals are going to have a reasonably short period of high danger, but there are a few animals that continue to shed the organism, maybe in very small numbers, which may be infectious to another cow in the herd for one to two years.

DR. RUSSELL: Thank you, Dr. Ray and Dr. Nicoletti.

Question Number (5): A number of non-bovine hosts have been reported to be experimentally susceptible to Brucella abortus. Which animal species are likely to be naturally infected and a reservoir of brucellosis for cattle? Which of these species are found in the southern United States and what is the prevalence of Brucella infection in these non-bovine species? I think everybody pointed out fairly well that the non-bovine hosts are insignificant for the most part. Dr. Plommet mentioned a survey done in the western part of France where they found a very small percentage of mice infected for a short period of time. Dr. Meyer mentioned that Brucella abortus has occurred in both sheep and goats, but the infections were self-limiting and apparently were not of danger of being transmitted to cattle unless there was a fairly close association or direct exposure between the different species of animals. Swine could transmit Brucella suis to cattle, which could cause a positive serological reaction to Brucella abortus but would not cause clinical disease as the organism would be located in the mammary gland.

DR. FRANK HAYES (University of Georgia): In a sense you might say I represent the big game animal interest of the southeastern United States. So, naturally there is nothing I would like better from this symposium than to get a clean bill of health for all wildlife to take back to my sponsors. So, I'd like to ask a few questions, starting with the bison in the Yellowstone National Park. A few years ago, there was a big uproar about the buffalo in Yellowstone. It's quieted down a little bit, but I remember that the American Veterinary Medical Association expressed great concern about the buffalo reservoir. There is also concern for the elk. In other words, brucellosis is primarily a disease of cattle from *Brucella abortus* infection, but it may affect such things as buffalo, elk, deer, rats, mice, fox, and other predators. However, wildlife are really inconsequential and pose no threat to the National Brucellosis Eradication Program. I'd like to see if I am interpreting the information correctly.

DR. RUSSELL: Thank you, Dr. Hayes. Dr. Meyer, you spoke on that earlier, would you like to add anything to that?

DR. MARGARET MEYER (University of California): I've consulted with Dr. Ray about this a lot, and we believe that the bison in Yellowstone National Park are infected, and have been as far back as 1930-31 when Marsh and Tunica did some work there. But there's no evidence that they are spreading the disease to cattle. There are a few bachelor bulls that wander out of the park; however, the reproductive rate is high, and brucellosis is one mechanism of keeping the population of the herds more or less under control. The only evidence that there's any transmission of *Brucella abortus* from the wildlife of Yellowstone is through some elk that may be in contact with the bison. There has been some evidence that some of the elk are infected with *Brucella abortus*. Whether the infection goes from cows to elk, or from bison to elk and then to cows is not known. There have been instances where pregnant elk have wintered over in cattle areas because they're not so stupid as to wander off in the snow when they can go into a barn. When they have aborted there, some cows have been infected by exposure to the infected elk. This is not a raging problem, but is a very isolated singleton type of occurrence. Perhaps Dr. Ray has some information about this situation.

DR. RAY: I deleted a page out of my comments because I thought Dr. Hayes would cover this tomorrow. We are concerned about the bison, as they are natural reservoirs of brucellosis. The infection rate in Yellowstone hasn't been determined for ten years or more, but the last test, which was done in 1965 or 1966, indicated that the prevalence was somewhere between 23 and 50 percent on the basis of the 800 animals tested. I don't believe I would agree with Dr. Meyer that the calving rate is high in that herd. The Yellowstone Park people don't want a high calving rate in the bison because of the population problem. The population is increasing and, as Dr. Meyer indicated, one of the population controls is brucellosis, the prevalence of which has increased. The reason for the testing back in the mid 60's was because they were going through a herd reduction program during that time. Since then, they have hired a new staff of biologists and implemented some new concepts to produce an entirely natural environment with no man made management factors imposed on the herd. The bison have overgrazed the range; however, the biologists feel this is fine because this provides some carcasses for the eagles, wolves and grizzly bears to feast on. So they are not concerned about overgrazing and the resulting high mortality in the bison because the biologists want to provide a natural environment. The elk situation, with the populations that have developed, does not seem to be a problem. We have sampled elk in various parts of the country with generally negative results - similar to the results we found in deer. One exception to this elk picture is in the Jackson Hole area of Wyoming in which the prevalence of serologic evidence of infection is quite elevated. One of the situations in Yellowstone is that they have essentially two elk herds, a northern herd and a southern herd. In the northern herd, which has been sampled several times during the last 40 or 50 years, we find about one percent reactor rate and these animals are in pretty intimate contact with the bison. In the southern herd, which ranges 75 to 100 miles south into the Jackson Hole area during the winter, the animals have been tested in at least two of the feed grounds for the past several years. The infection rate runs somewhere between 19 and 25 percent. One of the differences between the management of this herd and the northern herd is that in the Jackson Hole area the agricultural utilization of the land has reduced the winter feed ground area for the elk. The state of Wyoming and the federal government have established feed grounds to maintain the herd's population between 10,000 and 20,000 elk. In the concentrated feed grounds, the animals are supplemented with hay, which is fed on the ground where the animals are very densely populated; in fact, they are often feeding shoulder to shoulder. In these feed grounds, aborted fetuses have been recovered from which *Brucella abortus* has been isolated. The biotype isolated has been the same one that we find in the bison. Apparently we have altered the animals' behavior sufficiently to cause a brucellosis problem. We don't yet have a solution to that problem. This area is land that is commonly used for ranching and the elk are seen in contact with the cattle, eating off the same hay stacks, and so forth, during the winter. There has been no documented case of transmission from elk to cattle, but we have some infected cattle herds in that area in which *Brucella* could have been transmitted from infected elk.

DR. HAYES: Dr. Ray, you made reference to the dilution factor regarding the rivers, the streams and so forth, and there is no indication that insects transmit brucellosis. Considering elk and the bison, would you say it looks like the chances are really nil that these animals play any part or pose any threat to the National Brucellosis Eradication Program?

DR. RAY: The ranchers in the area surrounding the park are concerned because some of their cattle migrated into the park this past year. One group of cattle migrated several miles into the park and there were several bands of bison that migrated out of the park, including some females.

DR. HAYES: You really have a dilution factor compared to other possibilities, such as cow to cow transmission.

DR. RAY: I don't know what you mean by dilution factor. You have relatively few cattle that get into Yellowstone National Park, and you have relatively few bison that get out of the park. However, there are some stray animals that go in both directions, and the cattle that migrate into the park have an opportunity of being infected in some areas under the appropriate conditions at the right time of the year. The bison that come out of the park have an opportunity of exposing the cattle under certain circumstances. I'm not saying that this is a frequent occurrence, or perhaps may not be as significant as one of the other methods of transmission.

DR. RUSSELL: Dr. Ray, do you have any problem including the elk or bison in the wildlife reservoir of *Brucella abortus*?

DR. RAY: No. Only restricted populations of elk, though.

DR. AVERY: I'd like to comment on a couple of things on the wildlife situation. Along the foothills in Alberta, we had a significant incidence of brucellosis when we started the program. Without becoming involved in the wildlife, but merely by a test and slaughter policy using the standard agglutination test which we have had in Canada for a number of years, we were able to certainly certify all the herds in the foothill area. I'm not saying that we may have been lucky and there was no brucellosis in the wildlife, but from spot checks that we did a number of years ago, we certainly had indications that elk were infected. But it would appear, at least in that area, that if the elk are still infected then there has been no transmission from the wildlife to the cattle. As far as the buffalo are concerned, we had a very large herd in Wainwright, Alberta on an army area, and in 1927 somebody got the brilliant idea that we should establish Wood Buffalo National Park, which is just on the border of northern Alberta and the Northwest Territories. Certain people, including Dr. Cameron, were against this because they realized at the time that there was a high incidence of both tuberculosis and brucellosis in those buffalo, which were at the time called the plains buffalo. When the bison were moved into Wood Buffalo National Park we not only bastardized the two strains that we had, and I think you still have here in the states, that is the plains and the woods buffalo, but we infected the woods buffalo with both tuberculosis and brucellosis. There is no doubt from work done with the buffalo at Wood Buffalo National Park that we had a high incidence of positive animals and there is no doubt that it will spread from buffalo to buffalo. Fortunately, I think it is part of a population control program because we used to have 18,000 buffalo and then it came down to about 12,000 and then increased to 14,000. It fluctuates, and I'm sure that predators do play a part in this fluctuation, but I'm also sure brucellosis and tuberculosis play a part in controlling the buffalo population. We have, in contact with the buffalo, moose and some barren ground caribou, but it doesn't seem that the infection is spreading from the buffalo to any other wildlife in the area.

MR. MOORE: I have never been accused of being a candidate for a doctorate, so I easily qualify for the most unscientific person in this room, and I realize that my question may be very basic. Dr. Hayes, I do share your concern for the wildlife because I like to hunt, but I'm far more concerned about the survival of the commercial beef producer of Texas than I am about the wildlife. I'd like to ask, if we are not concerned about those reservoirs of infection in wildlife, how then can we reconcile that to a program that is called "eradication"? While I'm not scientific, I am a law school dropout and I understand the word "eradication" to mean total elimination, and I do not see how we can have total elimination of brucellosis and still not be concerned about any reservoir or even one *Brucella* organism.

DR. RUSSELL: Would anyone like to comment on that question?

DR. RAY: I think I will preface my remarks by saying that we are concerned about the bison.

DR. HAYES: Well, since it appears that I'm unsuccessful in getting the bison and elk off the hook, may I get all of the other forms of wildlife off the hook? May we go on record here today that all other forms of wildlife are inconsequential. A piece of the loaf is better than none.

DR. RAY: You have to include the caribou.

DR. HAYES: Let's say everything in Texas and the Southeastern states. Now, a half a loaf is better than none.

DR. RAY: You got 98 percent of the loaf.

DR. HAYES: I think Mr. Moore's point is well taken here.

DR. RAY: We have no evidence from our serologic surveys or epidemiologic events that species other than bison, caribou and limited population of elk are able to sustain an active biologic reservoir of brucellosis in this country. However, in Europe, the European hare is involved in the epidemiology of swine brucellosis, but we don't have a comparable situation that we are aware of in the United States.

DR. PAUL BECTON (USDA, Maryland): Mr. Moore, I would like to repeat what Dr. Ray said. We in USDA are definitely concerned about the incidence of brucellosis in the bison and in the elk and we have certainly not finished with that question. At times we do get stymied because of the people we have to deal with, but we have not finished with the wildlife situation.

DR. SARAH HURLEY (Madison, Wisconsin): I was just hired a month ago by the Fish and Wildlife Service as their Research Epizootiologist. One of the reasons that I'm here is that we are going to be setting up a project with the Jackson Hole elk population on brucellosis and also with the bison in the Yellowstone herd. There is some concern.

DR. RUSSELL: Thank you. Any other comments? Question Number (6): Are there any documented instances of breed, sex, or age susceptibility to brucellosis? Age susceptibility has been spoken of quite a bit by Dr. Meyer, who mentioned as age increases, particularly past puberty, susceptibility definitely increases. Breed susceptibility, as Dr. Meyer mentioned, especially in breeds that mature early such as the Jersey, does occur, but this would be more of an age artifact rather than a true breed susceptibility. I noticed that there was very little mention made of breeds today except that Dr. Plommet carried out his experiments in the Holstein breed, so maybe that's an area that needs to be looked at more closely. However, most current literature states that there is a lack of breed susceptibility.

DR. PLOMMET: On sex susceptibility, we made the assumption that the females were as susceptible as the males in our hypothesis. This was an easy way to estimate the ratio of infected females to males at birth. But I am not sure that's true, because from experiments done in guinea pigs and in mice we had sex susceptibility of fetuses *in utero*. The males are more often infected *in utero* than the females. This is very easy to measure in this species because you have 12 fetuses in a guinea pig, about half of them male, half of them female, so you can easily have sex susceptibility determined this way. And it's about the same in mice. So if the same is true in cows, our assumption was wrong.

DR. RUSSELL: Are there any questions?

DR. GODFREY ALTON (Parkville, Victoria, Australia): I wonder if the question of testing of steers is relevant in this question. The European Economic Community (EEC) regulations require that all animals over six months of age be tested. In other words, in your eradication campaign, if you haven't done this, then you're not free from brucellosis at the end of your experiments. Therefore, steers, castrated male animals, come into this. This is a very important point in countries who are intending to do business with the European Economic Community.

DR. BRINLEY MORGAN (Weybridge, England): As I understand it, steers are not yet classified as animals which are routinely tested. But the question is being pursued and I think Ireland is doing a great deal of experimental work on this, but certainly, at the moment anyway, they have not been included as testable animals in the eradication program. There's one point I would like to mention. We've talked about and heard a great deal today about the calf born of a reactor dam and this has been entirely on the question of its infective status. When a calf does ingest colostrum from the dam, in addition to the organisms, it also acquires colostral antibodies. And from our work we know that these tend to persist for very much longer than we had previously thought. Our own work shows that they persist for up to five months. This depends, of course, on the type of tests that you're doing. We asked ourselves what effect this would have when you come along at three or four months of age to vaccinate these calves. We did an experiment to try and separate the susceptibility of such a calf - these are its infective state and its passively acquired antibody state. What we did was to take the antibodies from the colostrum and inject these into the calves and then follow this by strain 19 vaccination. To cut a very long story short, what we did find was that these calves did have passively acquired antibodies that adversely affected their subsequent resistance. We had something like 70 percent protection with the routine strain 19 in ordinary cows and about half that in those cows which had passively acquired brucella antibodies. I think this is something we have to bear in mind when we are talking about the way we treat and handle calves from reactor dams.

DR. ALTON: Could I come back on this business of steers because I don't know what the EEC people do amongst themselves, but their third country directive, which is a regulation given to countries outside the market, says ever so definitely and clearly that you have to test all animals over six months of age. I don't know if this is of interest to the United States, but it certainly is to some other countries that might want to do business with the EEC.

DR. CUNNINGHAM: I was just going to comment on the EEC business requiring that steers, or bullocks as we call them, be tested. I think it affects us in Ireland far more than it affects anybody else in Europe, because an awful lot of our bread and butter and the cake on top of that comes from the export of bullocks. It has arisen, primarily at the moment with Germany, that the Germans believe that they are free of brucellosis and they seem to be sincerely worried that the people in Germany might contract brucellosis from the meat of steers. So in that belief, they quite rightly insist and have insisted now for some years that any steers that we export from Ireland to Germany must pass an export test - an agglutination test of less than 20 international units. We have fought this in Brussels very strongly ever since we went into the EEC, and I am very pleased to say that it's one of the things that Britain has really backed us up on as it does affect Britain too. Anyway, there was a proposal that we should carry out an experiment in Ireland; I think the procedure was that we should expose the bullocks to infection and see what happened and then try to culture Brucella from the bullocks at some stage later on. I think you will be in agreement with me that this was totally ridiculous as we believe that if the Germans want this sort of an experiment carried out then they should foot the bill for it, but they were not keen on doing this. I think the present state of impasse on the situation is that the experiment is not going ahead.

May I come back to another point? Dr. Morgan raised a very interesting one. I didn't know that he had also been working with calves on this question of interference to a vaccination with strain 19 in calves carrying colostral antibodies. We did considerable work on this about five or six years ago. As a matter of fact, I have graphs and all sorts of things prepared on this but I never got around to publishing the data. We got a lot of calves in those experiments which had colostral antibodies from negative dams. We have treated dams in different ways: we had cattle which had been exposed and sensitized, say to field strains; cattle which had been vaccinated with strain 19; and other cattle to which we had given killed strain 19 for other experiments and then 45/20 vaccines when they were late in pregnancy so that they had high blood titers. The cows were bacteriologically negative on calving and then these calves were retained and used in the next experiment to see what would happen when we injected them at different ages with strain 19. I'm interested, too, in that Dr. Morgan says than antibodies were detectable until about five months of age. In some of our calves we detected antibodies until they were up to nine months of age using the Coomb's test. We found that low levels of antibody in the young calf would prevent strain 19 from taking. And we found that in the calves from an infected herd, born of infected dams that had high levels of maternal antibodies, about 50 percent of these calves would fail to respond to strain 19 vaccine up to the age of four and a half months of age. To test this out further to see whether lack of a serological response was a good indication that the calves were not responding to strain 19 vaccine, when these calves got to about nine or 12 months of age, we injected them with 45/20. Where a calf had given a negative response to strain 19 vaccination and subsequently gave a negative response to 45/20 vaccination, I think it was fair enough to assume that this calf had not even been sensitized by a normal dose of strain 19.

There was one other aspect that we had to ascertain. We

had to ask ourselves if these calves were immunologically tolerant to Brucella abortus. I think we satisfied ourselves on this by giving them another injection of 45/20 to which they all responded. The cattle that did not respond to strain 19 vaccine because of maternal antibody responded quite normally to two injections of 45/20 vaccine, so that I think what we were dealing with were quite normal calves - they didn't have any defect in their immune system.

DR. RUSSELL: Thank you Dr. Cunningham.

DR. EDWARD SCHILF (USDA, Washington, D.C.): I'm a little concerned about the effect of the calf born in the infected herd and the fact that we don't develop the desirable resistance that we do with strain 19 in the completely negative animal. In some of the northeast states back in the early days of the program, the states did carry on a very extensive vaccination program with strain 19. The reactor animals were not removed from the herds and when we got around to testing these herds they ended up with a very low rate of infection. I realize that when we have the antibodies there that we should take strain 19 out of circulation, but I think on this observation that we got a better protection from strain 19 than we think we should.

DR. BERMAN: Dr. Schilf is quite right on the epidemiological circumstances, but I would remind him, however, that in those days we were vaccinating calves at six to eight months and consequently the colostral antibodies would be at a very low level in the offspring of such infected dams. It seems to me that this is a significant problem which again emphasizes the necessity of pressing on with doing research on problems as they emerge in the conquest of this disease problem.

DR. RICHARD HIDALGO (Texas A&M): Dr. Cunningham, would you care to relate the percentage of infection in your steers that are going to Germany; whether you do the testing in Ireland or in Germany, and what the infection rate is in steers?

DR. CUNNINGHAM: I didn't do the testing personally, of course, but it was done in Ireland and it is quite interesting. Our overall infection rate of positive titers in steers was less than two percent. In Europe for intercommunity trade, a bovine animal must show a blood titer of less than 30 international units so that any bullock showing a titer of over 30 international units can't be exported. So this is what I'm talking about, we had less than 2 percent of bullocks showing a positive titer.

The other mark, between 30 and 60 international units are the levels of interpretation for intracommunity trade, anything less than 60 international units can move. For the establishment of officially brucellosis free herds within a community, there must be no animals showing an agglitination titer of over 60 international units. This gets us into another ballgame all together, and I think you will agree with me if you have ever tested a herd or had a herd tested of over 100 brucellosis free animals. Did you ever get a completely negative test in a herd of over 100 animals; that is, all animals having titers of less than 30 international units? We find in Ireland that we do get some herds which will be free on one particular test. But even if Ireland were completely free of brucellosis, as is Denmark, we believe that we would have about eight thousand herds constantly locked up as being reactor or suspect reactor herds using these levels of interpretation.

DR. RUSSELL: Question Number (7): In view of the emergence of detection of new Brucella species in recent years, what is the probability that a new species could emerge in cattle after the elimination of Brucella abortus? Dr. Meyer spoke about this, in fact, she has some articles on this subject in the American Journal of Veterinary Research, Feb. 1976 issue. Dr. Meyer stated that chances of occurrence are fairly remote, and then only to another host species and it should not cause a problem in the bovine host. One wonders how this would play a part in Brucella latency or development of the L form? Has there been anything determined as far as the involvement of the L forms in latency?

DR. MEYER: I think in the aged cow that there may be L forms. This was reported in the papers that Dr. Nelson and I did several years ago on recovery of strain 19 from some singleton animals in herds that had been negative for a long time. One of the things that puzzled me, and I'm sure puzzled him, was that two or three of these animals were nine to 11 year old cows, calfhood vaccinated within the right age range, had been negative on all milk tests for eight or nine years, and then suddenly they were shedding strain 19. Now if, *in vivo*, there's the same mechanism of having an organism go into an L form by contact with the right physiological concentration of steroid hormones, then its conceivable to me that in an aging animal which is dropping in hormone production, that there could be a reversion back to an intact cell wall organism. And earlier in their life, where the animals have a hidden L form, then apparently they're not producing antibodies to that form at all. The organism then reverts back to an intact cell wall and the animal has antibody production and shedding of the organism. Now this is sheer speculation, but it would be a part of the answer to these long term negative "strain 19 animals" that have been in closed herds where there's no chance that they've had exposure to strain 19 again or been accidentally vaccinated as adult animals, and ten years after the fact, they're shedding the organism - so to me this is one possible explanation.

DR. RUSSELL: Question (8): There is evidence that the portal of entry of *Brucella* is either ingestion or through the conjunctiva - which route appears to be more probable in range cattle? In cattle in confinement? One would have to assume from what has been said this afternoon that the oral route is more important in range cattle. In confinement, where you have a heavy concentration of cattle, Dr. Plommet's work pointed out that the conjunctival portal may be very important because he did find a very high number of *Brucella* in the parotid lymph nodes as well as other lymph nodes in the head. Furthermore, he was successful in transmitting *Brucella* by inoculation into the conjunctiva of the bovine. Other routes of entry certainly should be considered; however, brucellosis is not transmitted venerally in cattle during normal service. The only other route that was mentioned was the congenital transfer, *in utero*.

Question Number (9): What significance can be associated with the various insects, (flies, ticks, lice, etc.) in regards to their role in transmission of *Brucella*? With the exception of the reindeer warble fly and possibly mechanical transmission by flies breeding on an aborted fetus, the likelihood of vector transmission seems to be very remote. Especially in view of the tremendous amount of work done on vector transmissions, it should have been shown to be important before now if vectors were a major method of transmission.

On the basis of what I remember of these three papers, that is the summation of the answers to the epidemiology questions. Are there any other comments? If not, at this time I would like to open the discussion to anyone in the room on any of the material discussed this afternoon or this morning.

DR. A. M. PICKARD (Raymondville, Texas): I would like to ask Dr. Nicoletti and Dr. Cunningham to explain the false negatives and false positives on the card test?

DR. NICOLETTI: I think from the standpoint of the false negative it is quite clear from the studies that have been done that false negatives largely do not occur - they do occur, but they are quite rare. From the standpoint of the false positive, it is a very difficult question to answer. You have to talk about the population in which the studies are being conducted. In Dr. Morgan's studies on which he spoke this morning (and I would certainly like him to elaborate on), I think he quoted a statistic of one percent of the population from which there was no evidence that brucellosis existed. Certainly in our own studies in New York, we found that in non-infected populations there was a significant over-condemnation of animals. However, I can't remember the statistics. So I think again, we have to come back, and it's very difficult to talk in terms of the percentage of over-condemnation, and describe the population in which you're doing studies. I'm sure Dr. Morgan would like to elaborate on his own data from this morning.

DR. PICKARD: You mentioned in New York that the over-condemnation would have been higher than one percent, is this correct?

DR. NICOLETTI: It was eight-tenths of one percent (0.8).

DR. MORGAN: I'm going to answer as far as our own evidence is concerned and I'm sure you can't remember the table I put up by now, but it was the one on the relationship between rose-bengal plate (RBP) test and the serum agglutination and complement-fixation (CF) tests. It was not related to the RBP tests and culture and this is the first thing that I want to make clear. Excepting that, we were then relating the RBP test with the agglutination and the CF tests in herds in which there was no infection; we found that there was one percent false positive rate. All our work, basically, is related to the relationship between these two serological tests. The only other thing we had, of course, was related to the abortion in cows which were culturally positive but negative to all the serological tests. And there is nothing you can do about that.

DR. DONALD PIETZ (USDA, Iowa): As we mentioned this morning, you have to look at the population you're testing. In most states they are using a surveillance procedure to detect a potentially infected herd. And these are the herds they are testing. If you go out into the animal population and test the entire population, the majority of animals are going to be negative. If you take the standard agglutination test, you're going to find a number of suspicious animals in the general population and occasionally find singleton reactor animals in herds with no other evidence of infection. The card test eliminates the majority of these types of reactions. In evaluating the card test, you're already using some type of system to detect the potentially infected animal. Then, you are evaluating over-condemnation on this basis.

MR. AVERY: There is one thing I haven't had very straight in my mind today; I think that when we were talking about false negative and false positive and everything to do with them, it would be well if we started out by defining some of the terms that we're talking about. I understand these in terms of sensitivity and specificity. Specificity being measured as the percentage of those that do not have the disease that give the negative reaction. So, false positives really are the converse of specificity. False positives, on the other hand, are very different than the things that we measure by noting the percentage of culture positives amongst those that give a reaction. On the tests we are going to do, I think it would be very useful to straighten out this entire problem. If we could address the problem in terms of some standard nomenclature I for one would know what we're talking about.

DR. PIETZ: There are a lot of problems in trying to determine this. Number one, how do you determine whether there's disease or no disease? When you start evaluating your tests, as I mentioned this morning, the common method is to isolate the organisms from the milk - but you have got to recognize the deficiencies of this. So there are a lot of problems in trying to simplify it, which would make it easy to determine the sensitivity and specificity of a test. But if you do have disease and a positive serologic result, you certainly have a true positive; and if you have a negative serologic result, you certainly have a false negative. If you have no disease and you have a positive serologic result, that's certainly a false positive; if you have a negative serologic result, that's a true negative. You can calculate the sensitivity by taking the number of true positives divided by the number of true positives plus the number of false negatives and multiply it by 100 to convert it to percentage. And you can calculate the specificity by taking the number of true negatives divided by the number of true negatives plus the number of false positives and multiply by 100 to convert it to true percentage. But what are we going to use as a guideline to determine disease or no disease?

DR. MEYER: The presence of the organism.

DR. PIETZ: How are you going to find the organism? I mentioned this morning that the only way you are going to find Brucella is to kill the animal and culture all the tissues and then compare one test with the other, until you calculate this percentage. The only thing you are determining with a single test is the status of that animal at that point in time - not two or three weeks later. The only way that you can determine this is to take the animal and isolate it and let time take its course, and some of those animals will remain infected and some will become negative.

DR. PICKARD: In the meantime, you have overkilled the rancher's cattle. What suggestion have you got to overcome this?

DR. PIETZ: If you leave those animals in the herd, you're exposing the rest of the animals; you're perpetuating the disease, and you're taking out more animals in the end. You have to make a decision some way or another as to what is the best approach to take. You can take a sensitive test, screen the animals, and move the positive ones to a separate herd so they don't expose the negative animals. You then retest the positive animals and take those reactor animals to slaughter. Follow the animals that were positive to the sensitive test to see what they do over a period of time. Continue to test the negative animals, because many of them are in the incubation stage; you have to repeat that cycle over a period of time.

DR. PICKARD: Dr. Cunningham, in a herd that has been calfhood vaccinated, what percentage of over condemnation would you expect from the card test?

DR. MORGAN: While Dr. Cunningham is getting his figures together, can I again make reference to the approach I made this morning quoting the paper which Davis did at my laboratory on the question of the sensitivity and the specificity of the card test. Again, I want to make clear that these are in relation not to the culture status of the animal, but to the agglutination and complement fixation tests status. In our tests these were undoubtedly reactor animals. He gives a figure, which I have in my written paper, that the sensitivity of the RBP tests was calculated at 96.2 percent and specificity of the test as at 97.1 percent.

DR. CUNNINGHAM: In Ireland we have no calfhood vaccination and we don't use the card test. All I can say about the card test is that some years ago we did a couple of surveys using the Brewer Card Test and one using the Rose Bengal Test and there was no difference between them. This was borne out by the results of our first survey on about four and a half thousand animals, because the results we got on the second survey were the same as we got in the first. And our figures agreed with what Dr. Morgan said a few minutes ago, during a similar survey in Weybridge at the same time. We compared Rose Bengal tests, tube agglutination tests, complement-fixation tests and Coombs tests, and there was somewhere around 95 percent agreement with the agglutination test over the whole number of animals. But when one looks at agglutination titers below 30 international units, we did get some false positive card tests and these animals were negative also on the CF tests. So we did get false positive card tests compared to the other tests. And at the other end of the scale we found that when the titer of agglutinating antibodies in the serum was up around the 200 international units, then we got complete agreement as one might reasonably expect, because both tests were positive.

DR. RUSSELL: Thank you, At this time I'd like to thank the speakers, Dr. Meyer, Dr. Ray and Dr. Plommet for their excellent presentations and for their participation in the discussions. I also want to thank the other speakers who participated in the discussions.

IMMUNIZATION

Moderator: Richard J. Hidalgo

Immunity to *Brucella abortus*

Claude Nelson

Nearly every nation which has embarked on a program to control or eradicate brucellosis in cattle has employed the use of vaccination at some time in the program. These efforts to provide immunity to this disease have utilized a broad spectrum of organisms: living and dead; virulent and attenuated; related and unrelated.

Only a few years after Bang and Stribolt first isolated *Brucella abortus* from infected cattle, Bang (1906) was attempting to induce immunity in cattle by vaccination with living virulent cultures. The United States Bureau of Animal Industry permitted the manufacture and distribution of live *B. abortus* vaccine as early as 1919. In 1932 this country discontinued the permits for virulent vaccine production. Strain 19 vaccine was officially approved for use in the United States brucellosis program in 1939 (U.S.L.S.A. 1936).

One could easily find many experts in the field of brucellosis who would differ in their opinions about what is a satisfactory or successfully immunized animal. What is successful immunization to the scientist may not be successful to the cattleman. What is successful to the cattleman may not be successful to the officials administering an eradication program. Most of the literature on this subject supports the fact that no vaccine developed to date has approached a 100 percent resistance to normal challenge. At this time we must accept as successful something less than total protection of all animals vaccinated against brucellosis.

Under natural and experimental conditions, strain 19 vaccination enhances resistance to B. abortus infection in cattle. This enhanced resistance has repeatedly been characterized as "relative immunity." If the acquired immunity is only relative, that is, if it is able to prevent active infection after exposure to small or moderate numbers of virulent organisms, but unable to prevent active infection following exposure to large numbers of virulent organisms (Manthei 1959; Annual Report BAI 1959), vaccination cannot be the only tool used in a control or eradication program.

It is generally agreed that vaccination with strain 19 by itself cannot eradicate brucellosis infection from our cattle population, but it can be used effectively together with other measures to lay the groundwork for eradication. Present evidence suggests that it raises the degree of immunity for the individual animal to a level at which replication of the virulent field strain is restricted following access to the body tissues by natural exposure. Unlimited multiplication in the uterus and in the mammary glands is prevented so that abortion and excretion in the milk are much less frequent than in a non-vaccinated population. This effect leads to a reduction of the infected material excreted and thus reduces the danger of infection to other animals of the herd and to the human population involved.

Huddleson, in 1946, developed the M-strain vaccine. Extensive field trials in midwestern states demonstrated a relatively low level of induced protection. McEwen and Priestly (1938 and 1940) reported a strain (45/20) of low virulence which was relatively non-agglutinogenic. This strain was later used for production of a bactrin now produced in Europe and Australia. The strain 45/20 vaccine has been used in field and controlled studies by USDA for several years.

Hendricks et al. (1956) reported that the protection afforded by killed strain 45/20 in adjuvant administered to calves in two doses at six and nine months of age provides comparable protection to that elicited by strain 19. His data supported that of McDiarmid (1966) in demonstrating the lack of protection provided by a single dose of 45/20 bacterin. Data (unpublished) obtained in USDA-sponsored field studies utilizing 45/20 bacterin as a diagnostic agent revealed a very high level of overcondemnation when following the protocol reported by Cunningham: 91 percent overcondemnation by Coombs, 75 percent overcondemnation by CF. The disease continued to persist for months after using this procedure as a diagnostic tool.

Today's advances in the field of immunology have clearly demonstrated that when dealing with an intracellular pathogen one cannot use the level of circulating antibody as an indicator for immunity. Most animals vaccinated in calfhood will exhibit a high humoral antibody level immediately following injection with strain 19. This antibody level will gradually decline to the point where six to eight months after vaccination it is rare to find IgG (7S) antibody present in the blood. This lack of circulating antibody has no direct relationship to the degree of resistance the cow may have to a challenge exposure to brucellosis.

Cell-mediated immunity is the area of primary research utilized today in attempting to develop resistant animals to intracellular pathogens. If immunity can be transferred from one animal to another without having to establish a low-grade infection or without the use of antigens which produce circulating antibody, the host defense mechanism can be stimulated quite rapidly without interference with the diagnostic test procedures.

Since this modern concept differs from the old classical theories on relating antibody level to resistance, we still hear people talk about the test and slaughter programs as used in most countries as being wrong. They claim the program which removes high-titered animals is actually taking away those with the most resistance. Obviously this is an erroneous concept.

Since immunity cannot be related to circulating antibody levels, controlled experiments involving known challenges have been employed to measure duration of strain 19 induced immunity. Wright (1942) vaccinated calves in 260 infected herds. There was no significant difference in infection rates or numbers of abortions for these cows when followed through five separate gestations. Manthei et al. (1951) found similar results under controlled experiments in five separate groups of cows vaccinated in calfhood and exposed during their first, second, third, fourth and fifth pregnancies. In fact, the old animals appeared to be more resistant to artificial conjunctional exposure. One can conclude that calfhood vaccination with strain 19 does afford immunity which is of a relatively long duration. Berman et al. (1952) found that there was no significant increase in resistance to challenge provided by revaccination.

When reviewing the literature to determine the effectiveness of strain 19 as an immunizing agent, one finds many articles covering this subject. Early literature and program directives provided for the use of strain 19 in adult cattle. Miller et al. (1944) observed that in one herd of 56 cows adult vaccination appeared to stop the spread of infection, but in another herd the abortion rate remained about the same after adult vaccination. Moore and Mitchell (1950) vaccinated serologically negative cows (1 to 11 years of age) in 14 infected herds. At the end of the first pregnancy following vaccination they determined that of the 73 animals which were not pregnant at the time of vaccination, 96.9 percent calved normally, but *B. abortus* was isolated from milk or uterine exudate of 27.5 percent. Of the 112 which were pregnant at vaccination, 85.7 percent calved normally and 21.4 percent were infected. Other earlier workers found adult vaccination with strain 19 to be of practical use in actively infected herds when combined with blood testing, removal of reactors, and calfhood vaccination.

The Montana livestock sanitary officials together with USDA (1959) conducted a survey of beef cattle in Montana to determine the relative protection afforded by strain 19 in the population. Their data covered initial area testing conducted between 1952 and 1958. Data on 951,000 cattle in 21,400 herds was presented. Some of the conclusions drawn from this study were:

1. In partially vaccinated herds, brucellosis occurred 65 percent less frequently within the vaccinated population than it did within the nonvaccinated population. This means a protection rate of 65 percent was provided by strain 19 in the face of a known exposure under field (range) conditions.
2. In infected herds in which all animals were vaccinated, brucellosis occurred 60 percent less frequently than it did within nonvaccinated cattle in partially vaccinated infected herds.
3. The herd infection rate was 7.28 percent in those herds in which all animals were vaccinated and was 9.5 percent in those herds in which none of the cattle were vaccinated. This meant a reduction of only 23 percent in the percentage of herds infected when total vaccination was practiced.
4. Vaccination alone cannot be expected to eradicate brucellosis or to free the majority of infected herds from the disease. Infected animals must be identified and eliminated.

5. Vaccination was useful in building the resistance of susceptable animals against brucellosis, but its limitation must be recognized.

Another excellent summary of the effectiveness of strain 19 was provided by the State of California (USAHA 1959, 1965). Their information disclosed that following a ten-year compulsory vaccination program in dairy heifers, they were able to achieve vaccination levels of approximately 90 percent in dairy breeds and 60 percent in beef heifers. Their overall cow population was approximately 1.6 million. Data obtained in 1946 indicated that 17 percent of the dairy cattle and 8 percent of the beef population were infected before the onset of the vaccination campaign. When the testing program was conducted ten years later (1969), the overall infection rate was 1.7 percent of the 1.8 million cattle tested. They concluded that the intense vaccination program reduced the overall infection rate by approximately 87 percent. Three counties with predominantly beef cattle on semi-range conditions disclosed the following data:

Herds % Vaccinated	Percent Reactors Cattle
0-25%	2.4
26-50%	1.3
51-75%	0.6
76-100%	0.2

With the lowered infection rate attributed to vaccination, California achieved Modified-Certified Status in six years and Certified-Free Status six years after that. They did have a very aggressive and well-enforced test and slaughter program.

Controlled experimental data by Hendricks et al. (1966) supported the observations of the Montana survey with respect to the protection provided by strain 19. Their study revealed that 69 percent of the calves withstood the challenge of $7.5X10^5$

organisms of strain 2308. This work demonstrated that three-month-old calves can be vaccinated with strain 19 without adverse effects and a significant degree of immunity was established. These data together with the work of Lambert et al. (1961) have provided the basis for our recognizing the official vaccination of female calves with strain 19 at the age of three months and over. Redman et al. (1967) reported up to 70 percent protection of calves vaccinated as young as two months of age. The number of animals involved was relatively small.

Several of the positive factors have been discussed relative to the use of strain 19; such as, degree of protection, duration of immunity, lack of significant adverse systemic reactions, lack of reversion to virulence and the need for only one immunizing dose. There are several disadvantages associated with the use of this product which should be mentioned. Some of the most common drawbacks are:

1. Calves must be gathered at young age--often before weaning time.
2. Protection is not as high as would be preferred.
3. Occasionally a residual infection of strain 19 is established which influences surveillance procedures.
4. Antibody titers of IgM antibodies persist for prolonged period if the vaccine is used in older animals.
5. Sterility problems occur if used in male calves.
6. Undulant fever has occurred in humans following vaccination accidents.
7. Proper care prior to administration is required or else it can loose its effectiveness due to loss of viability.

Since this strain does produce serum globulins similar to those of virulent field strains, there have been problems associated with diagnosis of brucellosis in immunized cattle.

Most persistent titers following the use of strain 19 were of the IgM(19S) fraction. The development of supplemental tests designed to detect and measure primarily IgG have greatly reduced this problem. This problem was also diminished by the use of strain 19 at the three to six-month age range. There are essentially no persistant IgG titers six to eight months after vaccinating at this age provided the heifers are not accidentally bred.

A review of test data involving nearly 10,000 cows in several large infected Florida dairy herds showed that approximately 95 percent of the card test positive animals were also rivanol and complement-fixation test positive. In subsequent tests of the five percent that were card test positive but negative to other supplemental test, about one-half of these revert to negative and the other half become positive to all tests, indicating infection (Hendricks unpublished). This would indicate that in known infected herds the card test does not significantly overcondemn. This is especially interesting in the face of a relatively high population of strain 19-vaccinated cattle.

The persistence of strain 19 infection into adulthood of cows has been reported by various workers. Jones et al. (1965) described the strain 19-like characteristics of isolates recovered from adult cattle which had been calfhood vaccinated. Meyer and Nelson (1967) described the recovery of twenty-seven strain 19 isolates from twenty-one dairy herds in California. Of significance was the fact that seventeen of these isolates were recovered from animals of the Jersey breed. It appeared evident that the Channel Island breeds, which are sexually mature at a younger age and are more susceptible to the initiation of early pregnancy, are more likely to establish localization of strain 19 in the tissues. They also reported that the ages of the cows at the time of isolation of strain 19 varied from eighteen months (an early bred heifer) to a seven-year-old Holstein cow. This investigation was over a three-year period and involved the monitoring of approximately 850,000 vaccinated dairy cows. This would support unpublished Wisconsin data that persistence of strain 19 infection in adult cattle occurs very infrequently.

The question of whether strain 19 can be spread from one animal to another is often discussed. Unconfirmed reports have been heard of bull calves becoming infected when penned closely with heifer calves which have recently been vaccinated. Mingle et al. (1941) demonstrated the stability of this low virulent strain by making seven serial passages in cattle.

Meyer and Nelson (1969) purchased eleven strain 19-infected cows from California dairies and allowed them to each nurse a calf for periods of up to eighteen months. This time period represented more than the normal cow-calf relationship under natural conditions. In each case the cow was determined to be shedding strain 19 in the milk before and during the nursing period. In no instance did any of the calves develop titers to the standard tube agglutination test or demonstrate any evidence of contracting strain 19 infection from the dam.

It seems clear, therefore, that when infection persists beyond the normal postimmunization recovery period, the animals cannot later clear their tissues of the organisms and they remain residually infected for long periods of time, perhaps permanently. This process does not pose a threat to the use of strain 19 in an eradication program.

At this time it would appear that strain 19 is the best strain available for an immunizing agent when considering the compatability of this agent with the livestock industry management practices and with the needs of the United States regulatory bodies.

References

Anonymous, 1940. Proposed policy involving official recognition of calfhood vaccination. Proc. 44th Annual Meeting of the U. S. Livestock Sanitary Association, pp. 100-102.

Anonymous, 1948. Report of the Chief of the Bureau of Animal Industry, Agricultural Research Administration, USDA, pp. 42-44.

Anonymous, 1959. U. S. Department of Agriculture. Agricultural Research Service Brucellosis vaccination survey, beef cattle - Montana (1952-1958). ARS-91-12 (1-7).

Bang, B. 1906. Infectious abortion in cattle. J. Comp. Path. and Therap. 19:191.

Berman, D. T and Irwin, M. R. 1952. Studies on repeated vaccination of cattle with Brucella abortus strain 19. The response of vaccinated and revaccinated cattle to conjunctival exposure with a virulent strain of Brucella abortus during the third gestation period. Am. J. Vet. Res. 13:351.

Hendricks, J. B.; Powell, H. S.; Roebuck, D. E.; and Ray, W. C. 1966. Determination of protection among calves vaccinated at various ages with either strain 19 or 45/20. USDA, APHIS, Veterinary Services, Hyattsville, Maryland.

Hendricks, J. B. (Personal Communication - unpublished data).

Huddleson, Forest. 1946. The mucoid phases of the genus Brucella. Amer. J. of Vet. Res. 7(22):5-10.

Jones, L. M.; Montgomery, V.; Wilson, J. B. 1965. Characteristics of carbon dioxide independent cultures of Brucella abortus isolated from cattle associated with strain 19. J. Infect. Dis. 115:312.

Lambert, G.; Amerault, T. E.; Manthei, C. A.; Goode, E. R., Jr. 1961. Immunogenic response of calves vaccinated at different ages with Brucella abortus strain 19. Proc. 65th Annual Meeting of the U. S. Livestock Sanitary Association, pp. 93-98.

Manthei, C. A.; Mingle, C. K.; and Carter, R. W. 1951. Duration of immunity to brucellosis induced in cattle with strain 19 vaccine. Proc. Am. Vet. Med. Assn. 88:128.

Manthei, C. A. 1959. Summary of controlled research with strain 19. Proc. 63rd Annual Meeting of U. S. Livestock

Sanitary Association, pp. 91-96.

McEwen, A. D., and Priestly, F. W. 1938. Experiments on contagious abortion: Immunization studies with vaccines of graded virulence. Vet. Rec. 50(35):1097-1106.

McEwen, A. D., and Priestly, F. W. 1940. The vaccination of guinea pigs against Brucella abortus infection with living and heat-killed suspension. Vet. Rec. 52(42):743-744.

McDiarmid, A. 1966. Vaccination against brucellosis with particular reference to the use of killed adjuvant vaccines prepared from the nonagglutinogenic strain 45/20 Brucella abortus. Agriculture Research Council, Institute of Research on Animal Diseases, Comptron Nr. Newberry, Berkshire.

Meyer, M. E., and Nelson, C. J. 1967. Recovery of Brucella abortus strain 19 from immunized cattle. Proc. U. S. Livestock Sanitary Association, pp. 96.

Meyer, M. E., and Nelson, C. J. 1969. Persistence of Brucella abortus, strain 19 infection in immunized cattle. U. S. Livestock Sanitary Association, pp. 159-164.

Miller, A. W.; Wight, A. E.; Crawford, A. B. 1944. Report of cooperative brucellosis control work in the U. S. Proc. 48th Annual Meeting of the U. S. Livestock Sanitary Association, pp. 48-57.

Mingle, C. K.; Manthei, C. A.; Jasmin, A. M. 1941. The stability of reduced virulence exhibited by Brucella abortus strain 19. J. Am. Vet. Med. Assn. 99:203-204.

Moore; Thomas; Mitchell, C. A. 1950. Vaccination of sexually mature cows with Brucella abortus strain 19 vaccine. Canad. J. Comp. Med. 14:209-213.

Redman, D. R.; Deyoe, B. L.; King, N. B. 1967. Resistance of cattle to Brucella abortus following vaccination at two and three months of age. J. Amer. Vet. Med. Assn. 150:403-407.

Stuart, J. E.; Bills, C. B.; De Mattei, J. D.; Macc, D. L. 1959. The results of eleven years' vaccinating with strain 19. Proc. 63rd Annual Meeting of the U. S. Livestock Sanitary Association, pp. 83-90.

Wright, A. E. 1942. Report of cooperative brucellosis work in the United States. Proc. 46th Annual Meeting of U. S. Livestock Sanitary Assoc., pp. 149-154.

Wixom, H. G., and Vanderwagen, L. C. 1965. Calfhood vaccination: Its relation to brucellosis eradication. Proc. 69th Annual Meeting of the U. S. Livestock Sanitary Association, pp. 141-148.

Experiences with Strain 45/20 Vaccines in Ireland

Brendan Cunningham

History

In the 1930's when the search for a suitable vaccine against bovine brucellosis was being pursued, Buck and his colleagues discovered a natural mutant strain which has since become widely known and used as strain 19. In the United Kingdom, McEwen pursued the line of producing a suitable mutant by passaging strain 45 through guinea pigs. On the 20th passage he found the strain recovered was rough and on testing this strain in cattle he found it produced a serviceable immunity and had the added attraction of being non-agglutinogenic. When used as a vaccine it did not interfere with the serum agglutination test (McEwen 1940, 1946). This was strain 45/20.

The vaccine was quite widely used in the United Kingdom until it was reported that it could revert to smooth form and full virulence (Edwards, de Ropp and McLeod 1945; Taylor and McDiarmid 1949) and it was then withdrawn from use as a live vaccine.

Later, using guinea pigs, McEwen and Samuel (1955) showed that: (1) the same strain, heat-killed and incorporated in a water-in-oil emulsion, provided "an adjuvant vaccine of higher protective property than did a smooth non-virulent (strain 45) or a smooth virulent strain (strain 544)" and (2) "the heat-killed adjuvant vaccine (K45/20A) conferred as high a resistance to infection as a living non-virulent vaccine". These findings were confirmed by McDiarmid and Sutherland (1957). In 1963 McDiarmid showed that, in cattle, two doses administered at six-week intervals conferred a "considerable immunity".

A number of trials have since been recorded, some controlled and some not. Ray (1975) assessed the results of five trials carried out in the United States. The K45/20A vaccine was judged to be not effective when used below six months of age or when only one dose of vaccine was given. Protection was good when cattle over six months of age were given two doses of vaccine at a 10 - 12 week interval and challenged during mid-pregnancy with 0.75 X 10^6 _B. abortus_ strain 2308 (this American challenge dose appears to be equivalent to the British challenge dose of 15 X 10^6 strain 544.).

McKeon (1975) compared the potency of two 45/20 vaccines in controlled experiments in cattle. Protection afforded by each vaccine was good (75 percent and 70 percent). Gaumont et al. (1973) in a controlled trial comparing nine different vaccination schedules found K45/20A vaccine to give 82 percent protection which was higher than the 71 percent provided by strain 19. Results of trials carried out in the mid-1960's were recorded by the author (Cunningham 1968). In these trials K45/20A vaccine consistently gave better protection in cattle than did strain 19.

Use of Vaccine in Ireland

In the Republic of Ireland we have used K45/20A vaccine since 1965, and this vaccine alone since 1968--strain 19 having been banned in 1967. In all, some 4.5 million doses of vaccine have been used, some by the Department of Agriculture in Official Programmes and the remainder by private veterinarians working in areas outside the specified Clearance Areas. In general prophylactic use it has satisfactorily controlled the disease. In official use it has been extremely valuable in bringing "problem" infected herds rapidly under control, and, as far as we are yet aware, it has been 100 percent effective in the diagnosis of latent carriers in problem herds. We define as "problem herds" those herds in Clearance or Accredited areas which: 1) in spite of test and slaughter methods continue to have reactors (disease still active in an unvaccinated population) and 2) herds which have been accredited for some time (1 or more years) and then break down with abortions and/or reacting cattle.

In Ireland we ceased using strain 19 in 1967 and as it is now eight years since, there are very few strain 19 vaccinates left - and these are old cows. Thus, when using K45/20A vaccine prophylactically in the field, where we come across post vaccinal titres to the serum agglutination test (SAT) or complement fixation test (CFT) these can be considered to be due to sensitisation by previous exposure to field strains. One may consider them: a) a nuisance, or b) a good indication of the true epidemiological situation which otherwise would have remained unknown.

The latter is often valuable information and can be useful in formulating plans to control the disease in a herd or in a suitable geographical area. This obviously would not be possible if cattle in which strain 19 had been, or may have been used, were present in the population. In assessing such situations one must bear in mind the importance of natural immunity versus the danger of latency in areas of differing prevalence and act accordingly.

Some comparisons between strain 19 and K45/20A vaccine are listed below:

Strain 19	K45/20A
Smooth strain - Agglutinogenic	Rough strain - Non-agglutinogenic
Must be confined to calves 3 - 6 months old. Herd vaccination not possible.	May be used in young or adult cattle (But not less than 6 months old). Vaccination of a herd is feasible at any time.
Live vaccine - Cheap to produce.	Dead vaccine - more expensive to produce.
For effective use almost all female calves in area must be vaccinated. Entails 2-3 visits per year.	Use may be restricted to herds where its use is indicated. It may be cheaper to use in the field as one annual visit for vaccination may be sufficient.
Live vaccine - dangerous to operator. In a small percentage of vaccinates strain 19 may persist as a low grade infection.	Dead - cannot infect operator or cattle (though adjuvant can cause a nasty reaction if accidentally self administered)
Protection approximately 70 percent	Protection approximately 70 percent
May take up to 7 years to obtain an immunised herd.	Herd immunity can be induced in 2 - 3 months.
Transient effect on BRT if given to adult cows (4-5 months).	No effect on BRT even when given during lactation.
Duration of immunity - five gestations (McDiarmid)	Duration of immunity - two gestations and in the absence of challenge immunity declines to about 30 percent after 4 - 5 years.
One dose of vaccine is maximum.	Two initial doses of vaccine, and a booster every 12 - 18 months is advocated if conditions still warrant it.
No persisting local reaction.	Local reaction is long lasting - though should not be unduly large.

In considering the use of vaccine in the field one must look at the serological responses to vaccination (with strain 19 and with K45/20A) and the serological responses to natural virulent field infection. The types of serological responses are associated with the types and doses of antigens present (R or S), the age of animal exposed, and whether the animal is pregnant or not at the time of exposure.

Serological Responses to B. Abortus Antigens

1. Strain 19 vaccine, (calfhood), (Figure 1).

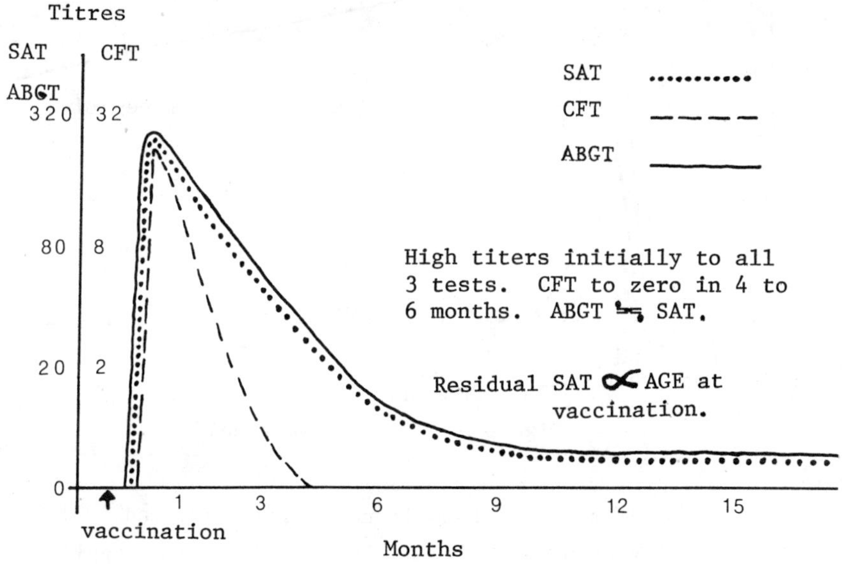

Figure 1. Strain 19 vaccine.

a. High SAT, CFT and antibovine globulin test (ABGT) withn 10 - 14 days (SAT = ABGT); CFT reverts to zero in four - six months.

b. ABGT remains within two tubes higher than SAT

c. SAT reverts to negative levels inside nine months when used in calves three - six months old. In older vaccinates a number of animals may never revert to below positive or inconclusive SAT levels.

2. K45/20A vaccine (Figure 2).

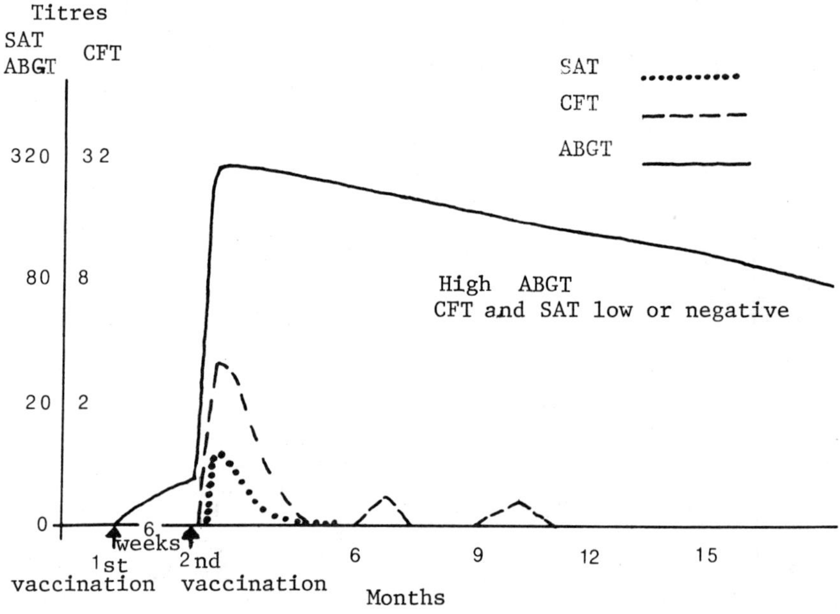

Figure 2. K45/20A vaccine.

a. First injection - Usually no SAT, no CFT, and ABGT usually below 4/40 (in adult vaccinates same applies except ABGT may continue to rise above 4/40 from about ten weeks after first injection, maybe to 1/80 to 1/320 levels).

b. Second injection - Characteristic secondary response occurs in about a month (rather delayed for a secondary response). High ABGT - usually 160 and over; SAT - usually nil - a small percentage may give temporary inconclusive/low positive response. CFT - not usually marked - most animals nil - some may show temporary titres up to about 2/8.

3. Exposure of unvaccinated females to field strains of B. abortus (usually smooth strains).
   a. Non-pregnant animals (Figure 3) - After natural

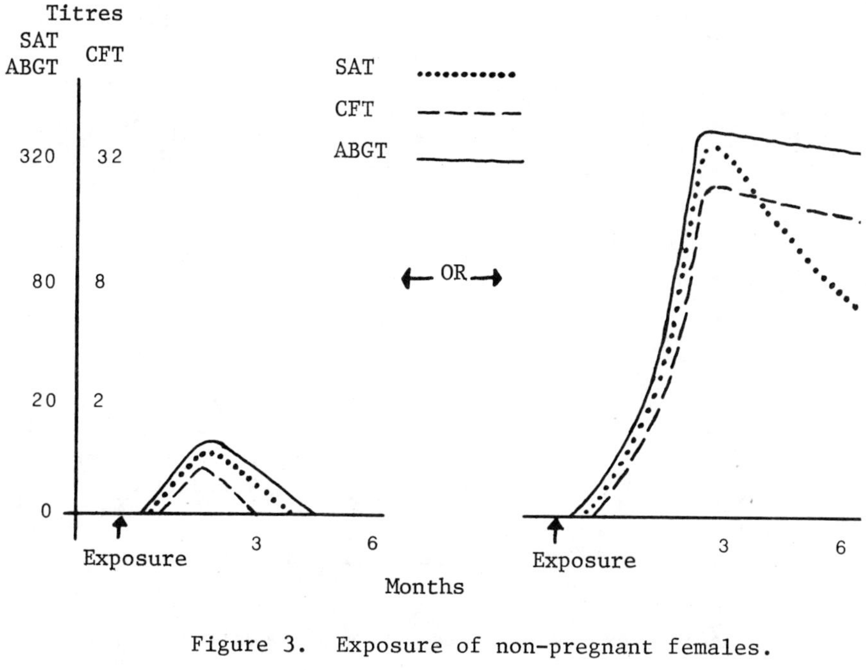

Figure 3. Exposure of non-pregnant females.

exposure (conjunctival or oral) serological responses are usually minimal and short lasting - low ABGT, possibly low CFT and low SAT - all may revert to zero levels in as little as three months (the time is somewhat dose-dependent). This exposure may result in natural immunity greater than 90 percent or latency (6 percent has been suggested as a figure for latency by Van den Born and Vervoorn 1965) (Figure 4). Of

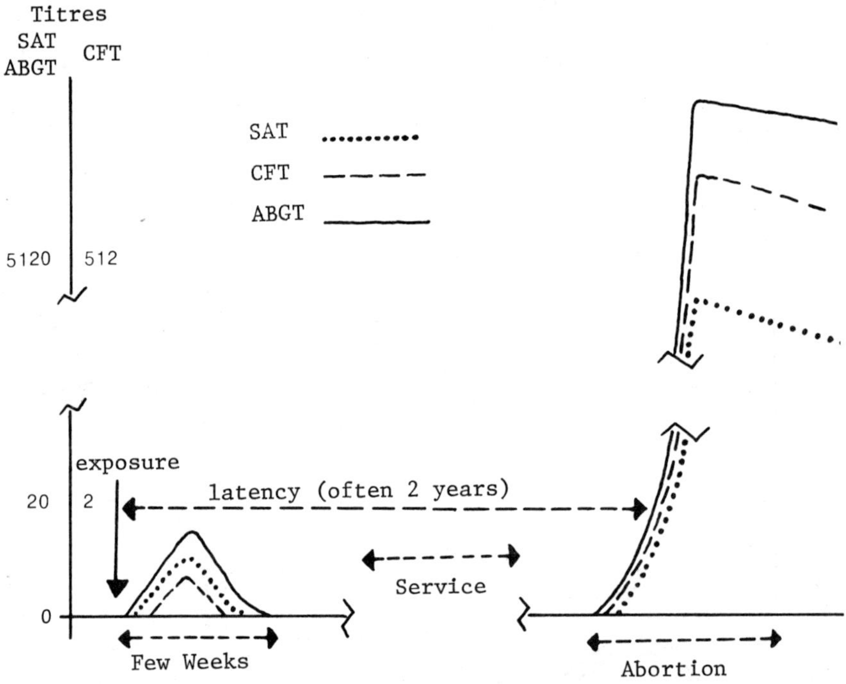

Figure 4. The latent carrier.

animals exposed in this way only a small percentage (probably only about 2 percent) progress to active infection and persisting positive titres.

b. Pregnant Females (Figure 5) - These animals may show the same serological picture as above as a direct response to exposure. Thereafter, they may remain negative even up to the time of abortion. Time from

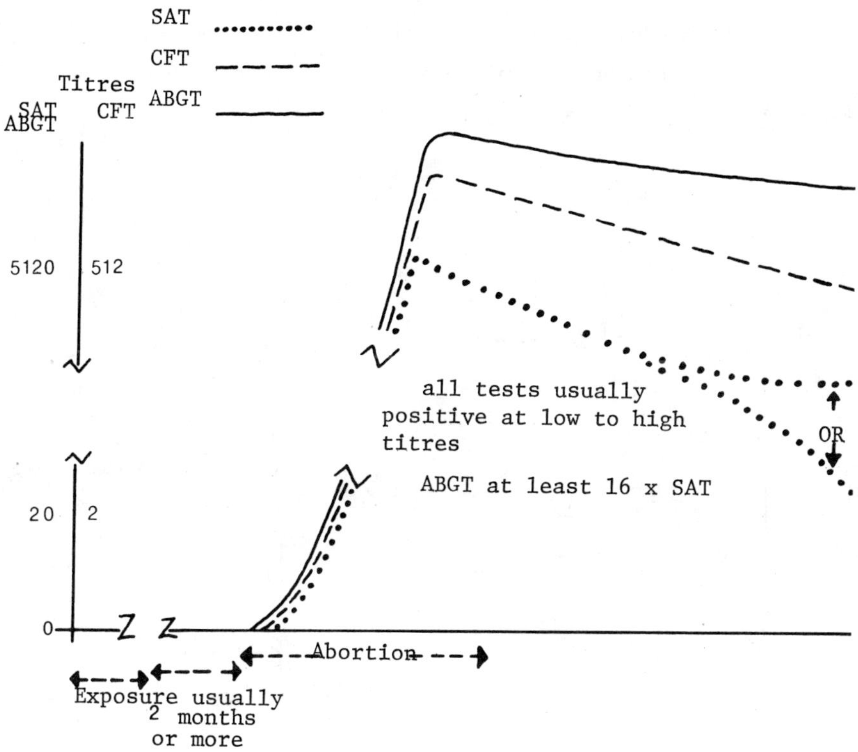

Figure 5. Exposure of the unprotected female during pregancy. This almost invaribly causes abortion.

exposure to abortion is usually at least two months (May be as little as one month if exposure is very heavy) (McEwen 1940). Pregnant unprotected females exposed to infection almost invariably (over 90 percent) abort and are particularly vulnerable up to the seventh month of gestation. Susceptibility during pregnancy varies. If challenge occurs in early pregnancy parturition is usually at or near full term but infected! When challenge occurs in mid pregnancy the incubation period is one to two months and abortion occurs at seven to eight months. Animals challenged in late pregnancy will usually carry to term but the parturitions are often infected (Thomsen 1950).

4. The Anamnestic Test (Figure 6).

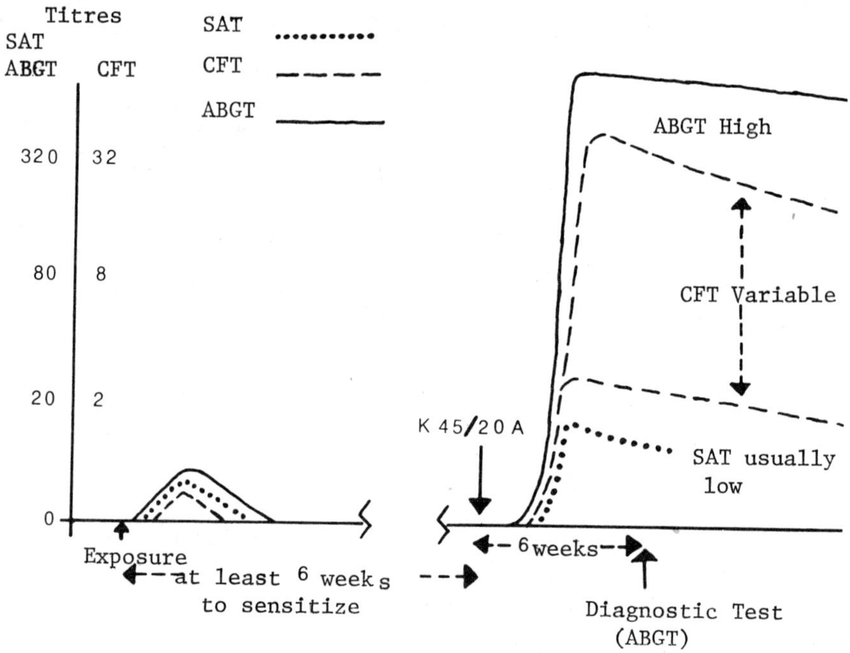

Figure 6. The anamnestic test. (This test is applicable only in animals which have not been vaccinated with strain 19 vaccine.

In animals previously <u>sensitised</u> to agglutinogens and CF antigens (of smooth field strains), one injection of K45/20A produces a secondary serological effect; high ABGT and usually high CFT but the SAT is not usually markedly increased.

In areas of high prevalence, one should in the early utilised as an anamnestic test to identify and remove possible latent carriers (provided strain 19 has not been used in the animals - if so this will cause false positive results). It has proved to be a very valuable procedure.

In areas of high prevalence one should in the early stages of control make allowances for vaccinal enhancement of blood titres - otherwise one might grossly overkill - particularly if the CFT were widely used.

In conclusion, if K45/20A is the only vaccine in use in an area or country:

1. The SAT is virtually uninfluenced by vaccination so it can still be used as the basic diagnostic test.
2. Vaccination of previously exposed (sensitised) animals will cause CF titres. Some such titres may persist for two years or so, but as it often takes two to three years to bring a large herd under good control such animals may eventually be culled to clear up the herd serology.
3. In brucellosis-free animals vaccination with K45/20A vaccine does not cause prolonged serological problems.

References

Cunningham, B. 1968. Proc. Int. Symp. Brucellosis I, Tunis, 1968, vol. 12, pp. 11-16.

Edwards, S. J.; de Ropp, R. S.; and McLeod, D. H. 1945. Vet. Rec. 57:259.

Gaumont, R.; Trap, D.; Thorel, M. F.; Gayot, G.; Pierre, F.; and Dhennin, L. 1973. Rapport 128, Session Generale XLI de O.I.E., Paris.

McDiarmid, A., and Sutherland, F. B. 1957. Vet. Rec. 69:1067.

McDiarmid, A. 1962. Ann. Inst. Pasteur 102:792.

McEwen, A. D. 1940. Vet. Rec. 52:97-106.

McEwen, A. D. 1946. Vet. Rec. 58:56.

McEwen, A. D., and Samuel, J. McA. 1955. Vet. Rec. 67:546.

McKeon 1975. Proc. Int. Symp. Brucellosis II, Rabat, 1975, vol. 31, pp. 343-350.

Ray, W. C. 1975. Proc. Int. Symp. Brucellosis II, Rabat, 1975, vol. 31, pp. 335-342.

Taylor, A. W., and McDiarmid, A. 1949. Vet. Rec. 61:317.

Thomsen, A. 1950. Brit. Vet. J. 106:1-15.

Vanden Born and Vervoorn. 1965. Bull. Off. Int. Epiz. 63:1531-1534.

Adult Vaccination

Paul Nicoletti

Several factors have contributed to the increasing difficulties of eliminating brucellosis from some cattle herds through test and slaughter methods. These include the decreased levels of vaccination, larger herd sizes, and increased cattle movements. In addition, there are technical problems such as variable incubation periods, sero-negative infected cattle which abort or calve normally and differentiation of vaccinal and infection titers.

In recent years there have been requests to re-institute adult vaccination in selected herds. In December, 1974, the Brucellosis Committee of the United States Animal Health Association approved experimental studies. These commenced in Florida in May of 1975. Several serologic procedures and methods of vaccine administration are being evaluated.

Vaccination of adult cattle has been studied by a large number of workers using a variety of immunogenic products in a variety of dosages and methods of administration. Some of the live products which have been utilized were strain 19, mucoid phases, Rev. 1 and 45/20. The inactivated agents were Pilet-Bonneau, 53H38A, K45/20A and field strains. *Brucella* cell fractions have been prepared. These and whole cell products have been sometimes combined with adjuvants. Routes of vaccine administration have included subcutaneous, intramuscular, respiratory, intracaudal, intradermal, and via the conjunctival sac.

It is impossible to compare all of the research studies which have been conducted and this paper will briefly summarize some of those related to strain 19. Preliminary results of some phases of the Florida experiments will be included.

Herd Resistance

Many workers have reported on the effectiveness of vaccinating adult cattle, both under field conditions and more controlled conditions. Berman, Beach, and Irwin (1954) found that two groups of cattle when vaccinated by different routes were significantly more resistant than unvaccinated controls. In a large problem herd, Berman and co-workers (1950) found that adult and calf vaccination contributed to the elimination of brucellosis after test and slaughter methods had failed. Other workers who have reported on the usefulness of vaccination in infected herds are Lothe (1943) in Wisconsin, Haring and Traum (1943) in California, and Lawson (1950) in England.

It is generally agreed that vaccination of adult cattle will practically eliminate clinical disease and this greatly reduces the degree of exposure to healthy cattle. It is also generally agreed that vaccination alone will not completely eliminate the infection.

In two large dairy herds vaccinated approximately one year ago, we have observed a great reduction in the incidence of brucellosis. It is hopeful that a combination of vaccination, diagnosis of infected cattle through special tests, and removal of these cattle will eliminate the disease where conventional test and slaughter methods had failed.

Individual Resistance

The responses to vaccination will vary in each animal depending upon many factors. Immunity is cell mediated and there is no satisfactory method for measurement of immunity.

Data from many sources suggest that from 65 to 75 percent of vaccinated animals will be completely protected against most kinds of exposure (Manthei, 1959). The immunity is relative and depends largely upon the virulence and numbers of the infective strain.

Route of Administration

Several studies have been conducted to determine the best method of vaccination to produce immunity and hopefully reduce post-vaccinal seroagglutinins. Those methods receiving the most attention were subcutaneous, intracaudal, and intradermal. Different dosage levels were evaluated and the results were summarized by Manthei (1952b). There was little difference in the degree of immunity to brucellosis in cattle vaccinated between 12 and 18 months of age with 5, 1, and 0.2 ml of strain 19 vaccine inoculated by the subcutaneous, intracaudal, and intradermal methods, respectively.

We have observed no apparent differences in immunity in a herd in which one-half of the cattle were vaccinated with 5 ml subcutaneously and one-half were given 0.2 ml intradermally of strain 19.

Studies are underway to determine if inoculating strain 19 in the conjunctival sac will produce immunity and reduce post-vaccinal agglutinins. These are based upon unpublished reports by Plommet and co-workers in France.

Dosage of Vaccine

The exact relationship between the minimal dose of vaccine and degree of immunity is not known. Results obtained on a limited number of cattle vaccinated with 0.2 ml strain 19 subcutaneously showed that the immunity was equal to that produced with the same dose inoculated intradermally (Manthei et al. 1952a). Recent studies in England (Report of Ministry of Agriculture, Fisheries and Food, 1975) showed no differences between a 5 ml and a 0.25 ml dosage of strain 19 administered subcutaneously in cattle which were later challenged with a virulent strain.

We have inoculated one large dairy herd in Florida with 5 ml and 0.25 ml dosages of strain 19 and will study the serologic and immunogenic effects of these procedures.

Postvaccinal Diagnostic Problems

There are many papers which deal with the well-known difficulties of differentiation of post-vaccinal titers and those developed from infection. This diagnostic dilemma is nearly always cited as the major reason for not using strain 19 vaccine at any age. Cattle vaccinated beyond the first months of life develop agglutinins which may persist for long intervals. The decline of titers on standard agglutination tests appears to be more related to age at the time of vaccination than any other factor.

Most of the research conducted on persistence of post-vaccinal agglutinins was prior to the development of qualitative antibody tests, now usually called supplemental tests. Field studies and controlled research have clearly shown the superiority of these supplemental tests in diagnosing brucellosis.

Few studies have been conducted on adult vaccinated cattle using supplemental tests. Worthington et al. (1973) concluded that the complement fixation, rivanol agglutination and mercaptoethanol tests were generally negative six months after adult vaccination in over 100 cows.

In the current Florida studies, five serologic tests are being evaluated in adult vaccinated cattle. These are the standard tube, mercaptoethanol, card and rivanol agglutination, and complement fixation tests. We have observed that the complement fixation test becomes negative after vaccination of adult cattle sooner than agglutination tests. Most cattle are negative on the complement fixation test within a few weeks. The rivanol agglutination test is also proving to be very useful in differentiation of vaccinal and infection titers. The other tests are of questionable value but additional studies will more thoroughly evaluate their future role and effectiveness in adult-vaccinated cattle.

Post Vaccinal Abortions

The abortifacient effects of inoculating strain 19 has been studied by many workers and a literature review was made by Manthei (1952b). Results have varied and depend upon inoculation dosage and route, stage of gestation and concurrent infection in the herd.

We have inoculated over 1000 cows in all stages of pregnancy and the reported abortions have been less than one percent.

Udder Infection and Public Health

Post-vaccinal udder infection due to strain 19 and its excretion in the milk occur infrequently. We have recovered organisms indistinguishable from strain 19 from less than two percent of over 700 lactating cows vaccinated from two to three months previously with 5 ml of the vaccine. In cattle vaccinated at least six months the percentage of cattle excreting strain 19 was less than one percent. Blood titers on supplemental tests have been used to detect possible milk shedders.

There is no evidence that humans have become infected through ingestion of strain 19 contaminated milk.

Systemic Effects

Manthei (1952b) summarized the reported systemic reactions in vaccinated cattle. He concluded that the majority of animals inoculated with strain 19 have a rise in temperature during the immediate four day post-vaccinal period regardless of the three routes of inoculation studied.

Several workers have reported varied and temporary decreases in milk production. All investigators observed that the maximum loss was two to three days following vaccination and production returned to normal within nine days. Our data have not been summarized in the several herds under study, but in one large herd there was a 11 percent reduction in milk yield and 15 percent reduction in feed consumption beginning two days after vaccination. There was normal milk production and feed consumption within a few days.

Conclusions

The use of strain 19 in adult cattle provides a means to rapidly elevate herd resistance to brucellosis. This will not eliminate the disease in infected herds and sound management practices combined with removal of infected animals will be necessary.

The diagnostic problems caused by vaccination with strain 19 can be largely overcome by the use of supplemental tests and proper interpretation of the results.

Different dosages and routes of administration of strain 19 have been studied and additional investigations are underway. These may assist in solving some of the diagnostic and other problems which are associated with adult vaccination.

The elimination of brucellosis from a herd is a challenge which is often difficult and veterinary expertise must be included in the efforts.

References

Berman, D. T.; Jones, L. M.; and Beach, B. A. 1950. Studies on repeated vaccination of cattle with Brucella abortus strain 19: II, Results in a large "problem" herd. Proc. 87th Ann. Mtg. A.V.M.A., pp. 171-176.

Berman, D. T.; Beach, B. A.; and Irwin, M. R. 1954. A comparison of the effects of subcutaneous and intracaudal vaccination of sexually mature cattle with Brucella abortus strain 19. Am. J. Vet. Res. 15:406-411.

Great Britain, Ministry of Agriculture, Fisheries, and Food. 1975. Diseases of Breeding Department, Central Veterinary Laboratory, Weybridge, Surrey, England, pp. 16-20.

Haring, C. M., and Traum, J. 1943. The effect of Brucella abortus strain 19 on cattle of various ages and its bearing on adult vaccination. Proc. U.S.L.S.A. 47th Ann. Mtg., pp. 42-46.

Lawson, J. R. 1950. Strain 19 and the control of brucellosis. Vet. Rec. 62:823-830.

Lothe, H. 1943. Clinical observations on methods of control of bovine brucellosis. J. A.V.M.A. 103:1-5.

Manthei, C. A.; Mingle, C. K.; and Carter, R. W. 1952a. Comparison of immunity and agglutinin response in cattle vaccinated with Brucella abortus strain 19 by the intradermal and subcutaneous methods. Proc. U.S.L.S.A. 56th Ann. Mtg., pp. 100-114.

Manthei, C. A. 1952b. Evaluation of vaccined methods and doses of *Brucella abortus* strain 19. Proc. U.S.L.S.A. 56th Ann. Mtg., pp. 115-125.

Manthei, C. A. 1959. Summary of controlled research with strain 19. Proc. U.S.L.S.A. 63rd Ann. Mtg., pp. 91-96.

Worthington, R. W.; Mulders, S. G.; McFarlane, I. S.; and Becker, D. 1973. A serological investigation on adult cattle vaccinated with *Brucella abortus* strain 19. Onderstepoort J. Vet. Res. 40:7-12.

Experiences with *Brucella* Vaccines

Godfrey Alton

Strain 19 Vaccine

In some states of Australia the use of strain 19 vaccine is prohibited and in other states it is used extensively. In one state the vaccination of female calves is compulsory. There is nothing illogical in this since conditions vary greatly from state to state.

There are vast areas in Australia where the carrying capacity of the land is less than ten cattle per square mile. In these areas the use of strain 19 vaccine becomes very difficult. There are many properties where the cattle are only mustered once or twice a year; this makes it more or less impossible to ensure that all female calves are vaccinated between three and six months of age. The actual handling of the vaccine by stockmen working in camps miles away from the homestead poses problems. The keeping qualities of lyophilized strain 19 vaccine after reconstitution are very poor. Therefore, 45/20 vaccine is generally preferred under these circumstances. In some areas they are able to bleed young stock at the time of the second vaccination and remove reactors.

Good results have been obtained with strain 19 in closely settled areas. In Tasmania its use in areas of high prevalence brought the infection rate down to levels around two percent and this facilitated progress of the test and slaughter campaign.

We consider that the decision to use strain 19 vaccine has a bearing on the choice of a diagnostic test for use in vaccinated cattle. The buffered brucella antigen test, which we call the rose bengal test, does seem to be overly sensitive for use as a definitive test in strain 19 vaccinated cattle. We believe that in such circumstances it is best used as a screen test. The evidence suggests that the complement fixation test is the best single diagnostic test for use in individual cattle and it has the additional advantage that it can be used in strain 19 vaccinated cattle without undue interference.

The work of Cunningham (1968) and others, undertaken to evaluate strain 19 vaccines, indicates that there has been variation in the quality of strain 19 vaccines that have been used. This should be borne in mind when the relative effectiveness of various vaccines is being considered. Perhaps those with the most experience on the problem would give their views on the best method of insuring that batches of strain 19 vaccine are up to standard and on the part that can be played by tests in guinea pigs.

Brucella Abortus Killed 45/20 Vaccine

Two vaccines of this type are manufactured and used in Australia. Reading the labels on the bottles, the purchaser would believe that the contents were the same whatever the brand selected, but at least judging by the effect they have on vaccinated cattle, they are not. One of these vaccines causes bigger local reactions, less antibody production and slightly less protection in laboratory animals than the other one. Furthermore, examination of different batches of the vaccine that caused the greater serological response showed variation from batch to batch in the amount of antibody produced after vaccination. We observed the reactions of Hereford heifers born on one of our brucellosis-free field stations to three batches of vaccine. I will describe the complement-fixation(CF) reactions of the highest and least reacting groups. Table 1.

Table 1

Brucella abortus 45/20 adjuvant vaccine

number of animals positive and negative at various intervals

following vaccination and revaccination

Titre	Weeks after Vaccination		Weeks after Revaccination							
	6	12	1	2	4	9	13	18	22	27
1/64				1						
1/32				3						
1/16			2	7						
1/8			8	3	8	2	2		1	
1/4	1	1	2			1		2		
Neg.	14	14	3	0	7	12	13	13	14	15

shows the CF titres of 17 heifers; after the second dose of vaccine the titres at two weeks varied from zero to 1:64. In the low responding group none of the six heifers gave a positive CF test at any time. Six heifers is a small group but the difference between 17 out of 17 and zero out of six is significant. A third group of heifers gave a serological response somewhere between the two extremes just described but not significantly different from either of them. We do not condemn this product on these grounds but feel that it is unfortunate that we have to adjust our diagnostic testing schedules to cope with the worst of these variables. Our standard rules require one year to elapse between vaccination with 45/20 and a diagnostic test, except when it is being used in an anamnestic test.

Dr. Cunningham has stated in one of his publications that the 45/20 vaccine, called Duphavac, was chosen for use in Ireland partly because of the lack of variation in the way cattle responded to different batches of vaccine. Cunningham found, as we have, that there is little CF antibody produced following a single dose of Duphavac, but much more following a second dose. By contrast Miller et al. (1976) using Duphavac and a similar CF technique and antigen obtained the same response following primary vaccination with 45/20 as following the second dose. This vaccine and diagnostic test could not be expected to be effective in an anamnestic test.

Our main criticism of 45/20 vaccines is the variable serological response we have observed in vaccinated cattle. We feel that a big research effort to find a more uniform product would be justified. Another criticism we have of 45/20 is that it interferes most with the test that we think is the most valuable in the diagnosis of bovine brucellosis, i.e. the complement fixation test.

Of great interest to us is the anamnestic test, as it was first used by Tacken, to pick out carriers or congenital or neonatally infected heifers that do not have positive serology but are destined to become infective when they first calve. We hope, by eliminating such carriers, to be able to establish brucellosis-free groups of young stock that will spend the rest of their useful lives together in an isolated group. If such groups could be established each year as replacement breeding stock, then older infected cattle would gradually be eliminated and a brucellosis-free herd would result. This method is now being tried in the arid areas of Northern Australia where conventional methods of test and slaughter are very difficult to apply. It is too early yet to know whether this system is going to prove to be a practical one, but enthusiasm among the people taking part is very high.

The Bacteriology of the Brucella Abortus Strain 45/20

We have in our laboratory two strains of Brucella abortus 45/20; both were received from commercial producers of vaccine. When observed by the usual technique for the direct observation of colonies, both these cultures look completely rough and completely homogeneous. They do not look at all like the culture described by Brown et al. (1972), who reported that their 45/20 cultures consisted of a 50-50 mixture of smooth, intermediate and rough colony types.

We have investigated the effect of passaging various cultures and isolates from the 45/20 strain in guinea pigs. I think it is important to describe technical methods in some detail when talking about passage of micro-organisms in animals. In the work I am describing the passages were initiated with a dense suspension washed off an agar slope; at least 10^9 cells were injected intramuscularly. The guinea pigs were almost always killed 28 days after they were infected and cultures made from their spleens and a few lymph nodes. Usually several hundred colonies grew and these were washed off the agar plates and one ml of a pooled suspension, always more than 10^9 cells, injected into the next guinea pig. One commercial culture produced a 50-50 mixture of smooth/intermediate and rough colony types from the second guinea pig passage. When this was repeated, starting again with the original culture, the same thing happened. The other commercial culture went to nine passages without any change from the completely rough type. We also passaged four cultures of 45/20 derived from single colony isolates taken at random from the original (unstable) commercial culture. Three of these reached the tenth passage without any change in colony type being detected; whereas the fourth produced a 50-50 mixture of smooth/intermediate and rough colony types at the seventh passage. This is a very unstable strain of B. abortus and one wonders how it ever became the choice for producing a rough vaccine. I feel that it should be possible to produce a non-agglutinogenic adjuvant vaccine from a rough strain of B. abortus that is more stable than some of the 45/20 cultures now being used for vaccine production.

Brucella Abortus 45/20 As A Live Vaccine

This vaccine was used in Great Britain in the early 1940's as an alternative to strain 19. It was non-agglutinogenic and was well accepted by dairy farmers. Its use was prohibited following laboratory investigations by Taylor and McDiarmid (1949). These workers showed that when the 45/20 strain was passaged by intravenous inoculation of large numbers of bacteria through a series of pregnant cattle, definite changes in the direction of greater virulence began to be apparent after the third passage. Strain 19 passaged similarly retained its attenuated characteristics through the seven passages of the experiment.

Necessary caution probably justified the withdrawal of this vaccine on the evidence and there was always strain 19 available. Furthermore, there was no eradication envisioned at that time in Britain. Conditions in many areas are now quite different from what they were in Britain in the late 1940's and one wonders whether a re-examination of 45/20 or, better still, a more stable isolate from it or another rough culture should not be undertaken with its use as a live vaccine in mind. After all, the conditions under which the original live vaccine was tested for stability were very far from those likely to operate in nature. It was not determined, for instance, whether the more virulent mutants that emerged were able to infect contact cattle.

Vaccines Other Than Strain 19 and 45/20 Adjuvant Vaccines

There is good evidence that a smooth vaccine of B. melitensis (H38), when killed and incorporated into an adjuvant, is capable of protecting cattle against infection with B. abortus (Plommet et al. 1970; Dhennin 1973). There is, however, some controversy over the level and persistence of antibody that results from the administration of this vaccine. Details are given by the above quoted authors.

The initiative of Pilet and Bonneau (1970) in treating a killed culture of strain 19 with anti-Brucella serum to neutralize the antigens that stimulate an antibody response was a very interesting development, but unfortunately this product does not seem to have had much success (Renoux et al. 1970; and Dhennin 1973).

The Need for a Better Brucella Vaccine

I don't think that anyone considers our present Brucella vaccines ideal. Requirements for the ideal Brucella vaccine are very exacting and, therefore, such a vaccine is likely to be very difficult to produce. We need a product that has good keeping qualities, needs only one dose, can be given to animals of any age, doesn't give rise to an unacceptable local lesion at the site of inoculation, and doesn't stimulate the production of antibody active in the diagnostic tests being used in the area. The ideal vaccine should also produce a solid immunity which lasts for a lifetime. All the vaccines available at present lack several of these desirable qualities and a new vaccine could be a great improvement on these without being ideal.

It seems to be established that protection against Brucella infection depends on cell-mediated immunity and is not dependent on the presence of humoral antibody; in fact, the work reviewed by Parish (1972) indicated that the presence of antibody could interfere with the development of cell-mediated immunity. Parish's work suggested that chemical modification of the specific antigen could leave intact that part that stimulated cell-mediated immunity while inactivating the component responsible for stimulating antibody-producing lymphocytes.

References

Brown, G. M.; Love, E. L.; Pietz, D. E.; and Ranger, C. R. 1972. A. J. Vet. Res. 33:759-764.

Corbel, M. J. 1972. Brit. Vet. J. 128:xlvii.

Cunningham, B. 1968. International Symposium on Brucellosis, Tunis. Symposium Series, Immunobiology Standardization. 12:11-16. (Karger, Basel, N.Y. 1970).

Dhennin, L. 1973. Bull. Acad. Vet. 46:171-190.

Jones, L. M.; Thomson, P. D.; and Alton, G. G. 1958. J. Comp. Path. 68:416-427.

Miller, J. K.; Kelly, J. I.; and Roerrink, J. H. G. 1976. Vet. Rec. 98:210-215.

Parish, C. R. 1972. Transplantation Revs. 13:35-66.

Pilet, C. H., and Bonneau, M. 1970. Rec. Med. Vet. 145:25-36.

Plommet, M.; Renoux, G.; Philipon, A.; Lorenz, C.; and Gestin, J. 1970. Ann. Rech. Veter. 1:189-201.

Renoux, G.; Plommet, M; Philipon, A. 1970. Ann. Rech. Veter. 1:225-231.

Taylor, A. W., and McDiarmid, A. 1949. Vet. Rec. 61:317-318.

Immunization Discussion

<u>DR. RICHARD HIDALGO</u> (Texas A&M): What I would like to do before I summarize what was said about strain 19 and 45/20 vaccines is to give summary answers to the questions. The first question which is basic to all of the discussion is: <u>What is the definition of a bovine that has been successfully immunized by vaccination</u>? I think that this question was diplomatically avoided by a number of people and I don't blame them. I think that Dr. Nelson put it in a very simple but good definition in that he said, "a successful bovine immunization was an immunization that was able to prevent active infection after exposure to small or moderate numbers of virulent organisms." I think that is, at least, a satisfactory working definition. Now, I would like to first ask our morning program participants if they would take exception to this definition or if they would have anything to add to it?

<u>DR. CLAUDE NELSON</u> (USDA, Maryland): I don't think that there is much that we can add to it except that any of the studies done to date have shown that, using high enough levels of challenge with highly virulent organisms, one can infect nearly 100 percent of the animals. So, we can have an effective immunizing agent and still be able to break down immunity with severe enough exposure. Therefore, we really are talking about relativity.

DR. HIDALGO: Do we have comments from the remainder of our speakers? Now I would like to summarize some of the things that were said, first about strain 19 vaccine and then about 45/20 bacterin. I would like to reiterate that everyone has said that immunity is variable and that strain 19 immunization does result in less than total protection. However, strain 19 vaccine is valuable in reduction of the numbers of organisms in the uterus and the mammary gland which results in less excretion at the time of parturition and this, in turn, results in less exposure to susceptible cattle and, of course, to humans. The second part of the question is: Are circulating antibodies of significance in determining the degree of immunity? I think we had consensus that they were not. Would anybody take exception to this?

Now let us consider the advantages and disadvantages of strain 19 vaccine. First, it was stated that a single dose is usually adequate to produce an immunity with a duration of approximately five years. Also stated was that a second injection was of no advantage. There is usually a lack of systemic reaction in calfhood vaccinated animals, but there is some reaction in the adult as observed by Dr. Nicoletti. Adult cows did show a drop in milk production and feed consumption a few days after immunization. It was stated that the strain 19 organism does not revert to virulence, which is a definite advantage, and that the degree of protection varied from experiment to experiment but is roughly 65-70 percent. Now, the disadvantages will be summarized. First of all, the handling of calves is not always an easy thing to do under some management systems. Of course, the big disadvantage is that protection is less than desirable. There are occasional persistent titers that interfere with serologic testing, but with the use of supplementals and the card test we are able to take care of a portion of these persistent vaccine titers. There are occasional persistent infections. The vaccine is not suitable for use in the male and it produces sterility in certain cases. It is a human health hazard to those administering the vaccine and, very important, it is a labile product that is subject to deterioration if not carefully handled. So, those are the advantages and disadvantages of strain 19 vaccine. Have we anything to add to this--first from our morning participants? Then from any of our speakers? Dr. Jones, would you like to make a comment?

DR. LOIS JONES (University of Wisconsin): We conducted a survey of the number of strain 19 isolations that were made in the years when the problem herd program was in progress in Wisconsin. Up to about 1962, there were 33 isolations of a strain indistinguishable from strain 19 made from cattle in 31 different herds. Fifty-four percent of these animals were of the Chanel Island breeds as was the finding in California. But, on the basis of the known number of calves which were being vaccinated in Wisconsin at this time, it was estimated that during the three year period over which the 33 isolations were made, persistent strain 19 infections occurred in approximately two animals per 100,000 calves vaccinated. So we feel that this level of infection would not be detected in an ordinarily heavily infected area. At this time, we are still getting strain 19 infected herds in Wisconsin. We have, at the present time, about eight to ten herds under quarantine in Wisconsin. Three or four of these herds are infected with virulent field strains and the rest are infected with strain 19 of a one reactor situation. We go in and remove the one cow and the herd is free. Of course, the administration finds it a great nuisance to have to do follow-up blood tests in six out of ten herds but if we didn't have any vaccination perhaps there would be 40-50 herds under quarantine and this would be quite a different thing. We have been able to keep our incidence down with careful checking at our borders and so forth.

I would like to also say a word at this time about the way the vaccine served to speed up our eradication program in Wisconsin. When we started in 1952, we had at that time the highest dairy cattle population in the states and we had a prevalence of 42 percent positive herds on the first ring test scores. The follow-up blood test showed that ten percent of the cattle were infected. Vaccination had actually been in progress before the eradication program began in 1952, so considerable numbers of calves had been vaccinated. It was stepped up so that we eventually reached the level of 60-70 percent eligible calves being vaccinated. But in four years from 1952 to 1956 the ring test herds dropped from 42 percent positive to five percent positive and the reactors dropped from ten percent to one percent. Now, we don't believe that this could have been done without the level of vaccination that was in our herds at that time. Minnesota, our neighboring state, had about the same cattle industry although their population is lower. They have never vaccinated more than 22 percent of their calves. They took five years longer to reach brucella-free status. It is always very hard to get these figures. These are the sorts of comparisons we are trying to make from the records that are in the literature. Thank you.

DR. HIDALGO: Thank you Dr. Jones. Don't leave just yet. Dr. Enright has a question to ask of you.

DR. FRED ENRIGHT (Louisiana State University): I just wanted to find out, on your recovery of strain 19 from 33 animals, what organs or tissues were you culturing?

DR. JONES: Those were mainly milk samples and I believe very often that they were confirmed at slaughter by culture of the supramammary lymph nodes.

DR. R. J. AVERY (Ontario, Canada): Dr. Jones, how did you determine that the seven or eight remaining herds that were not infected with field strains were actually infected with strain 19?

DR. JONES: Do you mean under the present circumstances?

DR. AVERY: The latter report that you made on your ten present quarantined herds.

DR. JONES: Over the years the epidemiologists in our Department of Agriculture are able to recognize the herd pattern quite well. We are not doing as much culture work as we originally did. If there is a ring test positive herd, then individual animals are blood tested and, as in the case of the seven to eight herds, there is just a single reactor. When they take a milk sample, isolation is made and the reactor is confirmed with the brucellosis ring test (BRT) which is often positive in one quarter only. So, this is the way it is done and isolations are still being made. Of course, as you know, we wouldn't be so sure that it was strain 19 if we hadn't discovered this erythritol peculiarity of strain 19. We can identify it so easily now once we isolate an organism because strain 19 is sensitive to erythritol. It will not grow on medium in the presence of erythritol, whereas every other *Brucella* strain that we have found will grow.

DR. AVERY: Actually your diagnosis was made on isolation either from milk or from organs after the animal was slaughtered.

DR. JONES: Yes, with the exception of the recent ones. They are not doing cultures presently, but if they remove the reactor then there is no longer a problem in that herd.

DR. NELSON: Dr. Avery, in most cases these animals were raised on the farm and they were just coming into their first lactation when the herd BRT reverted to suspicious. You go back and you determine that this is the only animal in the herd that had a BRT titer as well as a blood agglutination titer that is positive to supplementals. You look at the history of that animal and you will find that she was a replacement heifer raised in the herd. She just came into her first lactation. So these circumstances are indicative of what you are dealing with. And, in most cases, they have been able to confirm this by culture attempts when they have pursued it in that direction.

DR. AVERY: Dr. Nelson, were all of these animals vaccinated?

DR. NELSON: Yes, these were vaccinated animals. Now, I think that it is interesting to observe that in the data that Margaret (Meyer) and I have in California we had these animals ranging from young cows to quite mature. Why would an animal five, six, seven, or eight years old suddenly revert to positive if she has been lactating through the normal periods? Is the strain 19 laying in a dormant type of a situation? Dr. Hendricks, do you have a thought on this?

DR. J. B. HENDRICKS (USDA, S. Carolina): I think that there is another possible explanation for that. In some older animals that we found, and we found two in one herd on one occasion, there was evidence that there may have been udder injections for mastitis treatment with a syringe that was contaminated with strain 19. There is another way to get at that but Dr. Jones mentioned that we are finding an average of about ten to twelve of these animals per year per about 500,000 calves vaccinated. I would highly question the capability to diagnose strain 19 infections without culture. We were able to do this when we had a level of about 300 infected herds per year in Wisconsin. We cultured every initial reactor, or part of them, from every single herd. I see no reason why Wisconsin can't culture a dozen a year.

DR. JONES: I'm sure we could.

DR. STANLEY MARTIN (Ontario, Canada): We have a large number of herds under quarantine in Canada right now and my guess is that over 70 percent are singleton-reactor herds. Our difficulty is that no matter where you look at that cow you can't find a tag and you can't find any indication that the cow was ever vaccinated. So we are faced with a situation where there are virtually no cows vaccinated in a herd and we have a singleton reactor and that is pretty difficult to blame on strain 19. And, that is a very common feature in 70 percent of our herds.

DR. JONES: I think that it is a different situation altogether.

DR. DAVID BERMAN (University of Wisconsin): Our experience certainly has been that in dairy cows with a single pass at culture we can recover from approximately half of the reactor animals in the herds with this pattern. Going back another time for milk cultures we can reduce this again by half, so this is approaching the limit. You obviously don't want to get out and try to milk some of those wild Herefords in the western states.

DR. MARTIN: Those that I spoke of are good Holstein cows.

DR. BERMAN: Are you, in fact, culturing them?

DR. MARTIN: No.

DR. BERMAN: It is relatively easy to do.

DR. BRINDLEY MORGAN (Weybridge, England): In Great Britain we very rarely found these strain 19-excreter animals. In my own experience over some 20 odd years, I think that we had no more than two or three animals from which we have definitely isolated strain 19 from the milk. But, over the last three years, we had another kind of problem which is the persistent reactor heifer. We come across these in herds which have passed all herd serological tests when we go back and do qualifying tests that include heifers. We come across animals, usually one or two, in a herd which has otherwise been *Brucella*-free for sometime. We usually pick these heifers up on the rose-bengal plate test. They usually give us low or inconclusive reaction to the tube agglutination test and a positive reaction to the complement fixation test. We normally start testing these heifers at 18 months of age. We constantly test these every three months or so, and by the time they are 24 months of age only about half of these resolve themselves. And, we are finding that this is a very serious problem in herds that are otherwise *Brucella*-free and, therefore, restrictions are put on the animals. We estimate that something like just less than 0.5 percent of heifers that are vaccinated with strain 19 do become persistent serologic reactors. We have never been able to isolate *Brucella* from these at post-mortem examination.

DR. NELSON: We have had an interesting discussion on this little aspect of persistent infections of strain 19 but I would hope that we would keep it in its proper perspective. That being that it is a relatively minor inconvenience that is inherent with using a live vaccine and one that certainly in our program in the United States today we can well afford to live with for a number of years. We shouldn't use it as an item of such grave concern that we consider not using strain 19 because of this. I think that Dr. Jones mentioned the fact that we are talking about a handful of herds in a state of hundreds of thousands of herds. And, what would they be talking about without this protection?

MR. HILMAR MOORE (Richmond, Texas): I realize the difficulty and the problems that the strain 19 reactors cause as far as testing and clearing, but is there any evidence that those cattle that are infected with strain 19 can spread the disease throughout the herd.

DR. HIDALGO: You have heard the question, gentlemen.

DR. PAUL NICOLETTI (USDA, Florida): A categorical no.

DR. HIDALGO: Any exceptions?

DR. HENDRICKS: If it spreads it is not strain 19.

DR. NELSON: That's right. I think that Dr. Hendricks' comment that if it spreads it's not strain 19 is correct. We just don't have any information to that effect. We have got much data to support the fact that it does not, controlled as well as field studies.

MR. MOORE: So, the only problem is in the testing process?

DR. NELSON: That's right.

DR. HIDALGO: I would like to now summarize Dr. Cunningham's remarks on 45/20. Dr. Cunningham stated that protection afforded by 45/20 varied from a high of 82 percent down to 70 percent. There is a degree of protection roughly equivalent to strain 19. But, he did make the statement that 45/20 in his hands consistently gave better protection than strain 19. He said that "it was effective in controlling disease" to quote him directly. But, it did not completely control infection in a herd. Now let us list the advantages and disadvantages of 45/20. First of all, it is nonagglutinogenic, meaning, of course, that it does not cause a reaction in the agglutination tests. He said that it could be used to immunize entire herds. That certainly would be an advantage. The next great advantage is that it is a killed product and that it has no problem in producing infections. It is not a hazard to the person administering the bacterin. He felt that it had no effect on the ring test and, of course, that is extremely important in his country. In the range areas that would be less important, but I would certainly think that it would be very important to our dairy industry. It can be used in a dual role to produce immunity and as a diagnostic reagent. Of course, he definitely stated that the use of it as a diagnostic reagent should be employed with caution; its use would be indicated where the incidence is low. He also stated that the duration of immunity was roughly two years in his experience. This is somewhat contradictory to what we have heard in the past, so I think that this is notable. The disadvantages as he stated them are: it is a more expensive vaccine to process; it requires two injections; and there is variation in strains and batches. Of course, Dr. Alton spoke at some length on the variations in the strains. Dr. Cunningham, that is a summary of what I think you said. Would you like to qualify or amend anything that I said?

DR. BRENDAN CUNNINGHAM (Dublin, Ireland): No. I think that that's a fair summary.

DR. HIDALGO: Thank you. I will now summarize Dr. Nicoletti's presentation on adult vaccination. He stated that it eliminates the clinical disease but it does not eliminate the infection within a herd. He stated that subcutaneous and intradermal dose administration did not show great differences in degree of protection. He indicated that he was currently trying 1/20 of the prescribed dose and that this seemed to be working well. He is currently involved in a trial on conjunctival administration of strain 19 but he did not say much about it. Perhaps, we will ask him to make a short summary of the conjunctival vaccination trial.

DR. NICOLETTI: For the study of conjunctival inoculation in one herd of approximately 700 cows, we have divided the herd into 40 percent in which we gave a five cc. dose, 40 percent in which we gave a 1/10 ml inoculation in the conjunctival sac and 20 percent are being left as unvaccinated controls. Our protocol provides for a two month post vaccinal study of the herd in which we would do the five tests that I have previously described and at that time we would include bacteriological studies on sero-positive animals. I emphasize sero-positive in the respect that in the conjunctival group, we are largely culturing any cow with suspicious sero-agglutination titers. In the five cc. group, as you might expect, the numbers of animals responding to the more sensitive tests, such as the card and tube agglutination tests, after two months is so high that it is virtually impossible to do culturing on all of these animals. So, we are largely using rivanol and complement-fixation at that point as possible indicators of those from which we might possibly recover *Brucella*. We must remember that these are, in fact, all infected herds that we are studying, so that the probability always exists that we are getting animals that are incubating the disease. We feel that at that point if you can bacteriologically prove that the animals are infected it is best to remove them from the herd and this is, in fact, what we're doing. So, that herd has been tested at two months post vaccination. A serologic and bacteriologic study making a comparison between the three groups of animals in that herd has been made. And then, two months after this, that is at four months post-inoculation, we are again studying the herd serologically and bacteriologically and reinoculating those animals that got the conjunctival inoculation based on the recommendation of the French studies. It was suggested that two inoculations were necessary for satisfactory immunity by the conjunctival route.

DR. HIDALGO: Thank you, Dr. Nicoletti. You did mention that this was based on the French work. I wonder if Dr. Plommet would give us a brief summary of that work?

DR. MICHEL PLOMMET (Nouzilly, France): The first slide (Figure 1) shows results of two conjunctival vaccinations with strain 19. The first black point is a standard vaccination by the subcutaneous route. And you can see that the serological response is 100 percent for about 12 weeks. This is a primary response. In heifers, if the vaccination is done by the conjunctival route with 1/10 of the normal dose, the response is of very short duration and of a low level. The positive tests in this slide are either agglutination, complement fixation or rose-bengal plate tests. Some cows were vaccinated and you can see (the dotted line) that we observed a higher response on most of the cattle. The duration was very short, too. Figure 2 will show you the serological response of

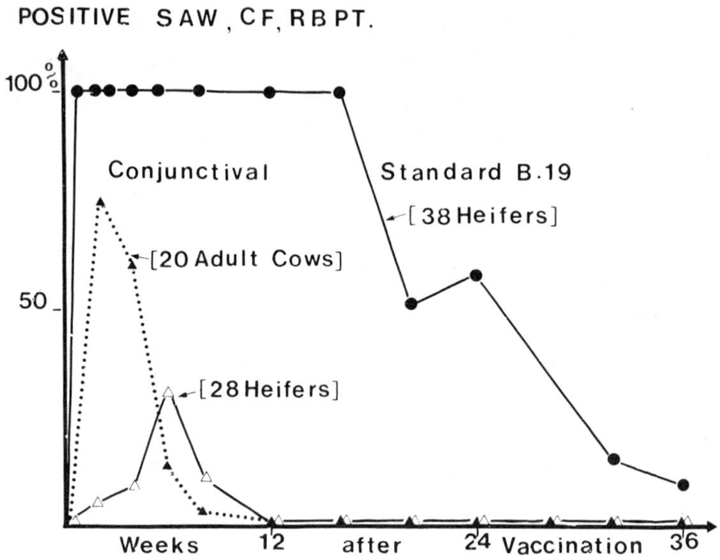

Figure 1. Comparison of the serologic responses of cattle vaccinated with strain 19 by the subcutaneous routes.

revaccination; the revaccination was made six months after the first one. All of the cattle that had been vaccinated by the standard method had positive responses for about two or three weeks following revaccination which then dropped to near zero in about two-three months. Conjunctival recall vaccination gave a positive response for sometime, but the response is very low, too. Table 1 will show you the results of challenge experiments done either on cattle injected subcutaneously with strain 19 at the normal dose of $9 X 10^{10}$ or heifers vaccinated at six months then recalled six months later by the conjunctival route with a $5 X 10^9$ dose. The third group includes heifers vaccinated twice, six months apart, by the conjunctival route with a $5 X 10^9$ dose. Then the last group is a control. You can see that protection is one out of 12 in the conventionally vaccinated group; six in 12 in the group after conjunctival recall; five in

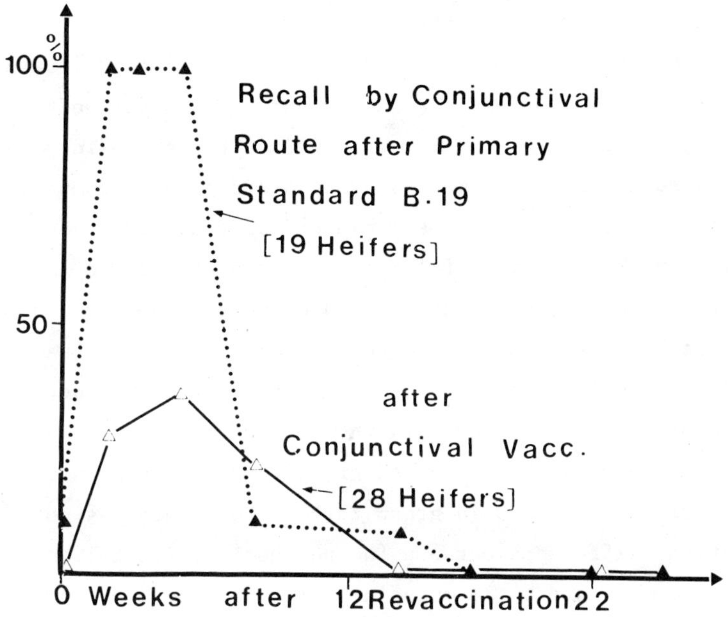

Figure 2. Serologic responses of cattle vaccinated with strain 19 vaccine by the subcutaneous and conjunctival routes and revaccinated by the conjunctival route.

Table 1

Results of Challenge of Cattle Vaccinated with Strain 19 Vaccine by the Subcutaneous and Conjunctival Routes

	Pregnant Cows Protected/Total	Term Calves
B.19 S/C 9 X 10^{10}	1/12	6/12
+ B.19 CR 5 X 10^{9}	6/12	8/11
B.19 CR 5 X 10^{9} TWICE	5/19	14/19
CONTROL	0/7	1/7

19 in the third group; and none in the control group. The groups are not very big because this was the first experiment done in cows. The protection afforded by the classical vaccination is quite low in this experiment but this is very often the case in our challenge system. This is not to be considered too bad of results in the normal vaccinated group. The comparison made clear that recall by the conjunctival route improves drastically the immunity of heifers and two successive vaccinations by the conjunctival route, which gave the low serologic response that you saw before, gave about the same immunity. The last column gives the number of calves born at full term: one out of seven in the control group; six out of 12 in the classically vaccinated group; eight of eleven in group two; and 14 of 19 in group three. So, there was no statistical difference between the percent of live calves in groups two and three. In my opinion two conjunctival vaccinations at a six month interval would give better protection than the classical vaccination. These data have not yet been published.

DR. HIDALGO: Thank you, Dr. Plommet. You see the basis for Dr. Nicoletti's work. I think that this certainly bears repeating with larger numbers because it looks very promising. Of course, Dr. Nicoletti also stated that the supplemental tests, particularly the rivanol and complement-fixation tests, were very helpful in his work in differentiating the serologic response to vaccination from natural infection in adult vaccinated cattle.

I will attempt to summarize the advantages and disadvantages of adult vaccination. The advantage is that it can be used as a remedial procedure where there is no calfhood vaccination and a severe problem exists within the herd. The disadvantages as Dr. Nicoletti stated them are: abortions did occur resulting from vaccination of pregnant animals, but this was less than one percent; infrequent udder infections were observed; and there was a systemic reaction occurring a few days after administration of strain 19 in adult animals resulting in decreases in milk production and feed consumption. And, of course, there was interference with serologic testing but with his battery of supplemental tests this problem was overcome. That is how I interpreted your presentation, Dr. Nicoletti. Would you like to add or amend anything?

DR. NICOLETTI: No.

DR. HIDALGO: I would like to summarize Dr. Alton's presentation and then open the discussion on immunization to the floor. Dr. Alton stated that in Australia both 45/20 and strain 19 were used and that there was some justification for this because of the conditions under which the animals were maintained. In the arid areas where the quality control of the live vaccine was not possible and where gathering of the cattle was not readily accomplished, 45/20 was used. He also stated that the use of strain 19 in Tasmania resulted in the reduction of prevalence down to two percent. He stated that the complement fixation test was the test of choice and that complement-fixation titers resulting from strain 19 receded faster than those of other tests but that he was concerned with quality control of strain 19 vaccine. He also stated that he was of the opinion that after the two percent level was reached by vaccination that it should not be discontinued. In fact, it should be continued until the infection rate was on the order of 0.2 percent, at which time the area is essentially free of the disease. He stated that 45/20 bacterin was used in the arid regions. Two brands were commonly used and they were not equal in efficacy. He also stated that there were batch variations within the better vaccine. There was some interference with the complement fixation reaction but the bacterin could be used effectively as a diagnostic reagent. He also made a plea for research to develop a stable rough strain for use in immunization whether it be 45/20 strain or some other. Dr. Alton briefly mentioned H38 vaccine and that was the first time we had heard about it up to this point. He concluded that it probably was not a real contender. This may be a point of controversy so we might open the discussion to our program participants on this subject. Does anyone feel that there is a candidate vaccine on trial at this point that could be used effectively whether it be H38 or Rev 1 or something else?

DR. PLOMMET: I would like to give you some information on the H38 vaccine. This vaccine was developed by Dr. Renoux while working in Tunisia and we have been working with this vaccine in cows in my own lab with Dr. Renoux. I should say first that Dr. Alton said that in regard to the serologic response to H38 vaccine there was some disagreement. There was no disagreement. In the first paper we published with Dr. Renoux we used one vaccination with H38 vaccine. After just one vaccination we had serologic responses that were about the same as strain 19 vaccination, lasting about six months. But, one vaccination is not enough to get a good immunity with this vaccine. So later we injected two successive doses two-three months apart. Under these conditions the serologic response is very high and very long-lasting so this is why there was some disagreement. Experimental data on the protection by H38 that I just gave you are data from Dana and Agomo who were working with the veterinarians in France and performed a very large experiment some years ago. These experiments were done with about 30 heifers per group and vaccination was accomplished with one injection of strain 19, two injections of H38 two months apart, or 45/20 vaccines A, B and C (the letters represent three different commercial brands). The protection expressed as the number of live calves with no detectable excretion of Brucella was best with H38 (Table 2).

Table 2

Results of Challenge with Brucella Abortus Strain 544 of Cattle Vaccinated with Strain 19 Vaccine and Strain H38 and Strain 45/20 Bacterins

Vaccines		Living Calf No Excretion %	Protected Cow %
Control		9	16
S.19	1 Injection	71	59
H.38	2 "	100	93
45/20 A	" "	52	62
B	" "	50	35
C	" "	82	76

Standard Challenge

B. abortus 544 15 X 10^6 From Dhennin, 1973

The strain 19 gave about the normal response (70 percent protection). Protection with 45/20 was from 50-82 percent in this experiment. The percentage of protected cows was expressed in the last column and you can see that H38 was the best vaccine.

DR. HIDALGO: Does anyone have a question for Dr. Plommet before he is seated? Before I open it up for discussion I would like to summarize Dr. Alton's characteristics of the ideal vaccine because I think that they are classical. First of all, it should have good keeping qualities. One dose should offer protection in animals of any age. It should produce no untoward reaction, no humoral antibody responses and produce solid, life-long immunity. That is quite a goal to strive for, Dr. Alton. Now, could we open up to questions directed to our speakers.

MR. JOHN ARMSTRONG (Kingsville, Texas): Dr. Nicoletti, in reporting on the work that you are doing on adult vaccination in Florida, I would appreciate it if you would give us more graphic comments with regard to levels of infection existing in those herds at the time you started this experiment, the percentage of abortions that were occurring and how those herds have responded to those vaccination procedures. What percentages of infection are you having subsequent to the vaccination and what percentages and exact numbers, if possible, of animals actually do react to the test afterwards?

DR. NICOLETTI: Mr. Armstrong, I did not bring with me the precise data on the results of those herds. The study in Florida, as I suggested in my paper, was authorized by the Brucellosis Committee of the United States Animal Health Association (USAHA). It is our feeling that the precise data should be presented to this committee at the Miami meeting in November. However, I think I can, in general, answer some of your questions. Two of our herds, as I mentioned in the paper, have been included in the studies now slightly over one year. In these two herds we have experienced something in the area of at least a 90 percent reduction of reactors. The reason I make that wording is that in neither of the herds were bacteriological studies made. Prior to the studies, they were simply using a diagnostic test, namely the card test, as an indicator of infection. Since that time we have not been able to use the card test exclusively as an indicator of infection simply because we are using strain 19 and there are, as you might expect, large percentages of cattle that are reacting to the card test and many of these reactions are persisting. We feel that we must use other tests, namely the complement-fixation and the rivanol tests. So, in terms of infection, this is what I am having to conclude. Initially infection was determined by agglutination titers and infection after the studies were begun was based upon bacteriology and serology. The two supplemental tests have both proven to be useful, supported by bacteriology. Perhaps you have other questions, Mr. Armstrong.

DR. NELSON: I think in relation to these data that Dr. Nicoletti just gave you, you want to keep in mind that these dairy herds had been infected for some time and they had ceased to carry on a test and slaughter program for an extensive amount of time prior to the initiation of the vaccination trial. Prior to the adult vaccination there was quite a period of time for build-up of reactor animals.

DR. NICOLETTI: I must correct my colleague. This is not true in some of the herds we are studying, only in two. The largest herd that we are studying had, in fact, not been tested and an additional herd had not been tested for one year. But, the other three herds that are included in our studies have religiously tested on schedule, including weekly tests of dry and wet cows, that is recently lactating cows. So, withdrawal from the program is not an explanation for the persistence of disease in these herds.

MR. ARMSTRONG: One point is still not clear to me. Are we to understand that you did have abortions in those herds prior to the time that you initiated this vaccination program?

DR. NICOLETTI: Definitely.

MR. ARMSTRONG: How many abortions did you have after you vaccinated?

DR. NICOLETTI: Well, in the vaccinated cattle in which we believe that the abortion was attributable to the vaccine there has been less than one percent reported abortion. In the herds in which the vaccine was used, the farmers tell us they have had no abortions attributable to brucellosis in vaccinated cattle since that time. Of course, we have to follow this up with cultural methods in cows that were reported to have aborted.

MR. NORMAN MOSER (DeKalb, Texas): In listening to the past people talk about 45/20, I haven't heard anyone state that it was dangerous from the standpoint of the livestock operator. Why is it prohibited or is it prohibited or is it just not available? It seems to me that the value is questionable but I don't understand why it is prohibited.

DR. HIDALGO: Dr. Nelson or Dr. Becton, would you like to field the question?

DR. NELSON: It is not prohibited; it is not available in this country commercially. There has been no license issued in this country for the production of it. I would imagine that if there were enough controlled study data that would support its efficacy and there was a biological firm that desired to produce it and it was approved by the Brucellosis Committee of USAHA as a recognized pilot program, it would be available. At this point there are no commercial firms that have requested license to produce it nor has there been sufficient data that it does have a greater or as good an efficacy as strain 19 vaccine. I think that is why we are still studying it in commercial herds and we still have additional herds going on study to determine if it will warrant licensing. However, at this time we have to get our 45/20 vaccine from Australia.

MR. MOSER: How does one go about importing 45/20 vaccine?

DR. NELSON: We have to get the special permit from a committee that deals with the importation of foreign biologics and vectors. It is an industry and scientific committee that we have to apply to. Dr. Ray can tell you about the committee. He makes the application and gets the approval to bring it in. I'm not sure of the makeup of the committee.

DR. WINTHROP RAY (USDA, Maryland): I don't know the full membership of the committee but it's the Agricultural Research Service, Veterinary Services and Veterinary Biologics that have a group that considers all applications for the importation of biologics to determine under which conditions they can be imported. We apply to that group and get a permit to bring it in under federal regulations.

MR. HILMAR MOORE: Dr. Nelson, in view of all of the testimony and papers that have been given, do you think that it is logical to say that 45/20 does have advantages and that it is a very useful tool that we could have in the U. S.? I mean, does it have to be proven in the U. S. that it is good or do you recognize that there are scientists in other parts of the world that are also quite capable? They seem to have progressed farther than we have in a much shorter period of time with the use of 45/20 than we have with strain 19 and, certainly, with the use of test and slaughter. In the meantime, they have not decimated their producers as we have in this country.

DR. NELSON: I think that we reported that there are a number of studies conducted in this country that confirmed data from other countries as to the degree of protection afforded by 45/20. We did report that. I think that you also heard differences of opinion with regard to the amount of post-vaccinal titer responses that were exhibited with 45/20. Dr. Alton gave some data that he had in his hand of more persistent complement-fixation titers following the use of the product than did Dr. Cunningham. Our studies have indicated that we also found some persistent titers but not enough to the point where it would be a detrimental aspect. However, Dr. Cunningham in his discussion and slides indicated that the use of 45/20 was not compatable or that he did not believe that it should be used in the program with strain 19. As I understood, it did not serve as a diagnostic tool compatable with the use of strain 19 and strain 19 has been widely used in this country for many years. We would have to then consider how we would use one in relationship to the other because it does evolve into a problem, a diagnostic problem, when you're using the two products, one over the top of the other or simultaneously. So, this is an area that must be given serious consideration. I think that Dr. Alton indicated that this is an area that they had problems with in Australia as well.

DR. HIDALGO: I'm glad that you mentioned that because we have skirted around the issue from time to time but I think that we must address ourselves to the question: Is there a place in a program for both immunizing products? We would like a response first from the participants of the morning session and then we'll open the discussion to the remainder of the speakers. The question is: Would it be possible and, secondly, advisable to use both products in a control or eradication program?

DR. NELSON: I would hope that there might be a possibility in this area. We don't, at this time, have this delineated. But, if we are talking about the primary advantage of it being used in an adult population, we would like to see some product available to our industry that we could go into a known adult population and do something to retard or reduce the spread of the disease. If Dr. Nicoletti's work proves out to be effective in the use of adult inoculation, we might have a product here. If it doesn't, maybe we need to look at 45/20. But with 45/20 when he did use it, in the few herds that he used it in, we did find a relatively high over-condemnation rate. And, I think that Dr. Cunningham supported this by saying that he found that in the areas of high disease incidence that he did not feel that it had as high a diagnostic value as it did in areas of low disease incidence. I think that it is supported by what we found in the few herds that we tried it in. But, I'd like to ask someone else to respond to the question as well.

DR. HIDALGO: Could we first have responses from our participants?

DR. CUNNINGHAM: A few minutes ago it was stated that Dr. Alton had put forward the suggestion that 45/20 raised difficulties in diagnosis. I think that he said that they don't test animals until 12 months after vaccination. There is certain logic in this and I think that the critical point is this: In Australia they are using the CF test as the determinant test. I would not entirely agree that you cannot go in and use the CF test something earlier than 12 months. However, one thing is certain, if you use 45/20 there is nothing to stop you from using an agglutination test of whatever type you prefer. Having gone into a herd and vaccinated with 45/20, one can carry on and use the tube agglutination test. We find that this vaccine has very little effect on the agglutination test even in known exposed animals (experimentally exposed). In a field situation where we have used it, as I mentioned this morning, we have found occasional animals in which agglutination titers "blew up" virtually sky high. Therefore, I don't think that anyone would have any doubt whatsoever as to whether these animals should be left in or taken out. Then, it's just a matter of deciding when you take them out. If they are cows that have calved down and are in the middle of lactation and not in calf, then obviously leave them in a vaccinated herd and get the lactation out of them. If they are heavily pregnant animals get them out quick before they spread more infection in the herd.

DR. HIDALGO: Dr. Nicoletti, would you like to add to that?

DR. NICOLETTI: No.

DR. GODFREY ALTON (Victoria, Australia): I agree with the remarks about using the agglutination test following the use of 45/20. One of the Australian states does this.

DR. NICOLETTI: Our limited experience with using 45/20 in the herds which I reported on yesterday is that certainly we believe the rivanol test is an excellent tool which you can use following the use of 45/20 in separating infected animals from those with post-vaccinal titers. I would support Dr. Cunningham's feeling about the amount of titers that are produced following two injections of 45/20. We have had some low levels of tube agglutination titers but again the rivanol test has proven very useful in differentiating infected animals from those that may have low levels of titers following two injections of 45/20.

DR. CUNNINGHAM: May I comment again, Mr. Chairman. There was another aspect raised there. The question was posed: Is it desirable to use strain 19 and 45/20 in the one eradication program? Personally, I would say that it is desirable not to use strain 19 where you propose using 45/20, simply because you are sensitizing animals with a smooth strain by using strain 19. Now, if things are being done as they should be done with strain 19 vaccinates, I presume they should be identifiable as strain 19 vaccinates. In this was you might be able to avoid some problems. Now, one of the problems is getting calves vaccinated. I imagine it is quite an immense problem in range herds of which I know virtually very little. Unless you make it compulsory that all calves are vaccinated with strain 19, I wonder if you are wasting your time. You call a thing compulsory, but unless you can make that compulsion stick you are out of business. In an area where it is even less feasible that all your heifer calves can be vaccinated with strain 19 it makes sense to me to use 45/20. I regret if I'm going against government policy, but it is my personal conviction. Why bother about strain 19 when you can wade in anytime there are indications for use of vaccine and just "plaster" a herd with strain 45/20?

DR. HIDALGO: We would now like to ask the opinion of all of the other speakers first and then we will open the discussion to the floor.

DR. PLOMMET: In our country 45/20 has been used for many years but if I could and had the power to do it, I would prohibit its use because we have too much trouble with this vaccine. There are big differences from one batch to the other; in serologic conversion and even in the degree of protection. In my opinion, a good vaccine should first be constant in production and until now most of the manufacturers are unable to get constant batches of 45/20. And, the second point is that any good vaccine should have a good method of control of efficiency. And, as far as I know, there is no such method for 45/20.

DR. CUNNINGHAM: Sounds like we are developing a European argument here. My experience dealing with vaccines goes back to the mid-50's when we were using strain 19 in Ireland. Really one of the main considerations in not using strain 19 anymore in Ireland was just as Dr. Plommet has said about 45/20 vaccine. We found a very wide variation in the efficiency of strain 19 vaccine. We had strain 19 vaccines that caused beautiful serological responses; bacteriologically in the laboratory they were beautiful but they wouldn't even protect guinea pigs. We tried it in guinea pigs and cattle and confirmed that this was so. Going on to 45/20 vaccines, again I would agree with Dr. Plommet that there has been rather varied history to 45/20 vaccines. We tried out four: one Dutch, one English and two French vaccines in Ireland and I agree that the results have been variable. Some of them have been very poor. One particular 45/20 struck me as though somebody had made the mistake in the laboratory and put adjuvant into strain 19 because we got serological responses that never ended. There was another batch of 45/20 vaccine that we got gross abscesses in 60 percent of the cattle we vaccinated. There was no difference really in the first injection and the second injection. As long as you had the batch number right you had 60 percent gross abscesses. What I'm calling a gross abscess is something that you see on a beast about half a mile away. When we opened up these abscesses a gallon of pus, more or less, was the norm. We also tried two French vaccines. One of them was a beautiful vaccine for use in the field. It gave absolutely no serologic response but it gave no protection either. One we tested more recently, Abortox, that I mentioned earlier this morning, appears, at least the batch we tested, to be a good vaccine. We got good protection from it.

Now, to my mind, and I put this in print some years ago, it doesn't matter what vaccine you are using to protect animals, it is well worthwhile and virtually incumbent on the state authority of the country in which that vaccine is being used to test batches of that vaccine every year or more. A rolling spot check on this vaccine should be done, not in guinea pigs or any laboratory animals, but in cattle. Well, one has heard or one will hear at times that to test vaccines in cattle is very expensive. Now, I don't swallow this at all because even if the vaccine you are testing is of no use at all you lose a batch of calves but you still have calved heifers that are still good meat. So you have lost a calf, but really, in a government laboratory that is nothing to lose any sleep over. There are plenty of other experiments carrying on all the time that are unproductive and quite wasteful. So, I have just put it quite simply that whatever vaccine you are going to use to protect your cattle, I think that someone should be employed to make sure that this vaccine can protect. And over a period of ten or eleven years we have consistently tested batches of the vaccine we use, which is actually Duphavac. We have tested this vaccine in cattle every year and we have not yet run into a batch that one could say that the vaccine was no good. I don't think that we have tested a batch of Duphavac in cattle where we got a protection rate as low as 50 percent. I could confirm all of this if I had figures with me, but right off the top of my head I can swear that we never got less than 50 percent protection with 45/20 vaccine.

Now, can I change the subject slightly to the topics that were raised earlier this morning on vaccines and, in particular, the application of strains by the conjunctival route? One of the differences I see in applying a live strain to the conjunctiva is quite an obvious thing that one does not get immediate serologic responses such as one gets when injecting a live strain. Instead of getting peak titers at about ten days, as one would obtain using injected strain 19, if one puts a challenge strain into the conjunctiva one doesn't get peak titers until about one month afterwards and at 10-14 days most animals will show no titers. So, it would appear to me that whatever dose you put into the eye that only a certain amount gets in and what you see in the serologic response is the multiplication of the organism in the challenged animal. A couple of years ago we set up an experiment and this again hasn't been published. We had two ideas in mind: (1) if we use the virulent strain, what extent are animals going to be infected and carry through this infection so that they abort and (2) we wanted to see again what sort of protection this virulent strain might give when the animals were challenged in mid-pregnancy in the normal way. The results we got were that out of ten animals which were given conjunctival exposure and then in mid-pregnancy challenged, nine out of ten were completely protected. I think that this was about the best results I ever got. And, it goes back to the days when McKeown in England and I'm sure somebody in America observed that the more virulent your vaccine strain the better is your vaccine. In the other group where we exposed them as yearlings to challenge and then put them in calfhood and let them ride through, one animal aborted so that one out of ten carried through the infection and aborted. The others calved down normally and were serologically negative. While on that particular experiment we may as well open it up. We compared the French vaccine, Abortox, and the Dutch vaccine, Duphavac. The protection rate was 75 percent (six of eight completely protected) with Abortox. With strain 19 we had 12 vaccinated and of these nine were completely protected so we got a 75 percent protection. Just to prove a point that we were challenging them, none of the eleven unvaccinated control animals withstood the challenge. They were all infected and out of that particular group of 11 there were only four viable calves. So, we were challenging them with a fair, effective challenge.

For some years we had the impression that where one is using a strong adjuvant like water in oil, why should we need two injections to protect? Now two injections make sense when one is using something like tetanus vaccine and your aim is to produce good titers of antibodies which is where the protection in tetanus lies. We had noted that where we give one injection of the 45/20 vaccine to cattle around a year old or older, that if we don't give them the second shot, somewhere around three-four months afterwards they build up their own secondary type response in that Coombs titers begin to rise after this time and they give the impression that they have been quite adequately sensitized, whether they are protected or not. So, in this experiment we included 12 animals that had gotten only one shot of the 45/20 vaccine and in this group nine out of 12 were completely protected. We had a 75 percent protection rate from a single injection of 45/20. As you know, from the first days that 45/20 was talked about in cattle by McDiarmid, it has always been suggested that you must give two injections of this vaccine to produce immunity. Even the manufacturer still goes along with the idea that the first just sensitizes and the second produces immunity. I feel that question is very, very open. Are we relying too much on other experiences and deducing that two injections are needed. I wonder if anyone else has anything to add to that?

DR. HIDALGO: Before we get into this I'm going to stick to the question of strain 19 and 45/20 together and am going to ask for comments from our participants. And then, I promise you I will open it up to the floor.

DR. MORGAN: Mr. Chairman, in Great Britain the 45/20 vaccine has been commercially available since 1967 alongside strain 19 which has been available since 1944. The latter has been used for the official calfhood vaccination scheme for calves between three and six months of age. Although 45/20 vaccine has been commercially available we have given very clear advice to veterinary surgeons and to farmers as to the circumstances under which the vaccine should be used. I have disagreed with my friend, Brendan Cunningham, about the serological response in animals following the use of 45/20 vaccine whether these have been previously given strain 19 in calfhood or not. We are finding that with the vaccine and the adjuvant that we have, there have been responses both to the tube agglutination test and particularly to the complement-fixation test. We have experimental data in previously unexposed animals where the CF titers have persisted for up to 18 months at diagnostically significant levels. Therefore, this is one of the first things that we had to bear in mind. We haven't allowed the use of the vaccine in herds which are undergoing eradication procedures. When we declare an area to be a Compulsory Eradication Area we prohibit the use of the vaccine for 18 months beforehand. This is again to take into account the serologic reactions that we are finding. I am hoping to say a bit more about this again tomorrow. We have recently reintroduced 45/20 vaccine into Britain in certain areas where there is a high level of animal population and of infection. I think only time will show really whether it has produced the effects I hope it will to reduce the prevalence of the disease to a level where in 1980 we can go in there with compulsory slaughter procedures.

DR. HIDALGO: Would any of our other speakers like to make a comment on that question? I apologize for the delay.

DR. HENDRICKS: I would like to make a couple of comments on 45/20, but first somebody brought up the differences between the countries. I would like to thank Dr. Cunningham for at least one similarity. The reason strain 19 hasn't worked in Ireland is the same reason that it has not worked in parts of this country. It is difficult to get immunity if you don't get it out of the bottle! We have done a small amount of work in this country with 45/20 a couple of times and gave an annual booster and then challenged these animals. We did get a reasonable immunity, somewhat comparable to that with strain 19. However, when we tried this in an infected herd where we injected 2/3 of the animals with 45/20 and left 1/3 as controls we got more infection among those that we injected with 45/20 than we did among the controls. Now, Dr. Cunningham has gotten 45/20 to work as a diagnostic agent in Ireland. Dr. Nicoletti has not been able to do that in this country. Dr. Nicoletti has also some experience where after attempting to use 45/20 as a diagnostic agent he gave a second injection presumably as an immunizing agent and apparently that was not terribly successful either. Certainly not to the degree that indications are with adult vaccination with strain 19. Could I end this with a question for Dr. Alton? We did get considerable differences between Duphavac and Bortin. I wonder if you would like to elaborate a little bit further on the differences of the products you have in Australia?

DR. ALTON: The three batches that have different serologic responses in vaccinated animals were Duphavac. The one that produces very little serologic response is a product called just 45/20 Adjuvant Vaccine. It is produced by a company called

Arthur Webster. It is said to be derived from Abortin that you mentioned but I think over the course of years it has lost any similarity it might have had.

MR. HILMAR MOORE: I think that partially answered the question I had for Dr. Alton. I cannot tell whether you disapprove of 45/20 or that you approve of it nor can I differentiate between the fact that some states or some sections of Australia use strain 19 and some 45/20. Do you have a comparison of the results of the two?

DR. ALTON: No, we don't have a comparison of the results. As a laboratory worker I would prefer not to have anything to do with either of them but it gets particularly complicated when animals are vaccinated with both. We realize that experience has shown that certainly strain 19 has a beneficial effect in reducing the prevalence of brucellosis at least in populations where the prevalence is over two percent. So far as Australia is concerned, Duphavac or 45/20 is generally used in areas where it is difficult to collect animals more than once or twice a year. The use of strain 19 in calfhood vaccination is not possible in these areas. I don't know of any figures for 45/20 but the people who use it find it acceptable to the owners of the animals. They are enthusiastic about it.

DR. WILSON WOHLER (San Angelo, Texas): We have heard that 45/20 is good and that it is not so good sometimes but generally it is said to be a good vaccine. And, we have heard that the serological response varies depending upon what test you are using whether it is complement fixation or the tube agglutination test. My question is: Has anyone experience using the card test as we use here in Texas after vaccination with 45/20?

DR. MORGAN: Well, not the card test but certainly the test that we are using, the rose bengal (RB) test, which I think in most respects is almost identical with the card test. After the second dose of 45/20 vaccine we are having reactions to the card test which do persist for up to a year after. This correlates fairly well with the complement-fixation titers as well. The tests become negative in the same sequence: the agglutination test, which if it does react does so at a very low level, is the first to become negative, then the RB test becomes negative after six months and the complement-fixation test is the last to become negative after about a year. The latter can be positive for up to 18 months.

DR. NICOLETTI: In our herds that we studied in Mississippi and one in Texas, following two inoculations with 45/20 we certainly did have interference with the card test. It is interesting that while we called the card test positive or negative and are not permitted to talk about the gray zone in between, in fact, this is what happened with the card test following two inoculations with 45/20. These animals did have what I'll risk calling trace reactions. They generally were not strong but you could see some reaction there. I would have to again disagree somewhat with my British colleague over the use of the complement fixation test following two injections of 45/20. This is not proven to be a serious problem with the CF test that we use. I would again emphasize that the rivanol test has been the best test in our hands for the differentiation of those titers that may have been produced by two injections of 45/20 from the disease.

DR. HIDALGO: Would any of the speakers like to comment?

DR. RAY: We have been using 45/20 in this country experimentally since 1963. We got, as Dr. Hendricks pointed out, comparable results from strain 19 as far as protection except in one study. I think that the difficulty that we have with 45/20 is what has been stated here over and over again. From trial to trial there is a great deal of conflict between the serological patterns and from one batch to another you are likely to experience difficulty or differences so that you just don't know what to expect after you use 45/20. In some cases you have persistent agglutination reactions and in some cases, which is more likely to happen, persistent CF titers even with the same batch of vaccine. We observed this in some cattle in South Carolina and also in some animals vaccinated at the University of Minnesota. We had wide discrepancies between the serologic results using the same batch of vaccine in different groups of cattle. So it opens up a tremendous question of: What do you do with these animals if you do test them a year later and you do find some positive serology? It is not only the card test that is involved. We also had problems with the rivanol and CF tests in some of these animals. We also had problems with the standard agglutination test in a percentage. So, it just causes a question of diagnosis. In some of these trials that have been conducted, we started out with cows that had been vaccinated as calves and revaccinated as adults with 45/20 and in the same trial we had cows of the same age that had not been vaccinated with strain 19 as calves but only subjected to 45/20 during the adulthood. Immediately in the postvaccination period we saw a great deal of agglutination reaction in the cattle that had been vaccinated both with strain 19 and 45/20. It was much more prevalent in that group than the other. After a period of six months, there was very little difference between the persistence of serologic reactions between the two groups; both had titered animals which were difficult to interpret in a field situation.

DR. MARGARET MEYER (University of California, Davis): I wanted to ask a question, not to make a comment. I wanted to ask Dr. Nicoletti a question on the adult vaccination in Florida. Did I understand that this was being done on herds that were already infected and having abortions? Could you tell me if you isolated strain 19 from these abortions and how did you tell they were from the vaccine rather than from natural infection that was there anyway?

DR. NICOLETTI: No. We have not studied any of these. The hypothesis that the abortion was due to the vaccine was based entirely on the period of time at which it occurred following the inoculation of strain 19, namely a few days later, the titer that was produced and the subsequent negative serology which developed in these animals. I cannot conclude that this was, in fact, abortion due to the vaccine. So, I'm concluding that abortion that followed administration of the vaccine may possibly have been due to the vaccine. The statistics that I gave you in terms of percentage of abortions following the use of the vaccine would include the possibility that there were abortions due to other causes.

DR. RAY: The same comment probably also includes the abortions occurring prior to vaccination in that we didn't identify the reason for the abortion prior to entering into the vaccine study. So, we don't know the "before and after" comparison.

DR. NICOLETTI: Not necessarily. What we do hope to do, of course, in retrospect, is to go back and to identify those cows that had aborted and see what they did serologically.

DR. RAY: Prove that the abortion was due to brucellosis.

DR. BERMAN: How can you evaluate this if you don't know what is going on before and after?

DR. NICOLETTI: The evaluation will be based entirely, not in terms of abortions, but in terms of reactors removed prior to the administration of the vaccine and infected animals removed following the administration of the vaccine.

DR. HENDRICKS: I just wanted to make a comment on what Dr. Ray was saying about the interference of 45/20 bacterin with the CF test. We did experience some animals that responded very similar to those Dr. Alton described in that we did get prozones or incomplete fixation even in a cold, overnight type of fixation. These were animals that were infected with field strains and were bacteriologically positive. Although they were reacting very high to some of the supplemental tests they did not respond to the CF test well. A few of them did not, anyway. Could I end with a question? Back to what the gentleman over here was asking awhile ago, we never did get an answer from Dr. Nicoletti. Do you have any accurate records as to the levels of abortions for each of the herds under the project in Florida?

DR. NICOLETTI: You mean prior or post?

DR. HENDRICKS: Prior to treatment?

DR. NICOLETTI: No, we don't. I would comment again on the question that Dr. Meyer raised about the conclusion that the abortions following administration of the vaccine may, in fact, be due to strain 19. I wonder how one may be able to determine this?

DR. HENDRICKS: You could take a culture.

DR. NICOLETTI: Of what? To my knowledge, the studies that have been done following the administration of strain 19 have not been very successful in isolation of the vaccine strain.

DR. HENDRICKS: In the work that was done by Manthei in serial passage of strain 19, in every case they gave an intravenous dose of strain 19, produced an abortion, and recovered the organism from the abortion. And, of course, in each case they had negative pregnant animals in the presence of the cow that did abort.

DR. NICOLETTI: In defense of what we are doing, the geography of the situation and the herd management would make it extremely difficult to get a fetus following the administration of the vaccine. We have studied milk but only after x number of weeks following the vaccination. And, in those cases we have not recovered strain 19 from the milk of any animal that may have aborted due to the administration of the vaccine.

DR. MEYERS: Have you been doing any milk tests or whey tests? Are you collecting enough milk and spinning it down and putting it into guinea pigs? I'm still baffled as to how you can go into a herd and not know if you are getting abortions due to Brucella, give adult vaccination, not collect fetuses and not know what is going on and still be able to draw conclusions.

DR. NICOLETTI: I thought we were talking about abortions specifically due to the vaccine. We certainly are doing a tremendous amount of bacteriological work on serologically positive animals.

DR. MEYER: Dr. Ray just said they did not know what the abortions were due to before you went in there. They may not be due to brucellosis.

DR. NICOLETTI: Well, that is quite true but if there were abortions occurring and large numbers of reactors being taken from the herd this is again what we had intended to do in terms of the reduction of the prevalence of the disease. In our studies I don't think we can make a comparison of the number of abortions occurring in the herd before and after the administration of the vaccine.

DR. MEYER: You have left the impression from your talk that strain 19 being administered to pregnant animals was, in fact, causing the abortions. I wanted to know how you knew that?

DR. NICOLETTI: Well, all I would like to suggest is that the number of abortions in the herd which have occurred for whatever reason following the administration of the vaccine has been less than one percent.

DR. HIDALGO: Do we have other questions from the floor?

DR. C. E. PAYNE (Bryan, Texas): I'm a practitioner here in Texas and I have been quite interested in the vaccination comparisons. Having been associated with the program and having used strain 19, I found it to be inadequate for our program. I would hope that we could find something better and it looks like it is going to take an act of Congress to ever see a dose of 45/20. We made a couple of references to H38 today. How much work is being done on this and how encouraging is it and what is the possibility that we might someday get this tested in this country? Is it far enough along and promising enough that it warrants looking into it at this time?

DR. HIDALGO: Well, who would like to answer Dr. Payne's question?

DR. NELSON: I'll just start handling it by saying that I don't know much about the European results with it, but I know that we do have an extensive evaluation of it going on in this country right now. Dr. Margaret Meyer at the University of California, Davis, has large numbers of animals under study with H38 vaccine at this time.

DR. PAYNE: Is there anything to report at this time?

DR. MEYER: We have barely gotten started really with the therapeutic aspects of it and the animals that will be on the prophylactic aspects of it have been vaccinated and will be bred this fall. So, we really will not have any results until at least a year from this August. And, the whole project will not be totally evaluated for another 18 months to two years until all of the data are ready to evaluate.

DR. HIDALGO: Would anybody else like to comment?

DR. PAUL BECTON (USDA, Maryland): I feel that we have listened to a tremendous amount of discussion from people who are very knowledgeable and have done a lot of work. I would like to speak just from our viewpoint as regulators, as that term has been used, and as someone who is searching for more effective means of dealing with the brucellosis problem that we have left in this country. Our interest, as you might gather, is certainly to find more efficient tools to benefit the owner of an infected herd and the owner of a herd that might be subject to infection or exposure so that we can more effectively deal with the problem. Now, you might say at this point we have a very liberal attitude toward the examination of any possible tool that may be available. On the other hand, we have a very conservative viewpoint regarding the possibility of approving something for use that might be leading you down the wrong road. As you can gather from the information that has been presented today, we are attempting to evaluate most of these products that have been used and have been discussed and we do intend to use them to the extent that they will be of value to us in eliminating the brucellosis problem as soon as we can get the information together.

DR. JOHN HOOPER (University of Texas, Galveston, Texas): I wonder if there were any data about the effect of these vaccines in cell-mediated immune responses of cattle? Isn't anyone looking at these?

DR. CUNNINGHAM: We are, at present, doing some work on cell-mediated immunity. One of the things we are using is a purified protein extract of *Brucella*, using it as brucellin. The question was: what effect does vaccine have on cell-mediated immunity? Both animals exposed and animals vaccinated give a positive skin reaction.

DR. MORGAN: I would challenge that. We have done a number of tests on vaccinated animals, both with strain 19 and 45/20, with brucellin and it is very exceptional for us to get any reaction. The only cell-mediated immune response to vaccine that I have seen has been in the guinea pig, where the strain 19 and the 45/20 adjuvant vaccine does give quite a marked cell-mediated immune response as determined by the skin test.

DR. ALTON: I would like to ask the question: Can you relate exactly the delayed hypersensitivity and cell-mediated immunity? How do you say "is anyone measuring cell-mediated immunity?"

DR. HOOPER: Well, I wondered if anyone was looking at lymphocytes, for example lymphocyte activation, not just skin test.

DR. ALTON: Our people are actually doing that but this is very much in the infancy. We find with guinea pigs that they can have a very good skin reaction (delayed hypersensitivity) and not be immune. You can't have the reverse. You can't have an animal that doesn't have delayed hypersensitivity and is immune. This question of activated lymphocytes is being pursued but this also is not a very simple procedure. At any rate, we don't have a pattern but they are trying it in my laboratory with 45/20 and strain 19 vaccinates and challenged animals.

DR. BERMAN: The history of studies of cell-mediated immunity in brucellosis can be divided roughly into three eras. The first, we will discard as primitive and ancient although there is a good deal of information in it. The second, we will call *in vitro* studies. I hardly presume to speak for him because Professor Elbery is in the room. There have been classical results of cell-mediated immune responses in brucellosis carried on in his laboratory over at least a 15 year period indicating very clearly that a cell-mediated response occurs following strain 19 and Rev 1 vaccination in laboratory animals and in livestock. This indicates very clearly that the dogma that has emerged in the hands of certain immunologists, since the intermediate period studies, that in facultative intracellular bacterial parasitisms the antibody-mediated immunity has nothing to do with the picture and that it is all cell-mediated is clearly erroneous. One day the pendulum will swing back toward an indication that we are dealing with total host responses. The antibody-mediated arm has a significant amount to do with the picture in total host immune response. Finally, what I would like to say is there is another group of studies which attacks a separate problem in the analysis of cell-mediated immune responses. This is the problem of differentiating between those responses, either *in vitro* or *in vivo*, which are attributable to: a T-lymphocyte interaction with antigens; those which are attributable to the whole set of consequences which flow from that; those which are attributable to interaction between *Brucella* lipopolysaccharide, antibody, B-lymphocytes and the complement system and a whole series of other kinds of problems that one deals with. Most of the antigens have been contaminated with lipopolysaccharide either in small or very large amounts. Most reasonable studies which have been carried out indicate: (a) that in appropriately vaccinated animals, there are antibody-mediated responses both to lipopolysaccharide and protein antigens and (b) in the same animals at the same time there are cell-mediated immune responses to the polypeptide antigens that can be demonstrated by appropriate means and (c) what we see in total host responses is a mixture of all of these kinds of things. In answer to the question: "Is anything being done with lymphocyte activation studies?", yes, but one must be very concerned about the kinds of antigens which are in use. In answer to the question: "Is anything being done with respect to other measures of cell-mediated immune response, such as MIF assays?", yes, these have been done and are being done. And, again, the issue of the type of antigen which is under investigation is one which is extremely important and one which is not easy to sort out.

DR. CUNNINGHAM: Mr. Chairman, I was just trying to get another short answer. It looks like another European dispute is brewing up here. We have been working with Brucella extracts for about seven or eight years. We tried them out as vaccines first and, as I mentioned before, these were remarkably unsuccessful. We also had extracts which when used as brucellin gave a quite good serological response as agglutinins. Of late, my colleague has produced a virtually purified protein and we have been getting very encouraging results with this product. In negative populations we get almost entirely negative skin reactions. In positive or exposed populations we are getting almost invariably positive reactions. And, on top of that, we are getting very little interference with any serological tests.

DR. THEODORE KRAMER (Auburn University, Alabama): Two or three of our speakers have mentioned the importance of cell-mediated immunity and, thinking about this in very general terms, there are three factors that affect cell-mediated immunity: one is the antigen about which we can do very little; the other is the adjuvant; and the third is the route of inoculation. Now, adjuvants were mentioned in connection with 45/20 and we know that certain antigens will give almost altogether cell-mediated immune response when given with a certain adjuvant or they may give an almost completely humoral immune response when given in other fashions. Similarly, the route of inoculation also has a bearing on what type immune response you will get. So, to bring this more into a question rather than a comment I would like to ask any of the speakers a number of sub-questions. One would be whether the adjuvant which was used with 45/20 in Ireland, United Kingdon, Australia and the United States was the same or whether these vaccines were separately adjuvanted? My second sub-question would be if there is a rationale for giving the live vaccine, such as strain 19, with an adjuvant or any other enhancer of the immune response. Now, I do realize that Freund's complete or, for that matter, any other water-in-oil adjuvant is not usable with a live vaccine but there are other possibilities such as endotoxin as is used with pertussis vaccine in human immunization, ion exchange resins and other new approaches to adjuvanting vaccines and I was wondering what, if any, attention is being paid to these possibilities.

DR. HIDALGO: Dr. Cunningham, would you like to respond to those questions?

DR. CUNNINGHAM: That's a big question but I'll have a go at it. The first question, I think was: Is the adjuvant in the different 45/20 vaccines the same? I can say definitely that it is not identical. They are similar in composition but the actual composition of some of these adjuvants are treated as sort of commercial patents. I understand that the one used in the Dutch vaccine, Duphavac, is the same one that they developed for use in a human killed influenza vaccine, if I'm correct. This adjuvant was found not to give undue reactions in humans. I'm reasonably familiar with the French 45/20 vaccine, Abortox, and the adjuvant is visibly different to that in the Dutch 45/20 vaccine. Dr. Alton may be able to say if the two Australian vaccines look alike but I'd say that this is possibly as far as any of us can go because the actual composition is treated as a commercial patent. As to the use of adjuvants in other ways, we have tried using a lesser adjuvant with extracts of *Brucella* cells and have tried them out as vaccines. The adjuvant used was aluminum hydrogel. It is difficult to say which of the components was of no use, whether it was the adjuvant or the extract, but in no case did we get any protection against challenge. As to the use of an adjuvant with a live vaccine, I don't think that I have any sensible comments to make on that I'll just leave that one alone to someone else.

DR. HIDALGO: Dr. Alton, would you like to comment on either of these two questions?

DR. ALTON: I was asked about the two adjuvants in Australia. I don't know. These commercial people don't tell you exactly what they are doing. Information on the Duphavac adjuvant was originally published in the thesis of Roerink, although I believe it has been changed. The two Australian ones look the same. I don't think that there is anything much in it. Dr. Kramer spoke about adjuvants in general. Now there are vast numbers of substances that have been investigated in this area and if there is any consolation to him, we have a biochemist in our group who is fairly familiar with this but it is a real jungle of things that you could try. Work has been done with live strain 19 and an adjuvant. I think that Dr. Renoux and possibly Von Dremlin in South Africa have done such work. Dr. Plommet has indicated that Dr. Renoux did not work in this area. I know it has been done without anything productive coming from it.

DR. DAN ANDERSON (Ft. Worth, Texas). I would just like to say a few words on my observations on thirty years of working in the wilderness with brucellosis. Really, in my position, I picture myself as an individual who is at all times interested in securing practical research work that can be applied out in the country. You might say that I'm one that carries the coal to Newcastle. As I have looked over this group for the last two days I have categorized it and have analyzed it. As I see it we have several different groups here who are vitally interested in brucellosis. One is this group of fine research people who have brought us information from all over the world. We have the "regulators", both state and federal. Then we have the "regulated" and interested ranchers and farmers. And, they are all important in this scheme of things. We know that. But, in thirty years of observing the problem of brucellosis, really I don't feel that we have made the proper progress that we should have and possibly it may be due to the fault of many of us. I feel that everyone along the line, the research people, the regulators and those of us out in the country are partially responsible. I know that I haven't followed the rules everytime. I'm not in jail yet but I was, at all times, interested in the welfare of my client and we tried to do the best we knew how. I know that right around the corner that brucellosis is going to be eradicated but I don't feel that it is going to be in my lifetime. Sometimes I hope that it won't occur in Texas because of the countries and states that we would have to protect ourselves against: Arkansas, Louisiana, Oklahoma, New Mexico and even Mexico. That would be a tremendous cost and expense in policing the areas. I want new tools for work in brucellosis. I'm speaking for the people of Texas. We see a credibility gap in this whole brucellosis program. Eradication and program are two words that we abhor because we are more interested in having a brucellosis control plan. I like the fellow's statement from Australia who stated "a plan that is acceptable to the agricultural community". I think that it was well put. That is all that we are looking for. Today I would like to challenge the research people to look into some of these newer things that we might have available. I do not feel that these areas have received proper attention. Let's look at the use of antibiotics and chemicals as a treatment for this disease. I know that it's terrible to even think about that because 50 years ago wood ashes and baking soda and everything else was sold supposedly to be used for the treatment of brucellosis. But, I think that we have come far enough along that we could look into those things that may have a practical approach. Hurriedly, there is another thing that we have not paid enough attention to and that is the state of nutrition of the animal. A lot of work has been done on deficiencies and I'm sure that a deficient animal is not going to be immunized with either 45/20 or strain 19 as well as a well nourished animal. One other statement, this 45/20 product and the possibilities of its uses really thrills me. I see in the great country of Ireland the eradication program is started in the North, but they are still vaccinating in the South. This applies to the U.S. We still have a few reactors from Texas clear across to Florida, but with these newer tools and the help of all you fine people we are going to make more progress in the future in our control program.

DR. HIDALGO: Thank you, Dr. Anderson, for those remarks.

MANAGEMENT AND PREVENTION

Moderator: Charles Boyd

Wildlife Reservoirs of Brucellosis

Frank A. Hayes

At the turn of the twentieth century, huntable populations of white-tailed deer (*Odocoileus virginianus*) had been virtually eliminated from the southeastern United States. The demise of this early food staple reflected the consequences of unrestricted market hunting and total disregard for wildlife conservation. Today, however, it is likely that more of these animals abound throughout this region than at the time of the first settlers. The return of this renewable natural resource resulted from changes in land uses and a more conservation-oriented populace.

Concerted efforts toward deer restoration commenced shortly before World War I and continued in a rather haphazard fashion until "black Tuesday" of October, 1929. During the depression years that followed, people of the southern states were confronted with a concern of much greater magnitude than wildlife restoration. Once again, the deer herds that had been reestablished were looked upon as a source of food for the protein-hungry human population. Earlier deer restoration efforts, therefore, were practically nullified until the late '30s.

Concomitant with emergence from the depression, the concept of wildlife management gained prominence throughout the Southeast and other regions of the United States. Public concern at a national level subsequently was reflected through passage of the Pittman-Robertson (P-R) Act of 1937, which is a sportsmen-sponsored tax bill, whereby hunters share the costs for wildlife restoration and conservation through self-imposed excise taxes on sporting arms and ammunition.

The P-R Act, therefore, represented a significant landmark for development of white-tailed deer resources of the Southeast and Texas. Game and fish departments also acquired stature as official governmental agencies and represented the actual foundation from which big game hunting would be reinstated.

World War II temporarily halted deer restoration. A precedent had been established, however, and after cessation of hostilities, efforts were intensified for development of deer restoration programs throughout the southeastern region. By the late '40s, the success of this undertaking reflected a feat for which many people were duly proud.

The summer of 1949 dates the first disease threat to this newly developing resource, whereupon in late August fishermen reported dead deer along streams and rivers of northern Georgia, western North Carolina, and eastern Tennessee. Deer mortality spread rapidly into several other southeastern states, wherein a 90 percent death loss was estimated on the Black Warrior Game Mangement Area of Alabama. The cause of death was not determined.

A few years passed without further incident, and in most localities where deer had died from the "mystery disease," natural reproduction gradually replenished the population. Game and fish agencies throughout the region simultaneously were conducting extensive trapping programs, and deer were relocated from Michigan, Wisconsin, Texas, etc. Increased protection paralleled restocking efforts, and sightings of these animals became commonplace. The public in general developed a high degree of pride in this new and expanding resource.

Then it happened again...in essentially the identical localities and at the same time of year..."deer plague" struck the second time in 1954, and for a second time preparations had not been made for pursuit of a diagnosis. Wildlife conservationists found this situation untenable, and grave concern was manifested for the future well-being of this highly prized outdoor recreational resource.

A recapitulation of this killing disease followed in the wake of the 1954 epizootic, when in 1955 KILLER-X hit with even greater intensity, expanding through much of the Appalachians and extending into the Ozarks. Thousands of deer were lost, but yet an organization was not in readiness for coping with this type emergency. For the third time within a decade, KILLER-X had come and gone without identification.

A general consensus was that the entire white-tailed deer resource was in grave jeopardy and could not withstand further assault by this mysterious disease entity. A pertinent question was proposed--"How can we hope to stop it when we do not know what it is?" Conservationists, sportsmen's groups, and the general public demanded action, and their representatives responded accordingly.

After a series of planning sessions, the Southeastern Association of Game and Fish Commissioners conceived an idea for coping with future crises of this type. It was recognized that an organization with the essential expertise and capabilities would be too costly for any one state game and fish agency to initiate and maintain. It also was realized that the problem in question was regional and not confined within state boundaries.

A cooperative approach, therefore, was developed for creating an organization that would afford diagnostic services to state game and fish agencies of the southeastern region. The program would be financed through annual pro rata funding and located in accordance with recommendations made by the Site Selection Committee appointed by the Southeastern

Association of Game and Fish Commissioners. After careful deliberation, the University of Georgia's College of Veterinary Medicine was chosen as the headquarters for what was to become the Southeastern Cooperative Wildlife Disease Study (SCWDS).

The early conception of the SCWDS was that of an organization primarily designed to wait for the recurrence of so-called KILLER-X. It was soon recognized, however, that many other problems involving white-tailed deer loomed just beyond the horizon.

Brucellosis, for example, was moving to the forefront as a potential clash of interests between this developing big game animal resource and the cattle industry. At that time, the United States Department of Agriculture (USDA), Animal Health Division's National Brucellosis Eradication Program was moving

about the status of wild deer as reservoirs of this multimillion dollar cattle disease. Clarification of this question, therefore, represented one of the earliest surveillance endeavors of SCWDS. Between 1957 and 1959, serums were collected from 6,710 hunter-killed or live-trapped deer. Through macroscopic plate agglutination procedures, initial testing was performed at an antigen:serum concentration of 1:25, and positive samples were titrated at 1:50, 1:100, 1:200, and 1:400 dilutions. If the serologic standards for testing cattle can be applied for evaluating tests with deer blood, 16 of the 6,710 serums would be classified as "suspicious" (1:50) and only nine as "reactors" (1:100).

Transmission studies conducted by SCWDS in 1961 showed that female deer acquired significant titers (1:100 or higher) to *Brucella abortus* within 42 days after inoculation, which suggested that the same standards for testing cattle could be applied to tests for deer serum. More recent information suggests that agglutination tests do not detect all animals infected with B. abortus. A combination of other tests as well as cultural procedures may have provided more reliable information on the role of deer in the epizootiology of brucellosis.

These data, nevertheless, agreed with accounts from other regions, which suggested that during that phase of the National Brucellosis Eradication Program, white-tailed deer did not play a significant role as reservoirs of bovine brucellosis. For the decade that followed, we in the Southeast were reasonably satisfied with this conclusion, which had been verified on several occasions by limited surveillance in which serums were collected from white-tailed deer in close proximity to infected herds of cattle. During the late '60s, an extensive study was sponsored by the Animal Health Division of USDA on the Ravenna Arsenal in Ohio, which reconfirmed our earlier position in the Southeast.

At this point, however, it should be emphasized that continued extrapolation from antiquated biological data often precipitates erroneous conclusions. More than two decades have passed since some of the earlier studies were conducted. At that time the population of white-tailed deer in the Southeast was far less than today. For comparison, the conservatively estimated current population of five million free-ranging white-tailed deer in the Southeast is at least ten times that of the population of these animals in this region 20 years ago. The number of cattle in the Southeast also has markedly increased.

As is the case with many other bacterial or viral diseases that affect domestic or wild animals, the increased degree of contact between cattle and deer, therefore, should be considered in the epidemiology of brucellosis. It subsequently is conceivable that sufficient contact has occurred between cattle and deer in some localities for bovine brucellosis to have become established in white-tailed deer. Further surveillance possibly could reveal an entirely different situation from that reported by SCWDS in 1958 and 1960.

If this has happened, simple arithmetic dictates that such a catastrophe would afford far more reason for concern than all combined accounts of this disease in bison, moose, elk, caribou, and reindeer. Frustration over these relatively few ungulates defies logical reasoning when paralleled by continued apathy for annually accelerating white-tailed deer populations in all states of the Southeast.

To further complicate this threatening situation, published records of susceptibility to brucellosis have been documented for a variety of indigenous small mammals, birds, and insects. A few examples include barnyard rats, wood rats, jack rabbits, hares, mink, foxes, coyotes, dogs, guinea pigs, English sparrows, American magpies, crows, pigeons, pheasants, domestic chickens, turkeys, ducks, geese, fleas, house flies, mosquitoes, bed bugs, ticks, etc. Indeed, in parts of Eurasia various rodents reportedly are intricately involved in the epizootiology of brucellosis in livestock.

When considering the mathematics of disease transmission as it now relates to the National Brucellosis Eradication Program, all potential reservoirs must be considered. The opossum and raccoon, for example, flourish throughout most of the United States where bovine brucellosis is so well entrenched. These particular mammals, as well as crows and a variety of other flesh-eating birds, often are closely associated with infected cattle and have ample access to aborted fetuses, placental membranes, etc., from cows infected with brucellosis. Yet, little is known about the role that these and other species of wildlife occupy as potential threats to future eradication endeavors in the United States.

An example of such hidden possibilities for reservoir status in wildlife was manifested through the Exotic Newcastle

Disease Eradication Program in southern California during 1972-73. As Wildlife Officer for the State/Federal Newcastle Disease Task Force Headquarters at Riverside, California, my primary responsibility was to determine whether viscerotropic velogenic Newcastle disease (VVND) virus had gained entry into the wild bird fauna of the quarantined area and the migratory waterfowl of the North American Hemisphere. Of the 9,446 true wild birds from which viral isolation attempts were made, VVND virus was retrieved from only three sparrows and one crow, which did not constitute a reservoir status. Mice on infected poultry premises, however, were significantly involved and warranted depopulation measures. This was contrary to existing concepts relating to the epizootiology of exotic Newcastle disease.

In conclusion of this small portion of the International Symposium on Bovine Brucellosis, it should be taken into account that since 1934 over 950 million dollars have been spent for controlling brucellosis in this country. Tremendous progress has been made, but the fact still remains that a long, expensive road lies ahead before total eradication is realized. To maximize the value of monies already invested and minimize that which must be spent before this goal is achieved, no stone should be left unturned. Since this nation's wildlife resources may represent a major stumbling block, this situation should be clarified at an early date in order to establish reliable parameters for the total program. Such may have a direct bearing on the number of cattle that may have to be slaughtered as part of the eradication effort.

Incidentally, the deer-killing disease to which reference was made during the early part of this presentation was diagnosed in retrospect during the summer of 1971. We now have reason to believe that the deer maladies of the late '40s and mid '50s were bluetongue (BT) and its companion entity, epizootic hemorrhagic disease (EHD). Evidence to date suggests these two viral conditions represent major emerging disease entities intricately involving cattle and deer in the Southeast. In a few more years, after each host species has been fully exposed to BT or EHD viruses, perhaps more attention will be directed along these lines.

Experiences with Brucellosis under Range Conditions in Northern Australia

William Slatter

The control and eradication of brucellosis is very much a joint effort between the producer, the veterinarian and the laboratory. Without co-operation between all parties, the scheme is most unlikely to succeed. From the outset the producer must be informed of the problems of the diseases; e.g. the effectiveness of the vaccines, the problems of residual titres after vaccination, the effect of parturition, etc. The veterinarian must be correctly informed on the level of security available, the normal management procedures, etc. so that a plan can be devised that will best suit that particular producer in his environment. The laboratory personnel should be informed of the problems of the herd so that they realise the type of cattle they are testing; e.g. vaccination status - whether recent or not and which strain - 19 or 45/20. In this way, a team effort will soon develop between all three parties. When this has developed, then progress will be much more rapid.

In any programme of this type, the importance of isolation and quarantine must be continually stressed and carelessness here is sure to eventually lead to breakdowns. The control and eradication programme at Brunette Downs will be used as an example of how we attempt eradication under range conditions in Northern Australia.

Brunette Downs is a property of approximately 3,000,000 acres (5,000 sq. miles) in the Northern Territory of Australia. It is situated at latitude 19°S and longitude 136°E approximately

250 miles from the Gulf of Carpentaria. The topography is that of rolling downs and interspersed between the downs are areas of semi-desert. The rainfall is predominantly summer (January-March), then a winter drought occurs until October-November when the early storms start. The average rainfall for the area is 350mm to 400 mm (approximately 15 inches) per year. Water is chiefly provided by means of 119 bores (bored wells) on the property. In the first few months of the year, there is abundant surface water, however by mid-year this has usually evaporated and the cattle are forced to the bores. Ideally, we aim to have approximately 500 cattle per bore. However, this ideal is seldom possible and it is not uncommon in the drier periods of the year to have 750 - 1,000 head of cattle watering at one bore. The bores are usually situated five to seven miles apart. Cattle leave the bores in the cool of the evening and return between ten a.m. and two p.m. to water. During this time, the cattle are in extremely close contact.

Brunette Downs is divided into three divisions:

1. No. 1 Stud. A herd of purebred and graded-up cattle which is now brucellosis and tuberculosis free. This stud contains approximately 4,000 cattle. This stud will be used as an example of how brucellosis can be eradicated under range conditions.
2. No. 2 Stud. This is a herd of 5,000 female breeders running with purebred bulls and is in the process of being graded-up to purebred status. This herd is now being managed to eradicate both tuberculosis and brucellosis. The present level of infection is 0.5 - 1.0 percent.
3. The Commercial Area. This contains approximately 50,000 head of cattle. By the end of the year, all females will have been injected with 45/20

bacterin and anamnestically tested. Testing is continuing and by the end of the year, the level of infection should be around one percent. At the end of the 1975 season it was approximately two percent.

Eradication of Brucellosis from No. 1 Stud

At the start of the eradication No. 1 stud contained approximately 2,500 head of cattle. The cattle in the herd are of considerable value. The main purpose of the stud is to produce replacement bulls for Brunette and an associated station in a brucellosis-free area of Western Australia. Because of the eradication programme being undertaken in the Northern Territory and Western Australia, it became obvious that unless a Brunette Stud could become free of brucellosis, no bulls would be able to go to Western Australia or any other free area. Hence the impending movement restrictions encouraged management to eradicate brucellosis.

In 1972, 2,460 head were subjected to both Complement Fixation (CF) and Rose Bengal Plate (RBP) tests by the government laboratory. A total of 370 cattle (Table 1.) reacted to the CF test for a reactor rate of 15 percent. It should be noted that this herd had over the preceeding years been subjected to various vaccinations including the following:

1. Calfhood strain 19
2. Calfhood strain 19 and adult strain 19
3. Adult strain 19
4. Calfhood strain 19 and 45/20
5. Calfhood strain 19 and adult strain 19 and 45/20
6. Single 45/20

It was suspected that a high percentage of the reactors would have been produced by the unusual vaccination

Table 1. Brunette Downs No. 1 Stud as of October 1972
Prevalence of Complement-Fixation Reactions
in Various Vaccination Groups

Type of Vaccination and Strain of *Brucella abortus*	Number	CF Positive	Percent
Calfhood - 19	767	131	17
Calfhood and Adult - 19	78	10	13
Adult - 19	43	9	21
Possible - 19	21	9	43
Calfhood - 19 and 45/20	144	25	17
Calfhood and Adult - 19 and 45/20	59	6	10
Single 45/20	241	120	50
Not known	132	18	14
Non-vaccinated adults	101	17	17
Non-vaccinated weaners	367	6	2
Bulls	507	19	4
Total	2460	370	15

procedures. However, a number of these animals were slaughtered and *Brucella abortus* successfully cultured (Alton et al. 1975).

The reason for the change to 45/20 was that in 1971-72 strain 19 was banned in the Northern Territory. The use of 45/20 was thought desirable because it was not logistically possible to vaccinate sufficient young heifers between three and six months of age in the extensive grazing areas of Northern Australia to produce a satisfactory level of herd immunity. Also 45/20, being a killed vaccine, has the further advantage in the Northern Territory of not being affected by climatic extremes (I.A.C. Report, 1976). There also is less danger to the operator when vaccinating with a dead vaccine.

In 1973 after detailed discussions with the management, it was decided to attempt to eradicate brucellosis. An eradication programme was thought possible because of the following points.

1. The stud occupies approximately 400 square miles of good country which is well watered and lightly stocked. This would allow us to maintain strict quarantine even in the face of severe drought. It is essential in any programme that clean cattle are always segregated from infected cattle whether vaccinated or not as we know that neither vaccine is 100 percent effective. In fact, the best protection we can expect is probably in the region of 70-80 percent (Cunningham, 1968).
2. The entire area is double fenced around its perimeter. The fences are spaced 12 feet apart. Brunette Creek bisects the stud area. This was considered to be a weak point in security because during the wet season the fences could be destroyed by floods or cattle could be carried into the stud by the floodwaters. To overcome this problem, it was decided to fence off an area of two to four miles on either side of the creek with a double fence. This would then aid the management of the programme in a number of ways:
   a. It allows the stud to be divided into three areas i.e. two female divisions separated by a buffer area of bulls. Because the bulls will be leaving the stud when they reach working age we have a continually changing buffer zone.
   b. If there is a breakdown in one of the divisions, it will be very unlikely that this would pose any serious threat to the other half of the breeding females.
   c. If animals were carried into the No. 1 stud area,

due to unusual seasonal conditions e.g. major floods, the only animals that will be exposed to infection will be the bulls that are destined for the Commercial Area. Hence, the breeding females should be isolated from any challenge beyond management control, except for wild animals e.g. dingoes dragging an aborted foetus or placenta through a double fence, etc.

d. It would allow security during and outside the breeding season, i.e. control of bulls.

e. It would also allow, during the dry season, a secure area where suspicious reactors could be held in isolation from the main herd until subsequent tests are performed.

3. All cattle within the stud are individually identified. The method of identification is as follows:

a. Shortly after birth, the animal is ear tattooed and its tattoo number is noted on the dam's card.

b. At weaning, the animal is then branded on the ribs with a fire brand and ear tagged with different coloured ear tags (with its number again written on the tags). Hence, the animals are permanently and easily identified.

4. The vaccination histories, as complex as they are, are known. This is a great aid when one in interpreting laboratory results.

In April 1973, Brunette Downs established its own laboratory and appointed a permanent technician. The tests used are the standard Rose Bengal Plate (RBP) Test and the Complement Fixation (CF) Test run in parallel on all sera. The CF Test is performed using the micro-titre technique and warm fixation. The microtitre system is based on the Cooke dynatitre. The CF Test is performed by the technique advocated by Alton et al.

Using this automated system, one technician can comfortably perform 600-700 tests per day. In fact, in excess of 1,000 tests have been performed on a number of occasions.

Prior to the commencement of the programme, it was decided to dispose of the foundation group of breeders. These cattle were either unvaccinated or the vaccination status was unknown, and by the previous tests had been shown to be highly infected. Hence all cattle going into the programme had been vaccinated prior to the commencement of the programme. As each paddock was mustered, all cattle were tail bled and each serum was subjected to RBP and CF tests. Any animal with a strong RBP reaction and/or CF titre of 1:4 or above was removed from the herd for retesting. Those animals were then subjected to two retests and if negative to both, were allowed to return to their group. However, if an animal was again positive, she was removed for slaughter (Figure 1).

Prior to the cattle returning to the paddock, all numbers were checked to guarantee all animals had been tested. If it was found that some animals were missing, the cattle were kept in hand until the missing animals were located. It is imperative in any eradication programme that all animals are tested. The beast that is left behind with a young calf or because she is calving or whatever the reason is the animal which might ruin the programme. Any animal that could not be tested was destroyed.

The herd bulls in the stud were left with the females all year. This also presented difficulties as it has been shown that animals that are pregnant or have just calved may give false results, i.e. negative and later become positive (Morgan and Richards 1974). However, on Brunette Downs, one finds that a high percentage of calves are naturally born in the first few months of the year. This is because of the seasonal conditions. The animals usually are putting on weight in March-July after

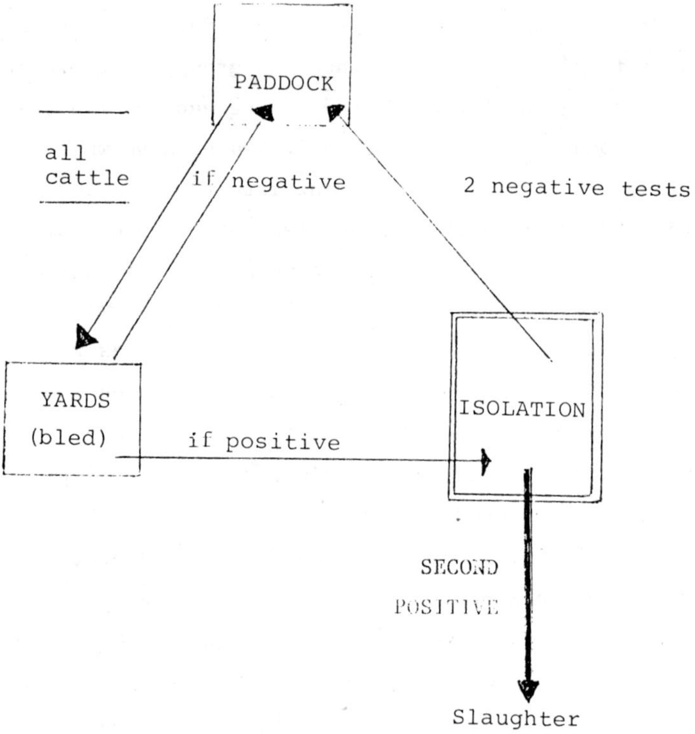

Figure 1

Brunette Downs No. 1 Stud: Testing procedure for Brucellosis

the summer rains. From then on, as the pastures deteriorate, the cattle are only able to maintain their body weight and then from September-January are usually losing weight, hence conception rates under these latter conditions would be markedly reduced. Therefore, the main calving period is January-May.

It is widely recognised that the bovine foetus may become infected with *B. abortus* in utero or during parturition and that colostrum or milk from any infected cow can be an abundant source of infection to the calf. There are two schools of thought regarding the subsequent course of disease in the calf. One school of thought maintaining that persistent infection does not occur and that there is, therefore, no danger in rearing such calves as herd replacements, provided they are removed from the sources of infection after the first few nursing periods (Fitch et al. 1941). The second school holds the opposite opinion that infection acquired at birth or in early life may remain dormant for months or even years, only to emerge as frank disease in an unknown proportion of cases (Plommet et al. 1973). Because of the danger of breakdown due to latent infection, all calves of reactor dams were also culled from the herd.

It has recently been shown by Lapraik et al. (1975) that, in an unknown proportion of calves born of infected dams, localised foci of viable organisms remain even though serological test titres return to negative levels. In this case, *B. abortus* biotype 1 was cultured from a calf that had been negative to the RBP, serum agglutination tube and CF tests for the last eight weeks of its life. *B. abortus* biotype 1 was also isolated from the dam at parturition.

Table 2 lists the number of tests performed and the reactors removed. On the first test, 133 reactors were removed for a reactor rate of 4.6 percent. Of these 133 reactors, 43 were condemned on the first retest and ten on the second retest. Hence 80 were allowed to return to their respective groups. The groups that had contained reactors were bled again late in 1973. From the results of this test another 20 reactors were detected for retest. Because of the impending wet season, it was decided to slaughter these cattle without retest. During 1973 all weaner heifers were subjected to the anamnestic test using an injection of 45/20 bacterin in an endeavour to locate any animals with latent infection. At the end of 1973, it was decided that we would stop vaccination. We felt that we had

Table 2. Brunette Downs No. 1 Stud Brucellosis Testing Programme

Date and Test	No. Tested	Reactors	Comments
April-October, 1973	2912	133	Reactors removed for retest.
Retest No. 1	133	43	43 removed from Stud area.
Retest No. 2	90	10	10 removed from Stud area.
October-December, 1973	826	20	Not retested due to impending wet season. 20 removed.
April-May, 1974	2454	10	
Retest No. 1	10	1	This animal was removed from the Stud area.
Retest No. 2	9	-	
May-June, 1974	867	10	All 10 were only suspicious reactors and were removed from the Stud area without retest.
July-August, 1974	2417	-	Official Test - NIL reactors.
March-May, 1975	3113	-	Official Test - NIL reactors.

the disease under control and any further vaccinating would only result in vaccination residues which might interfere with our aims to get the stud classed as brucellosis free.

In April-May 1974, 2,454 animals were bled and this resulted in ten suspicious reactors being detected. After subsequent tests, nine of these animals rejoined the herd. In May-June, the paddocks where the suspicious reactors had been detected were rebled. Another ten suspicious animals were detected. These were removed without further tests. The cattle that returned to negative levels were usually animals that had been previously vaccinated with 45/20. However, some may have been animals that had been exposed to but resisted infection (Morgan and Richard 1974). The problems of vaccination residues may be reduced in the near future with the use of a saline extract antigen prepared from Brucella abortus strain 45/20. This should allow the differentiation of uncomplicated 45/20 vaccinal reactions and natural infection (Miller et al. 1976).

In July-August 1974, 2,417 head were tested by the government and no reactors were detected. In April-May 1975, 3,113 head were again tested and again all animals were free. The stud will undergo another test this year to determine if it is still free.

The eradication of brucellosis has been achieved in No. 1 stud because:

1. The management was motivated.
2. Security is excellent.
3. All cattle are permanently identified.
4. All vaccination histories are known.
5. Clean musters are possible in this area and were achieved.
6. All reactors once identified were permanently removed from the herd.

7. The calves of all reactors were also removed from the herd.
8. The use of B. abortus strain 45/20 diagnostically.
9. The maintenance of strict quarantine within the area.
10. The use of CF and RBP tests on all sera.
11. The team effort of management, the laboratory and the veterinarian.

The No. 2 stud area is now in the process of being double fenced and this division is now also undergoing an eradication programme. The method of attack and the problems associated with it are similar to those of No. 1 stud.

The problems associated in the commercial area are different from that in No. 1 and No. 2 studs. In this area, it is impossible to maintain the same level of security and it is not possible with a herd of this size in the present economic conditions to work the cattle more than once per year. Because of this, it was decided that the method would involve a two tier level of attack, i.e. control of the disease in the adults by routine testing and also segregation of the weaner heifers and the development of a two herd system.

Vaccination of the herd commenced in 1968 and between 1968 and 1972 approximately 17,000 head were vaccinated with strain 19. In 1971-1972 strain 19 was banned in the Northern Territory and an additional 21,000 head were double vaccinated with strain 45/20. Since then the heifer weaners have had two vaccinations with strain 45/20 and all heifers have been anamnestically tested (Table 3).

During 1971-1972 a number of surveys were conducted and these showed a level of infection as high as 30 percent in some areas, however, this was probably also markedly affected by vaccination residues. In 1973, it was decided to attempt a two herd system and at the same time, maintain pressure on the adults so that in the event of a breakdown in security, we

Table 3. Brunette Downs Commercial Area: Brucellosis Vaccination History

Year	Number Vaccinated	Group
Strain 19		
1968	7290	Adults & heifers
1969	395	Heifers
1970	4350	Heifers
1971	4278	Heifers
1972	644	Heifers
Total	16957	
Strain 45/20		
1971	24388	Adults
1972	24322	Adults and includes 3144 heifers vaccinated twice.
Total Vaccinates	21178	Double vaccinates: 1st injection 1971 2nd injection 1972

would have the minimum of challenge to our clean heifers.

Prior to mustering all fences are checked and a road around the holding paddock is graded. This allows for quick daily checks of paddock security. The cattle are then mustered into the holding paddock. To aid our efforts for clean musters over the last two years, extensive use has been made of helicopter mustering. This speeds up the mustering process as well as ensuring a clean muster. Any animal that cannot be brought in for testing is destroyed. These are usually old bulls or injured animals. The cattle are then allowed to settle down for a day or so. One day before testing commences 600-700 adults are mustered from the herd.

Day 1, A.M.: Inject tuberculin and blood sample all adults. The weaners are then drafted off and trucked to the double fenced holding paddocks close to the station headquarters. Males are in one paddock and females in another.

P.M.: Muster the next day's cattle.

Day 2: Repeat

Day 3: Repeat

Day 4: The original mob is re-examined and the tuberculin and brucellosis reactors are removed and identified (permanently) or destroyed. The young calves are branded and the negative cattle are returned to their original paddock.

Day 5: Repeat

Day 6: Repeat

Wherever possible the calves of wet reactors are removed with their dams because of the danger of latent infection.

Different coloured ear tags are used and these can be marked so that they form a rapid means of identifying the vaccination and testing history of the animals. The TVI system of paint branding has also been used and in experienced hands is successful (Figure 2). We have found the use of back tags to be the most successful means of identifying cattle during testing. The retention rate is in excess of 95 percent and they are easy to read. Tail tags were originally tried, however 10-20 percent of the tags were lost and the tags, when soiled with excreta, were very difficult to read.

We find that under our conditions the level of infection in weaners from vaccinated adults is independent of the level of infection in the adults. Even when the infection level of the adults was around 10 percent the level of infection in the heifers rarely exceeded one percent. Table 4 gives the level of

Table 4. Results of Initial Brucellosis Testing in Adults in Commercial Area at Brunette Downs

No. Tested	Percent RBPT Positive	Percent CFT Positive	Percent of Reactors	Percent by Sex	
				bulls	females
2238	3.21	3.66	4.24	3.70	4.27
3640	1.48	1.78	1.92	6.66	1.71
1498	8.34	6.40	7.00	4.96	6.47
1783	7.01	5.21	5.21	6.45	5.17
1206	12.60	9.95	9.95	5.00	10.50
993	7.15	4.02	4.12	5.08	4.06
663	9.65	5.88	5.88	No bulls tested	5.88
3883	7.45	3.93	3.93	4.41	3.91
1034	2.99	1.83	1.93	5.55	1.87
16943*	5.80	4.17	4.34	5.11	4.30

*805 bulls tested.

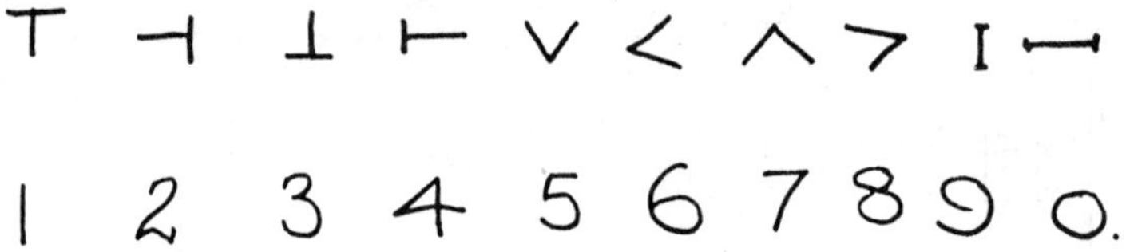

TVI - System of Identification

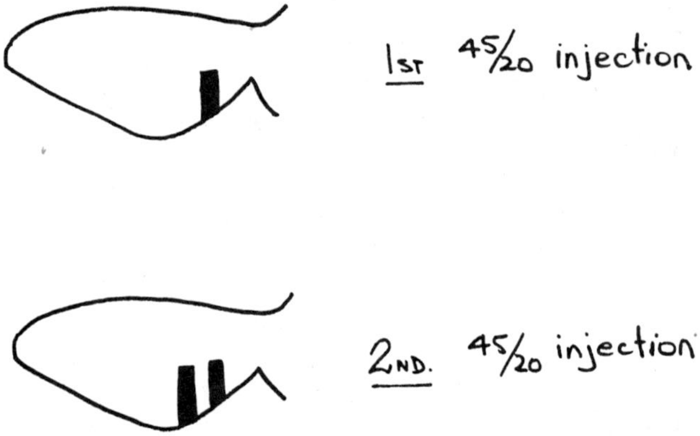

Vaccination Ear Marks

Figure 2

Brunette Downs Identification Systems

infection in adults. Table 5 gives the level of infection in heifers.

The heifers are tested at the station and all clean cattle are given the first strain 45/20 injection and notched on the bottom of the off ear (Figure 2). These heifers are then held in isolation until their retest in six to twelve weeks (Table 6).

Table 5. Results of Initial Brucellosis Testing in Heifers in Commercial Area at Brunette Downs

No. Tested	Percent RBPT Positive	Percent CFT Positive	Percent Reactors
1152	0.95	0.86	0.86
574	1.56	1.21	1.39
380	0.52	0.26	0.26
1593	0.87	0.62	0.69
743	0.53	0.67	0.67
559	1.25	1.25	1.25
1874	2.08	1.06	1.12
1368	1.4	0.7	0.8
1917	1.4	1.4	1.4
998	0.20	0.20	0.20
1383	0.50	0.36	0.43
12541	1.10	0.84	0.86

Table 6. Results of Second Test (Anamnestic) on Weaned Heifers in Commercial Area at Brunette Downs

No. Tested	Percent Reactors
3640	1.92
2165	3.69
1437	1.46
1229	2.61
1440	2.08
9911	2.36

This is an anamnestic test. All animals that give a strong (3+ or 4+) reaction to the RBT and/or a CF titre of 1:4 are removed as reactors. This is more severe than the criteria advocated by Cunningham and O'Connor (1971). However under the conditions that prevail in Northern Australia in the commercial beef cattle areas, it is not practicable to hold animals over for retest. The clean heifers are then given their second 45/20 injection and notched again on the bottom of the off ear. These cattle are not retested for approximately 12 months.

In 1974, the largest floods on record were experienced and 800-1,000 square miles of country were submerged. The years 1975 and 1976 have also been unusually wet seasons and this lake area has been maintained at 800-1,000 square miles. As the water dries back during the year we get very good feed. In 1974, it was decided that we would use the lake as another source of security. After the heifers are tested anamnestically, they start their way around the lake. Successive mobs of heifers follow them and older cattle are removed. We feel that it will not take two to three years for the lake to go dry and hence in the worst drought we should be able to carry the cleaner cattle without any breakdown in isolation.

In the northern part of the lake area, the clean heifers are isolated from the rest of the herd by a steer or bullock paddock. The northern neighbour has also agreed to place steers in his boundary paddock that adjoins our northern boundary.

It can be seen from Table 4 that the level of infection under our conditions in the bulls was higher than that in the females. Because of the shortage of bulls it was decided that any bull without any obvious clinical abnormality e.g. orchitis, hygromata, etc., after being permanently identified, would be used in the infected old herd and then culled with these old breeders irrespective of serological status. This procedure was based on the changing serologic picture that has been shown to occur in bulls.

During the last two years, the cattle market in Australia has been critically depressed. Because overstocking can endanger the whole programme, it was decided that all older cattle would be culled. This also will have a tremendous effect on the disease levels in the next year or so.

Under the extensive conditions found in Northern Australia, it is usual to find the first calf cows have reduced fertility (believed to be due to stress of rearing a calf under unfavourable conditions). Therefore, it was thought that a large increase in younger breeders might result in slightly smaller calf crop. However, to date this has not eventuated. In fact, the branding percentage has increased (possibly due to the reduced loss through brucellosis). Improved management and seasonal conditions could also be responsible for the increase.

Seasonal mating would be of considerable value because of the effect of parturition on immunoglobulin status. However, at the present time, this is not thought possible. It may be introduced when the economic situation improves.

I feel it is most important, where possible, to have

neighbouring properties undergoing a similar programme. Each property can then have clean cattle on their common boundaries and, therefore, reduce the chance of reinfection. This definitely leads to better relations with one's neighbour.

Conclusions

The control and eradication of brucellosis under extensive range conditions can be aided by the following points:

1. The development of a two herd system based on weaner heifer segregation.
2. Maintain testing pressure on adults to reduce the chance of re-infection of the clean heifers.
3. Isolation of clean weaner heifers from infected old herd by means of buffer areas of steers, bullocks, spayed cows, or cull non-pregnant females.
4. The use of strain 45/20 diagnostically to detect latent infection.
5. Identification of animals by means of ear marks, fire or freeze brands and the use of coloured ear tags.
6. Calves of reactors wherever possible should be removed.
7. The area chosen for the clean cattle should be secure with respect to feed, water, and fences and where possible should be kept understocked so that in the event of adverse weather conditions, the cattle will not have to be mixed with infected cattle.
8. Only bulls or semen from free herds should be used in the clean area.
9. Seasonal mating.
10. Culling of old cows.
11. Co-operation between neighbouring properties.

Precautions Necessary for an Individual Buying Replacement Stock to Prevent the Introduction of Brucellosis

There are numerous reports in the literature stating that it is very difficult to determine the brucellosis status of individual animals by serological testing or other means. Because of this, great care should be exercised when buying replacement stock. It has been shown recently that 10 percent of the herds receiving negative-exposed cattle developed infection as a result of those cattle (Schilf 1972). Therefore, consideration of the following points may aid in preventing accidental introduction of brucellosis:

1. Origin: Is the property where the animals are being purchased free of brucellosis? If so:
   a. How long has it been free?
   b. Is security good?
   c. Is the herd vaccinated?
   d. How long has it been since the last free test?
2. Vaccination Status: Because vaccination with strain 19 or 45/20 can affect a number of the serological tests used in the diagnosis of brucellosis, the following points should be determined:
   a. Are the replacement animals vaccinated?
   b. If so, at what age were the animals vaccinated?
   c. With what vaccine were the animals vaccinated?
   d. How long since the last vaccination?
   e. If vaccinated, are they identified?
3. Age and Pregnancy: Brucellosis may often have a long incubation period. The length of the incubation period depends on the size and virulence of the challenge dose, the resistance of the animal, and the stage of pregnancy at the time of exposure (Morgan et al. 1969). In pregnant animals shortly before

parturition when IgG_1 is depleted by transfer to mammary secretion, prozones may occur due to increased ratio of IgG_2 to IgG_1 (Plackett and Alton 1976). This may lead to a negative CF titre, however, in such cases the RBPT may be positive. Sexually immature animals may be serologically negative for considerable periods of time and subsequently be shown to be infected after they have calved or aborted (Plommet et al. 1973). Hence it is important to determine the following:

a. Are the animals sexually mature?

b. Are the animals pregnant?

4. Bulls: Evidence in the literature suggests major problems in the diagnosis of brucellosis in bulls. Reliance on serological tests alone will result in some infected bulls being regarded as uninfected. Infected bulls may be serologically positive or negative and may or may not be excreting _B. abortus_ in their semen. Antibody titres both in serum and semen may be negative or weakly positive in infected bulls and similar titres may be found in animals from which _B. abortus_ cannot be isolated. Lesions may be confined to the seminal vesicles and/or ampullae and may not be readily detectable except at autopsy.

These facts suggest that all bulls from known infected herds should be viewed with suspicion irrespective of their serological status. Since brucellosis can be transmitted to cows from infected semen used for artificial insemination (Bendixen and Blom 1947) it has been suggested that bulls from infected herds should not be used in artificial insemination programmes particularly when eradication programmes are in progress (Plant et al. 1976).

5. Tests: A wide range of serological tests is available for the serological diagnosis of brucellosis (Morgan 1967). Most of these tests have certain limitations. Therefore, their accuracy in the following situations should be considered when replacement animals are being purchased. Are the tests accurate in the following cases:
   a. Detecting early infection.
   b. Detecting chronic infection.
   c. Detecting latent infection (e.g. anamnestic tests).
   d. Differentiating between infection and vaccination residues.
   e. Are the tests affected by pregnancy?
6. Transport:
   a. Because of the danger of cattle trucks or railway wagons etc. being infected, it would be advisable to only use transports that come from a clean area or have been recently disinfected.
   b. If animals have to be off-loaded or rested, make sure that this area has also not been recently infected.

   Both of these points should be borne in mind as the stress of handling and transporting is often responsible for precipitating impending parturition. If an infected animal calves during transport we have a ready source of infection for the other animals in the shipment.
7. Isolation: Once on the property, isolation would be wise as we know no test is 100 percent accurate. The cattle should be kept in isolation until after calving, and they should then be retested. This can often be easily achieved by separating the clean cattle from the new arrivals by a buffer area of steers, bulls,

spayed cows or non-pregnant cull cows.

8. Contamination of Pastures: If there has been a breakdown, clean cattle should not have access to the pasture until sufficient time has elapsed (depending on the environment concerned) for the organism to have been destroyed. In the meantime, the affected area could be grazed by steers or other culled non-pregnant animals.

Treatment

It appears from a search of the literature that the treatment of brucellosis under range conditions at the present time is not practicable. The drugs cited include streptomycin, oxytetracycline, chlortetracyline and sulphonamides used either singularly or in combination. However, the results from their use have been indifferent. Recently, however, it has been shown in experimental trials in France by Plommet (1973), that micronised tetracycline given intra-peritoneally, either before the animals are exposed or within a short period after exposure gives satisfactory results. The micronised form of the drug has been suggested because this particle size allows uptake by the macrophages. In man, many treatments or combinations of treatments have been tried. Recently trimethoprimsulphadiazin has been tried with apparent favourable results. However, because of the problems with diagnosis (both serological and cultural) in the live animal, especially in sexually immature females and in bulls (where they can be serologically negative for a considerable period of time whilst still harbouring infection), it would be difficult at the present time to guarantee freedom from infection after treatment. Therefore, it would appear that animals after treatment should be kept in isolation until definitely proven to be free of brucellosis.

However, as techniques improve, it may be possible in very valuable animals to subject them to ovum transplants. In this way, the producer may be able to get a reasonable number of progeny from his elite cows. However, it should be realised that brucellosis can result in infected cysts being produced in the ovaries and the uterus. In these cases it would probably be unwise to subject these animals to ovum transplants as they may infect the recipients. Therefore, in these cases all animals should be judged individually. In Australia, the treatment of known brucellosis reactors is not permitted.

Vaccination - Should it Cease After the Elimination of Brucellosis

Whether vaccination is to be continued or not after the eradication of brucellosis will depend on the environment involved. It is hard to generalise because what might be the correct approach in a herd in an arid, lightly stocked area is not necessarily the correct approach for a dairy herd in Ireland. Hence, each area or property should be looked at individually. If vaccination is to be discontinued, the following points should be considered:

1. What level of security is available?
2. Can quarantine procedures be effectively enforced?
3. Are adjacent areas free?
4. Are there any problems with wild or feral animals?
5. Will it place unnecessary strain on the producers involved?
6. What is the normal degree of movement within the area e.g. do animals come or leave the area for summer grazing?

If vaccination is to be continued, the following points should be considered:

1. Will continued vaccination interfere with the serological tests that will be used to monitor the freedom from infection?
2. Is there any possibility that vaccination may lead to infection in a percentage of animals that have been vaccinated at the correct age (e.g. strain 19) (Schilf, 1972).
3. Could vaccination lead to a prolonged incubation and hence delayed diagnosis of the disease?

I feel vaccination should only be discontinued once we are sure that security is such that unvaccinated animals are not going to be challenged.

Acknowledgements

Without the interest and help of the management of King Ranch Pastoral Company, notably Mr. P. L. Baillieu, Managing Director and Mr. C. Weiss, resident General Manager, the eradication and control programmes at Brunette Downs would not have been possible.

I wish to thank Mr. G. R. R. Murray, V. B. Sc., Mr. R. W. Gee, B. V. Sc., Mr. D. Newton-Tabrett, B. V. Sc., and Mr. P. D. Claxton, B. V. Sc. for their helpful advice and criticism. Mr. F. P. Sheil has been responsible for the excellent laboratory work.

References

Alton, G. G.; Maw, J.; Rogerson, B. A.; and McPherson, G. G. 1975. Aust. Vet. J. 51:57-63.

Alton, G. G.; Jones, Lois M.; and Pietz, D. E. 1975. Laboratory techniques in brucellosis. W. H. O. Monograph Series No. 55. 2nd edition.

Anonymous. 1975. I. A. C. Report, Brucellosis and Tuberculosis. Canberra: Australian Government Publishing Service, pp. 11-12.

Bendizen, H. C., and Blom, E. 1947. Br. Vet. J. 103:337.

Cunningham, B. 1968. Irish Vet. J. 22:130.

Cunningham, B., and O'Connor, M. 1971. Vet. Rec. 89:681.

Fitch, C. P.; Boyd, W. L.; Kelly, Margaret, D.; and Bishop, Bucille M. 1941. J. A. V. M. A. 99:413.

Lapraik, R. D.; Brown, D. D.; Mann, H.; and Brand, T. 1975. Vet. Rec. 97:52-54.

Miller, J. K.; Kelly, J. I.; and Roerink, J. H. G. 1976. Vet. Rec. 98:210-215.

Morgan, W. J. Brindley. 1967. Vet. Rec. 80:612-621.

Morgan, W. J. Brindley; MacKinnon, D. J.; Lawson, J. R.; and Cullen, G. A. 1969. Vet. Rec. 85:639.

Morgan, W. J. Brindley, and Richards, R. A. 1974. Vet. Rec. 94:511.

Plackett, P., and Alton, G. G. 1975. Aust. Vet. J. 51:376-377.

Plant, J. W.; Claxton, P. D.; Jakovljevic, D.; and de Saram, W. 1976. Aust. Vet. J. 52:19.

Plommet, M.; Fensterbank, R.; Renoux, G.; Gestin, V.; and Philippon, A. 1973. Ann. Rech. Veter. 4:3,419.

Schilf, E. A. 1972. J. A. V. M. A. 161:1525.

Management and Prevention Discussion

DR. CHARLES BOYD (Texas A&M): We do have some questions which we feel would be appropriate for our visiting friends to answer. This one is directed to Dr. Morgan. In cattle that have been calfhood vaccinated with strain 19 vaccine: 1. What is the earliest date recommended for blood testing replacement heifers? 2. Which test would you use in this situation to detect infection in heifers?

DR. BRINLEY MORGAN (Weybridge, England): Thank you, Mr. Chairman. I can elaborate on how we do it and demonstrate what we are doing and leave it at that. I will compromise by saying that when we started the voluntary eradication of brucellosis in 1967 we tested calfhood vaccinated animals at 24 months of age. To put this into its correct context, at that time we were subjecting dairy herds to three milk ring tests at three month intervals. The milk ring tests were followed by the official herd blood tests and we sampled not only the animals in milk but heifers and bulls as well. We found through experience that we were finding reactors in the heifers at 24 months of age and when we modified the scheme in 1970 we reduced the age at which heifers (official vaccinates) were tested from 24 months of age to 18 months of age. The reason for the change was that we felt, due to the management circumstances in many of the herds where the young stock and heifers are often kept quite separate from the rest of the milking herd, that by monitoring the adult animals only we were not getting the correct situation of the whole herd. By this procedure we can pick out animals which we believed to be reactors to the test at a much earlier stage and to pull them out of the herd before they have had time to calve and become a danger to the other cattle in the herd. By doing this we have made problems for ourselves. We are finding that in a number of otherwise clean herds some animals are reacting to the test at 18 months of age. We are not able to resolve these and, therefore, are having to slaughter them as reactors although we are not able to recover Brucella from them at post-mortem examination. The answer to the first question is we test at 18 months of age. Another question which you didn't ask me is: At what age would we test non-vaccinated animals? We test these at 12 months of age, and again we feel that this is an important part of the control program especially in herds in which there have been breakdowns or in infected herds to pick up these animals at an earlier stage before they can do any harm. Whether these are animals which have acquired infection in utero or which have picked up infection during the course of their lives alongside other animals is something that I cannot answer. But I think it is important to keep the whole position of heifers in perspective.

The other part of your question was which tests we would use. The tests that we are using are the rose bengal plate test as a screening test and if that is positive, we follow it with the agglutination test and the complement fixation test and assess the results depending on whether the animal is a vaccinate or not. We have found by this method that we are picking up far more animals as heifer reactors than if we are relying on the agglutination test alone.

DR. BOYD: The next question is: At what age should replacement bull calves be blood tested for brucellosis?

DR. MORGAN: We test bull calves at six months of age.

DR. BOYD: The next questions then would be for Dr. Nicoletti. Is it necessary to have all animals vaccinated to bring brucellosis under control by vaccination? What is the lower limit of percentage of vaccinates needed to influence the spread of the disease in the herd? How should this level of vaccinates be attained-by compulsory vaccination or otherwise?

DR. PAUL NICOLETTI (USDA, Florida): I think it is generally agreed by epidemiologists that you need a high level of vaccination in any population in order for vaccine to be effective for control. Since the vaccine is not 100 percent protective, I feel that we should recommend the vaccination of all female replacements being added to a breeding herd. However when talking about the percent of cattle in a region that need to be vaccinated, I think Dr. Jones stated this morning that vaccination of 60-70 percent of the eligible calves in the state of Wisconsin was associated with a reduction of prevalence of infection from ten to one percent in four years. I would feel that 70 percent of the population vaccinated would probably be the lower limit for an effective vaccination program.

DR. BOYD: Would there be a comment from the audience?

DR. FRANK MANN (Wharton, Texas): In regard to the question of calfhood vaccination, how long was this calfhood vaccination program in effect in Wisconsin? My question is: Would a one year or a two-year intensive calfhood vaccination program be effective or would it have to be a five, six, or seven-year program?

DR. DAVE BERMAN (Univ. of Wisconsin): We administered the first doses of strain 19 vaccine in Wisconsin in 1938 on an experimental basis. In 1941 when I arrived in Wisconsin it was very common to go down the road and see abortions. By 1946, we were vaccinating calves in approximately 30 to 40 percent of our herds. By 1951 approximately 50 percent of the eligible calves were being vaccinated. Of course, a lot of them then go out and don't remain in the herds. We are not quite sure how many of them remained in and how many went out. In 1951, when we began the ring test surveys, 42 plus percent of the herds were ring test positive. And in the ring test positive herds approximately ten percent of the animals were reactors to the tests. At that time our herd owners were given the option of putting their herds on Plan A or Plan B. Plan B required vaccination with gradual removal of reactors but compulsory vaccination of all calves. By 1953 the whole herd was to be on Plan A which was test and slaughter and so forth. By that time we were vaccinating better than 70 percent of our eligible calves and we continued to vaccinate better than 60 percent of our eligible calves up until a few years ago. It is going to obviously take three years of intensive calfhood vaccination before the vaccinated animals come into production. It takes a relatively short period of time if you discontinue vaccination before the population of vaccinated animals drops down below levels which are going to give you protection. We have had recent importation of infection into the state from time to time. We find a striking difference in the number of tests necessary to clear those herds again based upon the proportion of vaccinated animals remaining in the herd at the time of the new introduction of infection from outside.

DR. MANN: We have talked about how long this immunity from strain 19 lasts and in my area of Texas we have Brahman cattle that are blessed with longevity. We palpated some 18 to 19 year old cows yesterday. These cows were calfhood vaccinated with strain 19 eighteen years ago. Are these cattle immune? Dr. Nelson mentioned five gestations. They have had many, many more than that and they have also had no boosters. They are serologically negative. I have wondered, are these cows immune and what should be done to protect them against brucellosis?

DR. NICOLETTI: I am sure no one has done any statistical studies on a population of eighteen year old cows. The only one that I know in the room who has probably done more work in the longevity of vaccination immunity than anyone else is Dr. Berman.

DR. BERMAN: I think you ought to frame those Brahman cows. I don't think any of us can tell you. As to what to do with them, the answer really is, what is going on around you?

DR. NICOLETTI: It seems to me that the second question in the series here is related to the first, that is, what lower level of percentage of vaccinates is needed to influence the spread of the disease in the herd? Again, I plead ignorance; but, again, I would have to believe that you would have to have a fairly significant percentage of the animals vaccinated. I think I can go on and talk a little bit about this third one: How should the level of vaccinates be attained? I particularly like to talk about compulsory vaccination and emphasize what my friend from Ireland pointed out this morning. I think all of us resent that word "compulsory" in any area. It seems to me that in the area of brucellosis, compulsion has generally implied an inclusion of public services, that is, publicly financed services. So, if we are going to include that word compulsion, it probably suggests that this vaccination is going to be financed out of public funds. As it exists now, this is largely not available so that if the services are provided-fine; but then even including this you have to have method for enforcing that word compulsion. I can see great problems. It's nice to pass laws or regulations or whatever calling for the compulsory vaccination, but its quite another matter to service that compulsory vaccination. I haven't answered the question, but I think I have raised some very serious points that have to be considered in a compulsory vaccination effort.

DR. BOYD: Are there further questions for Dr. Nicoletti?

ANONYMOUS: I just want to make a comment about the length of time to develop a fairly high percentage of the herd as vaccinates. There was an article about a year ago in the Livestock Breeder's Journal giving some different recommendations for herd culling procedures because of the over-population at that time and which persists today. I don't recall exact figures, but they were recommending that people cull a relatively high percentage of the brood cows and save the heifers. Then go back into a standard procedure of culling, maybe ten or fifteen percent a year, which would be the replacement rate. Projecting this over five year period, even if you had culled very severely and considered the fact that a relatively high percentage of the herd in the first year would go into the herd as non-vaccinates because they would be too old for calfhood vaccination, at the end of five years you would have about 60 percent of the herd vaccinated. I think it is a general consensus that 50 percent of the herd vaccinated does not give you necessarily 50 percent as much benefit as 100 percent of the herd vaccinated. I believe the Montana group concluded that about 70 percent would be the minimum where you would get reasonable benefit from calfhood vaccination.

DR. BOYD: The next question is directed to Dr. Margaret Meyer. What management principles have been documented to reduce the transmission of Brucella from infected animals to susceptibles - both intra and interherd?

DR. MARGARET MEYER (Univ. of California): In the interest of time I'll just go over these very briefly. Included in the interherd prevention of transmission is the purchase of animals from certified-free and modified-certified-free areas and from brucellosis free herds; blood testing the animal at the time of purchase; selection of official vaccinates and quarantine, or at least isolation, and blood testing after arrival and before addition to the herd. On the intraherd spread, the owner should be sure to obey the age limits on calfhood immunization; separate the dry, lactating and pregnant animals; use separate calving pens as parturition becomes imminent and test the animals at the specified times. Especially for animals that have undergone parturition and maybe are negative at the time, a 15 or 30-day test should be conducted thereafter to see if you can detect one of these latent carriers and also separate the titered animals from non-titered animals. If the titers are in the suspicious range the animals need to be re-tested, along with the proper and prompt removal of reactor animals. In cases of herds that have suspicious and titered animals an increased frequency in the testing program is advisable.

DR. BOYD: Will there be any other comment from the other speakers relative to this question?

ANOMYMOUS: California has a situation with very large herds and I think this requires some special management. Dr. Vanderwagen is in the audience and he has had some experience in handling these herds since some of them became infected a few years ago. I wonder if Dr. Vanderwagen would be willing to discuss this?

DR. L. C. VANDERWAGEN (Sacramento, California): In California we never worried about herd management when it came to brucellosis control. We were fortunate. Thirty years ago the livestock industry went to the legislature and said we need authority and we need funds to vaccinate and we need a program that will be enforced. We got authority, we got funds, we enforced a vaccination program, not compulsory but mandatory, in dairy heifers and optional in beef, and we did this for ten years. In the late 50's and early 60's we had a testing program that went through the state like a dose of salt. We started up north and moved south and they told us that when you get down south to those big dairies, those Dutchmen are going to kick you out; you will never clean them up. Within two years they had cleaned up. It was the people up north that were having trouble. The big dairies didn't seem to give us any problem. They averaged about 200 cows. Vaccination levels were close to 100 percent. We thought we had the world by the tail. We didn't worry about reintroduction of disease because we could whip it, we could clean it out. In 1973 we got the chance. It came back with a vengeance. We found we weren't near as smart as we thought we were. We now have 1000 cow herds on an average. Right now we have about 30 dairies infected and they average 861 cows per herd. The vaccination levels were at 50 percent not 100 percent. We had to do some rethinking and change our thinking as to management in these big dairies because they did not respond as they had earlier. You might have 50 cows in each of these pens or you might have 400 in each of the pens. Some of these dairies have 2,000 or 3,000 animals. We had to take a look at herd management because testing just didn't get the herds to respond. Before, with a 30-day testing interval or a two-week testing interval, there were no problems and within seven months there wasn't a herd that didn't respond and clean up. Some of these herds now have been infected four years. We are gradually getting the vaccination levels back up to 100 percent and when we get the management incorporated into the program we start getting some response. In an average operation the owner goes out once a day and looks in the dry pen. He brings in any cows that have calved. There might be 400 or 500 cows in here calving, aborting, or whatever. There is one variation. Sometimes they have a little pen that they call the close-up pen where once a day they bring heavy springers up and let them calve in very crowded conditions. One other variation, because it is so far from the house to the dry pen, quite often when they dry cows off, instead of putting them in the dry pen right away, they like to put them in the close pens so they can observe them. Cows are going in and then going to the dry pen, and cows are coming from the dry pen into here. If there is any contagious disease it goes back and forth. We recommend two basic management procedures. Get some calving pens and let the cows calve in them and stay there until the placenta has been cleared and then transfer the cows into the milking string. That's the number one procedure that we feel is essential to clean these herds up. Secondly, start a new dry pen. If you have infection in the dry pen its going to cook and boil and simmer there forever. As the cows dry off, start a new dry pen. Get a portable fence that can be moved across the lot. As the old dry pen is phased out the new dry pen theoretically contains all tested cows. We are testing every 30 days or every two weeks. So we have what we call a clean dry pen and a dirty dry pen. This has worked on some herds. Here again it's no better than the manager.

DR. BOYD: Dr. Hayes was able to tell us he has no data that shows specifically any incrimination of the deer population as a reservoir host. It was interesting to me that of 6,910 hunter killed deer and a few trapped deer (mostly bucks) that these were negative or yielded negative results with the exception of nine reactors at a 1:10 dilution. No deer samples reacted at 1:100 dilution or higher. They were using the same standard that was used on cattle so we would assume that it would be comparable. Having answered those questions that Dr. Hayes did in his presentation, I would like to call on our speakers and ask if someone here would care to share any information that he might have from his country relative to reservoir hosts for cattle population of *Brucella abortus* or other *Brucella* organisms? Dr. Meyer, would you care to elaborate, please?

DR. MEYER: I would like to make a few comments about wildlife and possible reservoirs for brucellosis. The comment was made that rodents in Russia were intimately involved in the transmission of brucellosis. During the last 20 or so years there have been several isolations from rodents in separate parts of the world. There have been isolations from rodents in North Queensland, Australia, in Kenya and in Russia, all of which seem rather out of the way places for having contact with domesticated livestock. The follow up on this has been that the rodents in Australia were in an area where feral swine were hunted. The type of *Brucella* isolated from them was closely related to type III *suis*. The same is true in Kenya where they had isolated type III *suis* from rodents and it was in an area on the banks of a river where game frequent so that transmission from rodent to rodent was ruled out but transmission from game to rodent was not. The literature indicates that the isolates from Russia are unidentifiable strains. As a matter of fact, one of the strains from rodents was the Brucella suis type IV and three or four of the strains were of a closely related biotype that had a B. melitensis antigen. One strain was Brucella melitensis. These strains were isolated where livestock had been present some six or seven years ago. However, the Brucella melitensis could conceivably have come from the Saiga antelope because Brucella melitensis has been found in the Saiga species. The type IV strains were in an area where the caribou or the reindeer are found. There has been no evidence whatsoever that the rodents can transmit brucellosis back to large animals. There have been sporadic instances of Brucella suis, melitensis, and abortus in rodents trapped in farm yards. The Russians have wanted to say that the rodents were a natural reservoir for brucellosis and that the Brucella they were finding in rodents in Russia came from an antique and ancient natural foci of infection. However, there has been some very recent work done on die off of rodents. There is an argument about whether the population density of rodents is sufficient enough so that you could have an indefinite transmission of Brucella in the rodent population. In the Scientific American in 1974 there is reported a cyclic die off of rodents where there can be a drop from 100 to 200 per acre down to one or two per acre. This occurs every four years and the cycle is synchronous in communities of rodents that are fairly separated and the cycle has been found to occur in Asia, in Russia and in the Americas. It has not been found in South America. So, the possibility of an indefinite transmission of Brucella in the rodent population with these being a hazard to domesticated animals is extremely remote.

The other possibilities of wildlife that have been mentioned are raccoons and opossums. In northern California near some infected swine herds we did trap some raccoons and opossums that had a titer to Brucella. We have not been able to isolate an organism from them. In some experimental work on infecting them, we could not establish that they could transmit it. I think that is essential. If you are going to say that you have a reservoir of infection, you have to not only find the organism, you have to show that it is transmitted from animal to animal in the reservoir and from the reservoir to domestic animals. Foxes have been incriminated and they seem to be susceptible to the organism into whatever environment they happen to be near. Foxes have been found infected with *Brucella abortus* when they have been caught near infected cattle. The same is true of foxes that have been trapped near infected swine. All the evidence indicates that the disease is self-limiting in foxes and it is not transmitted from fox to fox nor is it transmitted from foxes back to domesticated animals. Feral swine are a problem. There are feral swine in northern California that have been found to be infected with a type III *suis*. And it is also known, of course, that feral swine will breed with domesticated swine given the chance. In the southeastern United States there are feral swine and I understand that there has been an isolation of a *Brucella suis* type I cultured from feral swine in that area. You have feral swine here in Texas. Most of the reservoir in wild animals seems to be a greater hazard to swine than they are to cattle with the exceptions we discussed yesterday-the elk and the bison.

There have been several studies in the United States on deer and most of them have established that there are serological titers. To my knowledge there has been only one actual isolation of *Brucella abortus* from a deer in Arkansas. Again, it has not been established that it can go from deer to deer and from deer to cattle. This is a distinct possibility that is as yet an unproved one.

The jackrabbit has been incriminated and we all know about the problem they have in central Europe, particularly in Denmark, with the infection of the *Lepus timidus* (European Hare) and

Lepus europaeus species with Brucella suis type II. Surveys in this country have shown that an occasional culture can be isolated from a jackrabbit. There have been isolations of Brucella suis and one of Brucella melitensis. There have been serological surveys where rabbits have had titers but there is no evidence that in this country we have a problem like they have in Europe where you have this massive reservoir. Brucella do not seem to go from animal to animal within the species in jackrabbits nor do they persist and go back to domesticated animals.

The fact is that I am ready to say that, except for bison and elk and a possible local and temporary situation, in the United States we can give wildlife a clean bill of health as far as being reservoirs of brucellosis. There could be a possible contact source occasionally and this is more apt to be around swine.

DR. BOYD: Thank you, Dr. Meyer. Would there be other comments from the speakers?

DR. GODFREY ALTON (Parkville, Victoria, Australia): Could I fill in the situation a little bit about Brucella in wildlife in Australia because there is some confusion. I think I have it straight in my mind. In Queensland the domestic pig population is infected with Brucella suis biotype I, not very common but it occurs. There are feral pigs in this area and there was a scientific letter in perhaps the last issue of the Australian Veterinary Journal describing the isolation and identification of Brucella suis biotype I from these feral pigs that have some contact with domestic stock. Some years ago a type of Brucella (suis) was isolated from tree climbing rodents in Queensland. Cultures were sent to Dr. Meyer for identification, and these were identified as Brucella suis biotype III. Dr. Meyer has often been quoted in Australia as saying that this is due to contact with livestock and so forth. Brucella suis biotype III has never been isolated from any species of animal in Australia, to my knowledge, apart from these woodrats. I think that this ought to be made clear that there is no evidence of transmission of type III between wildlife and domestic live-stock in Australia.

DR. MEYER: Were the isolates from the feral swine from the same geographical location as the rats?

DR. ALTON: No. Some confusion has arisen about this. I feel that these rodent strains or so called biotype III have only been isolated from wildlife. This is the point that I am try-ing to make.

DR. MEYER: The point that I am trying to make is that at the time Brucella were isolated from the rodents who had contact with feral swine, were the feral swine looked into at that moment, not 20 years later?

DR. ALTON: Not to my knowledge.

DR. BOYD: Dr. Morgan, about England, sir, have you something to put into the pot?

DR. MORGAN: Happily, I can say there is no wildlife reservoir of Brucella at all in our country. We have made surveys in deer and there is no evidence at all in them.

DR. BOYD: Dr. Hayes has some definitive statements and I have one question for him after that.

DR. FRANK HAYES (University of Georgia): It really isn't definitive. I just want to correct a few things that I misled you on. We have isolated *Brucella suis* from one deer that was in very close contact with feral hogs. Inidentally, all of the joints of this animal were swollen and we obtained the culture from the joint fluids. As far as the titers in the nine out of 6,710 serum specimens that we processed, we did have reactions up to a 1:400 serum dilution. We considered 1:100 positive. We observed reactions in dilutions up to 1:400. I would like to reiterate the fact that our collections were made primarily from hunter-killed animals in November and primarily from bucks. I would like to ask Dr. Meyer one question: Has anyone studied cottontail rabbits?

DR. MEYER: Not extensively, but I think Dr. Thorpe in Utah has looked into some cottontail rabbits and found them to be negative.

DR. HAYES: I would like to make one more point clear on this particular disease. I would like to be able to speak with confidence and to get up in front of an audience with a clear conscience and say, "they ain't got it". I can't exactly do that now; I wish I could.

DR. BOYD: Would there be other comments relative to wildlife reservoirs? Then we will move forward with our next question. What precautions are necessary for an individual buying replacement breeding stock to prevent the introduction of brucellosis? I think I took from Dr. Slatter's paper that first would be replacement with vaccinated animals. At what age were they vaccinated; what was their capability of response and were they from clean herds? Does anyone have any comments to add? Should vaccination be stopped after elimination of brucellosis from a herd? To quote Dr. Slatter "it depends on the situation on the premises and the locale and whether those premises adjacent to him have been cleaned up."

DR. BOYD: Is treatment sufficiently reliable to permit its use instead of slaughter in valuable breeding cattle? If so, what drugs are recommended? Streptomycin, oxytetracycline and chlortetracycline were discussed and I drew from Dr. Plommet's presentation that you use micronized tetracycline given intraperitoneally. Would Dr. Plommet care to comment?

DR. PLOMMET (Nouzilly, France): Terramycin (oxytetracycline) was injected by the peritoneal route and we injected ten gm - one, two or three times. First, in experimental brucellosis the treatment was administered ten days after challenge in both pregnant or non-pregnant animals. I showed you these data yesterday. In pregnant animals one-half the cows were considered as cured. In non-pregnant animals 20 of 22 were cured. The cure was assumed from negative bacterial finding at slaughter. At lease 20 samples of lymph nodes or organs were taken from each cow and when no Brucella were found we considered this cow as cured. So you can see that when terramycin is administered ten days after challenge it is possible to cure quite a lot of the animals. In the second part of the experiment 21 cows that had aborted and were naturally infected were treated with one, two or three injections. We observed that four cows were completely cured. So, the conclusion of this research is that at the beginning of an epidemic of brucellosis it is possible to protect most of the animals that are definitely contaminated. If these cows are not pregnant you can expect about 91 percent success. In pregnant animals the success would be lower. But in natural infections of brucellosis which were long standing the percentage of cured was so low that it is of absolutely no interest in my opinion.

DR. BOYD: Thank you, Dr. Plommet. Would there be further comment relative to the treatment of selected cases of *Brucella abortus*?

DR. WILLIAM SLATTER (Brunette Downs, Northern Territory, Australia): In Australia you are not allowed to treat brucellosis reactors and they are supposed to be sent straight to slaughter.

DR. BOYD: What management principles can be employed on herds maintained on range conditions to hasten the elimination of brucellosis infections? From Dr. Slatter's paper I noted the following points: serologic examination of cattle with removal of reactors immediately; disposal of infected material and isolation of infected animals; maintenance of fences in good repair to prevent the intermingling of herds; managment of water and, if possible, elimination of common ground water sources and prevention of overpopulation and overstocking. Is quarantine and the limitation of movement of cattle mandatory in preventing brucellosis?

DR. WINN RAY (USDA, Maryland): There are a lot of connotations to this question. When we are talking about cattle in known infected herds or cattle that have been associated with known infected animals, certainly I think if we would poll the group we could agree on one thing. That is, you have to quarantine the animals that have been exposed and you would have to limit the movement. I am not sure that this mandatory requirement on the quarantine and limitation of movement of such animals is going to prevent brucellosis in every case. It's going to be mandatory in order to prevent brucellosis but there are some animals that you are not going to identify and, therefore, will not be able to interrupt the movement sufficiently to prevent all reintroduction or movement from all newly infected herds. So, certainly quarantine and the restriction of movement of exposed animals is a fundamental aspect of preventing the disease but, by itself, may not be enough.

DR. BOYD: Are there comments from any of the other speakers relevant to this question? Dr. Cunningham, there are two questions directed to you. How important is controlled breeding versus year-round calving in eliminating brucellosis from an infected herd? Are there instances or circumstances in which reactor animals may remain in the herd or on the premises and still not endanger the remaining non-reactor breeding cattle in the herd?

DR. BRENDAN CUNNINGHAM (Dublin, Ireland): The first question is pretty self-evident. It is extremely difficult to do anything with a herd when you have got year-round calving. For the simple reason that there is no time during the year when you can test the herd and be confident that you can interpret the tests most accurately. In the pregnant sector of the herd, you can never be sure whether a negative test means that the animal does not have brucellosis. A lot of our herds are spring calving herds. And we aim to test them mainly after calving has been completed. At this stage one can interpret tests quite accurately. And also, if the herd happens to be infected one has a number of months to carry out the tests in relative safety. By this I mean that you're safe that there isn't going to be a cow aborting in the middle of the test period. However, one can do an agglutination test at any time if it is considered desirable. Another point I would throw in here is that in our system of dairy management it has been well established by the dairy husbandry people that synchronized breeding makes economic sense. You see, we have grass growth during Summer and nothing much in Winter. So that normally our cows tend to throw their calves in the Spring. It is cheaper to produce milk from grass and that is why in Ireland the breeding to calve in the Spring makes economic sense. The second question is: Do we know the circumstances in which reactor animals may be retained in the herd? We have been looking into this for the past two years in six commercial dairy herds. To give a very short answer to this, it is possible to keep reactor animals in these herds. These are vaccinated herds and it is possible to keep them there quite safely as long as you segregate animals for parturition. I think my California friend has just made this very clear on the board. I was delighted to hear Dr. Slatter bring in management very forcibly. And I would like to compliment him on his description of how he managed Australian herds. I wonder myself, not being terribly familiar with either of the situations, if he can do that in Australia, why you can't do it here? I'm being impudent now, but I do think and I feel strongly that management is absolutely essential. If I am called into a herd as a veterinary surgeon to advise on getting rid of brucellosis and if the manager is either unwilling or is incompetent to follow management principles, he is wasting his time and he is wasting my time. It doesn't matter in those circumstances if you have got 100 percent vaccination or not because its quite possible to infect vaccinates.

DR. BOYD: Thank you, Dr. Cunningham. Will there be comment from any of you other speakers on these two questions? The next question is directed to Dr. Plommet. What effect do corticosteroids have on the animal exposed to or infected with Brucella abortus?

DR. PLOMMET: This is an extraordinary question which should have been directed to Dr. Wesley Spink of Minnesota, because they have been working with this matter 20 years or more. The conclusions have not been changed. The conclusions were that cortisone injected into mice before challenge induced little disease. And this has been used in some countries, Britain in particular, as a test for control of immunity in mice. If cortisone is injected after challenge there is practically no change in the course of the disease. In my lab we have experimented with cortisone in mice and in bulls. We used cortisone just in mice to stimulate latent infection. After treatment of the mice we wanted to know if there is some latent infection left. Therefore, we treated the mice for three weeks with cortisone and some of these latently infected mice would develop an acute infection which is far easier to detect. So, we tried the same treatment in bulls. Sometimes in the artificial insemination center the bulls have low levels of agglutinins which are considered non-specific and we wanted to induce a change in the titers in the bulls. Cortisone treatment neither reduced the agglutinin titer nor stimulated any detectable latent infections.

DR. BOYD: Will there be further comments on this question?

DR. MORGAN: We have in the literature in 1970 an article describing the effects of corticosteroids on the residual titers in animals which were showing inconclusive reactions to the diagnostic tests. In our work there was no effect whatsoever on the titers. We also have given corticosteroids to cows or heifers that have given us inconclusive reactions to the diagnostic tests hoping to mimic what happens if you give corticosteroids to animals with Infectious Bovine Rhinotracheitis (IBR) antibodies as they are supposed to stimulate the excretion of the virus. Again we have found that the administration of corticosteroids to such cows has had no effect either on the titers or the ability to detect actual living Brucella organisms at post-mortem examination.

DR. BOYD: That concludes our list of questions on this sheet. There will be some further discussion form the floor. Dr. Hayes has a question.

DR. HAYES: While our distinguished panel is intact I would like to get back to the bison in the Yellowstone National Park and request that a vaccination program be recommended.

DR. RAY: Dr. Hayes, you are about 13 years too late. In 1962, I believe, we tried to get vaccination in the Yellowstone bison. We managed to vaccinate eight bison calves, six of which were immediately slaughtered. So, we wound up with a net total of two vaccinated bison on the Yellowstone range. The game biologists at Yellowstone have considered the vaccination program in more recent years and are not in favor of such a program because it would mean rounding up the bison. That is one thing that they don't care to do.

DR. BOYD: This does not conclude the program. It concludes my part. I'm going to turn the program back over to Dean Neville Clarke who has some pertinent information and let him take it at this time. Dr. Clarke ....

DR. NEVILLE CLARKE (Texas A&M): Thank you, Dr. Boyd. I'm not sure it's informative or pertinent, but I'd like to try to bridge the gap. I admit to being party to helping with the formulation of these questions. As we get to this stage of our discussion and particularly as a result of discussing how we are doing and where we are going with our overall orientation with some of the producers in our state, it seems to me that we sit now at a position where we are finishing up our discussion of the management aspects of dealing with brucellosis in an individual herd. Tomorrow morning we are going to get into a situation where we are talking about the national programs of the various countries and we will be talking at a very broad level or national level about these kind of programs. The sort of hiatus that I believe we may have inadvertently left in our thinking here, which I would like to try to lay on now and ask a few questions about, is that situation that exists between the management of the individual herd and the overall national program. Let us come back and see if there are some more general concepts that we might explore, perhaps pretty much in summary, considering that we have pretty well discussed all of the aspects of diagnosis, immunization, epidemiology and management and prevention and see if we can bridge this gap. Perhaps if I tell you a little more specifically what I'm talking about it will make better sense. I would like to start by saying that I'm not trying to get into the mechanics of the regulatory program nor am I trying to address the question which has been asked of eradication versus control. I am, as I mentioned to our speakers the other night, hoping to reflect some of the concerns that we have across an extremely diverse group of producers. We run all the way from a group of dairymen who have been operating pretty much as you have heard about dairymen operating in Wisconsin and other countries, through registered and commercial beef breeders who have good fences and open pastures, down to the small time or part time rancher and farmer in the northeast part of our state who may do a lot of his cattle tending on the weekends, to the large operations in the brush country in south Texas. Some of these areas you have heard discussed during the last couple of days from a standpoint of economics, and logistics are having difficulty, at least in their own view, at this stage of the game, in making this a workable situation. Scientifically sound, economically feasible, and logistically feasible are three aspects of the program. The last two that I have mentioned seem to me to fit into the management arena and perhaps might be discussed a little bit more. I personally am very much encouraged over some of the conclusions that have already come in the form of a consensus from the discussions that have gone on here in the last two days. The use of supplemental tests on a routine basis have been endorsed by almost all of the speakers that we have heard talk here. We have talked about the need for improved epidemiology on a systematic basis. The resources that are required to do this are considerable. If there are to be programs actively engaged in with the endorsement and support of our industry in Texas, it is clear that it is going to take additional resources, sponsored from either federal or state levels, to support this with adequate and improved staffing to do a better job of epidemiology in the field. We have talked about a number of opportunities for improved program management here today, all of which are feasible within the bounds of the present federal program. We have also talked several times over the last day or two about trying to design a program that would build into it those features which would allow the producers in our state to be able to get behind the program. As Dr. Becton from U.S.D.A. has said, and as each one of the major organization officers from our producer groups have said, that's the keystone in getting something going that people can live with. Well, all of those things to me can be at least improved if not significantly improved using some of the precepts and some of the management concepts that we have developed here in the last day or two.

Some of the things that are not so easily agreed to and which I hope perhaps the panel could help us with by some additional insights and comments would be some of the other possible management alternatives that we would have, on an interim basis, to address some of the problems that we see here in Texas. One of the most significant things that would be of help to us in getting at this would be to discuss the fairly consistent opinion that we have heard expressed from the speakers that it is now feasible to use serologic testing to distinguish between the vaccinate and the infected animal. If this, in fact, can be done on a practical, economical basis at this stage of the game, then it seems to me that we opened up the question: *Is it feasible to use one of the two major adult vaccination programs that we talked about, and still fall essentially within the testing and slaughter program, but at the same time provide improved protection during the time that this program is going on?*

The second major question which is extremely controversial is the one which I think perhaps our European and Australian visitors can help us with. In most of the programs that we have heard discussed, we have talked about an ultimate goal of eradication. We have talked about an ultimate program of test and slaughter but in most of these cases we initiated those programs in other countries with situations that allow one to get ready for a test and slaughter program. The question that remains in my mind at least is: *Are there situations that remain in our state now where something short or a test and slaughter program as an interim measure would be a profitable and feasible way for us to be moving?* The kind of a specific question I believe comes to mind is: *What percent of reactors should you have in a herd before you transition from some kind of a vaccination program without test and slaughter into the test and slaughter program?*

As far as eradication and control is concerned, as many of the speakers have said, we perhaps know enough to proceed with an eradication program now. However, I feel that the question our producer groups are asking is: Can we afford to do it and if not are there other ways that we can do it and still attain the same goal? Perhaps our speakers can help us get at these.

DR. CLARKE: Would it be appropriate to ask our speakers: What would you define as the situation which would justify the vaccination of adult animals in advance of a test and slaughter program?

DR. MORGAN: We have a dual thing going on; one is a voluntary eradication scheme, and the second one is a compulsory area eradication scheme. There are certain parts in Britain where the population of cattle is very high, that is, very densely populated areas, with a high prevalence of infection. These would naturally be the last areas that we would entertain as being compulsory eradication areas. The area that suffered quite badly from the foot and mouth epidemic in 1967-68 where there was a lot of slaughter of animals is one of these areas. This came just a little bit too early in a way, because our voluntary scheme had not gone on long enough to have known negative replacement animals to repopulate this area. They have been buying animals and, as you would expect, the level of infection due to *Brucella* is still very high in this area. There has been a clamor for us, the government and the veterinary profession, to do something or another to help. At that time, of course, we had two things available anyway; one was the strain 19 calfhood vaccine and the other was 45/20 vaccine. What we have decided to do in this area is to encourage the use of strain 19 vaccine in calfhood and at the same time to allow the use of 45/20 vaccine in these areas as well. This is being provided free by the government, but there are restrictions. Before the vaccine is allowed to be used we insist that a herd blood test be done. It is quite amazing that one of the spin-offs from this is the number of herds in this area with a high total prevalence of infection that are in effect Brucella-free. Secondly, if there is evidence of infection, we then allow the use of the vaccine under controlled conditions and we stipulate that there must be two doses of strain 45/20 vaccine given within the period of six weeks, followed by annual vaccination and they must promise to do this for a period of three years. Now, if you ask me back in four years time, I should be able to tell you whether this has really worked, or whether it hasn't worked. But we do have evidence in Britain that given this kind of situation where there is a high level of infection in infected herds, that the use of the vaccine as part, and only as part, of the overall approach to the control of the disease can be quite effective. We find that as long as we stipulate how the vaccine should be used and that there must be prevaccination herd blood tests done, this gets the farmer and the veterinary surgeon thinking in terms of controlling the disease. If you go in there blindly and only use the vaccine, they will use it for awhile, then animals will be missed, and the repeat vaccinations won't be done. This is not as effective as a controlled voluntary program for the use of 45/20. We have very strict regulations governing the movement of animals into the eradication areas, and, therefore, animals from these high prevalence areas would not be allowed to be moved in. We would allow movement of animals into the clean areas only from other clean areas and we do have very rigid control over movement of animals in Britain because of the danger of introduction of disease. This has been a most invaluable tool in tracing origin of infection, thinking particularly of foot and mouth disease.

DR. RAY: I would like to make a comment. Dr. Clarke, in your question you asked what should be done before the test and slaughter program. I think it's important to review the status of Texas since that is what we are talking about. I would certainly second Mr. Moore's comment about the evidence of progress that has been made in this state. He pointed out that in his county, that the infection rate has dropped from ten percent to five percent, and out of the 254 counties in Texas, 75 percent of the infected herds were found in 86 of these counties. On the first area test of those 86 counties which occurred over the period 1958 to 1973, approximately 21,000 infected herds were identified. In April of this year in those same 86 counties there was a 90 percent reduction in the number of infected herds; it was now down to 2,000 infected herds. That population still constituted approximately 75 or 80 percent of the total infected herds in the state. So there has been a great deal of progress that has been achieved in Texas from what it was 15 to 20 years ago. I don't think we are just embarking on a test and slaughter program, we are just embarking on a new program.

DR. CLARKE: Thanks very much for the statistics and I understand your point. I guess my question really was not very precisely stated and would you address the question a little differently then. Are there individual herds or individual counties within this situation that we have in Texas that you would see being worked with any differently than with the standard program?

DR. RAY: Well, I think the question of adult vaccination and whether we should use it or not use it is a little premature at this point. We are trying to assess strain 19 in adult cattle and after we use strain 19, can we resume a test and slaughter program to eradicate the disease in those particular herds? We are also doing the same thing with 45/20 to see how it would fit into the program and what kind of complications we might experience if we did it on a wide scale. We have not finished our evaluation of these products in that particular context, and I think that until we have that kind of information it is a little too early to say that it would be a good thing to move into or not to move into.

NATIONAL PROGRAMS

Moderator: Archie I. Flowers

The National Brucellosis Programme of Australia

Godfrey Alton

The Commonwealth of Australia (Figure 1) is divided into

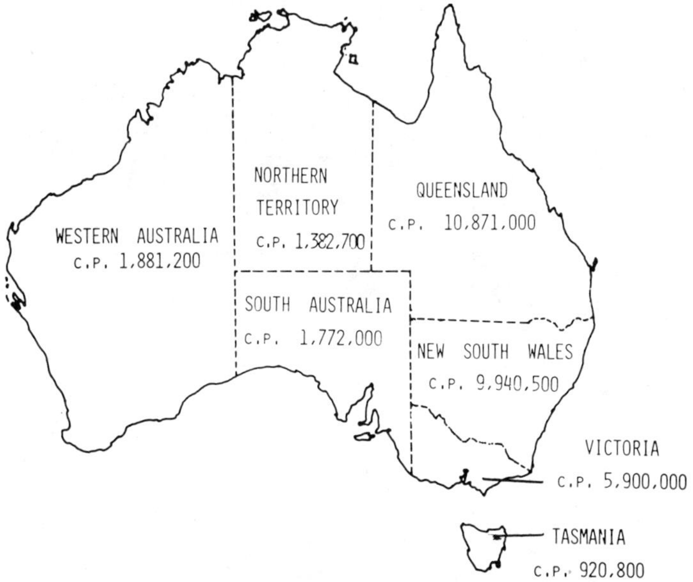

Figure 1. Australian States and Cattle Population (c.p.)

six states plus the Northern Territory. The central government is often called the commonwealth government and is situated in Canberra in a small area called the Australian Capital Territory. The organisation I work for is the Commonwealth Scientific and Industrial Research Organisation (CSIRO). The autonomy of the states and territories in national disease campaigns is less than that experienced in the United States. The Australian states are responsible for the day-to-day organisation of the campaigns, but policy and co-ordination is achieved through the Animal Health Committee which is made up of the Chief Veterinary Officers from each state, and representatives from the Australian Bureau of Animal Health and the CSIRO. The national brucellosis program is a joint Commonwealth and State Government venture with the commonwealth government providing at present about 70 percent of the finances for the campaign.

Figure 2 indicates the distribution of dairy cattle. The

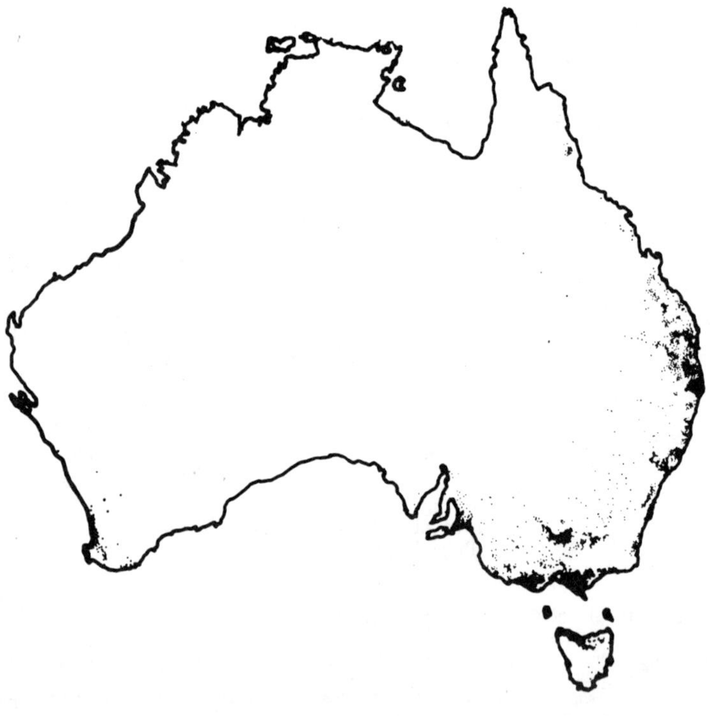

Figure 2. The Distribution of Dairy Cattle in Australia. Each dot represents approximately 5,000 animals.

dairy cattle are primarily concentrated in the eastern states not far from the coasts. The beef cattle (Figure 3), on the

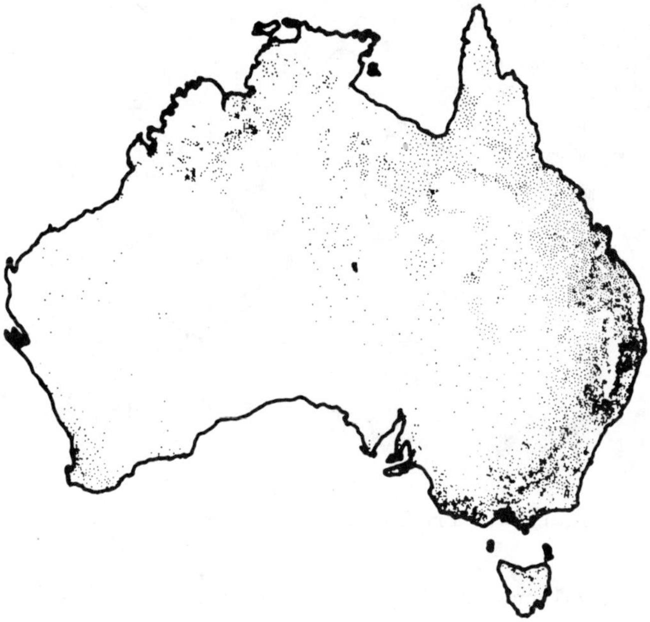

Figure 3. The Distribution of Beef Cattle in Australia. Each dot represents approximately 5,000 animals.

other hand, are more widely distributed and in many areas the density of cattle is very low, often about four animals per square mile. Conditions in some of these areas are such that eradication of diseases is very difficult. Figure 4 indicates the approximate prevalence of brucellosis in the different areas.

Tasmania began trying to eradicate brucellosis as long ago as 1930 when a voluntary scheme was launched which aimed at the establishment of accredited brucellosis free herds. This scheme had some success but was completely disrupted by World War II. After the war, strain 19 vaccination was introduced into areas

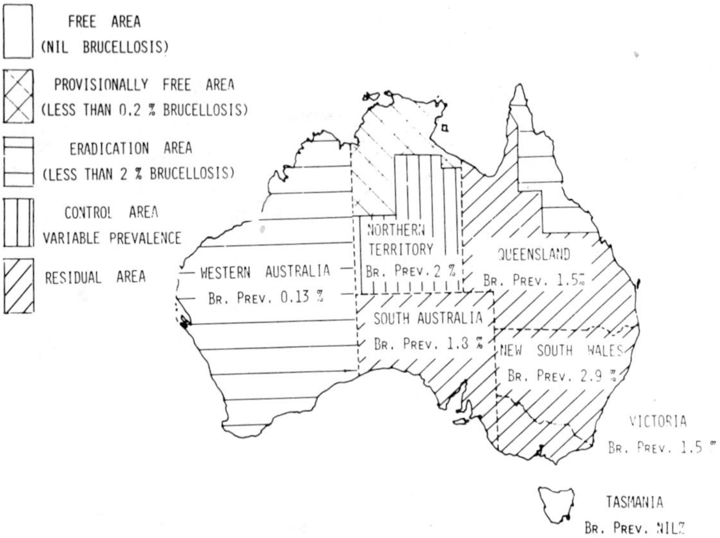

Figure 4. Prevalence of Bovine Brucellosis

of high prevalence and in one such area the prevalence fell from 13 percent to 2.6 percent over a period of 14 years. In the post war years eradication by test and slaughter was re-introduced using conventional methods. This process was gradually successful and Tasmania is now brucellosis-free. Strain 45/20 vaccine was used in the terminal stages as an anamnestic test and, in the opinion of the field staff, it appeared to be beneficial although detailed statistics are not available.

In Western Australia strain 19 vaccination was introduced in 1946. Eradication, however, did not begin until 1970 when a monitoring system was introduced and test slaughter begun in known infected herds. Strain 45/20 vaccination was introduced in 1968 and a few years later the use of strain 19 was prohibited. The prevalence of brucellosis in Western Australia is now estimated at 0.15 percent in breeding cattle. The remaining infected herds are concentrated in the southern part of the state. The northern beef-producing areas are judged to be brucellosis-free and perhaps always have been.

In the Northern Territory a survey carried out in 1969-70 indicated an overall prevalence of about two percent. The "top end", i.e. the northern third of the state, was found to be almost free and has since qualified as a provisionally-free area. There are about 100,000 feral buffaloes in this area that appear to have escaped infection altogether. The incidence further south is higher, especially on the Barkley tableland which is the principal cattle-breeding area in the territory. In the areas not designated provisionally-free, known infected herds are subjected either to 45/20 vaccination or to test and slaughter or both. In these areas, the regular mustering of cattle is sometimes difficult and at other times impossible. The search for alternative methods of eradication has already been described (see Slatter - Experiences with Brucellosis Under Range Conditions in Australia - this symposium).

In the other states (Queensland, South Australia, New South Wales and Victoria) the incidence of brucellosis is somewhat higher. Until recently, control has been mostly calfhood vaccination with strain 19.

A national program aimed at reducing the prevalence of brucellosis has been in operation since 1966. The prevalence of brucellosis has been reduced to such a degree that all states and territories can now embark upon and continue with the final phase of eradication by test and slaughter.

The Commonwealth Government has recently agreed to continue its funding of the campaign for an additional eight years, provided the states agree to embark upon eradication plans which will result in Australia achieving provisional freedom from brucellosis within the eight year period. The Commonwealth

Government has also agreed to provide funds to compensate owners for the slaughter of reacting cattle. The Commonwealth Government will provide 75 percent of compensation costs in the states and 100 percent in the territories, beginning in 1976-77.

The Animal Health Committee has published a document called Standard Definitions and Rules, which is very similar in intent to the USDA's Recommended Uniform Methods and Rules. These are minimum standards and the states are free to adopt more rigorous methods. The standard definitions and rules cover, amongst other things, monitoring systems for the detection of infected herds, methods of testing infected herds, definition of areas in the process of eradicating brucellosis, movements of animals, and standard methods for diagnostic tests.

When areas are taken into the eradication scheme they become declared areas as opposed to residual areas where eradication has not yet started. There are four different classes of declared areas, leading by stages to a brucellosis-free area. There must be a monitoring system in operation in all the different categories of declared areas consisting of at least periodic milk ring tests for dairy herds and abattoir trace backs for beef herds. Briefly the requirements for the different classes of declared areas are:

1. The Control Area status requires that all infected herds be placed in quarantine and all confirmed reactors be identified. Compulsory vaccination may be in force.
2. An Eradication Area must be so declared by the Brucellosis Sub-Committee as do the areas yet to be described. The prevalence of the disease as disclosed by monitoring must be not more than 2 percent. All infected herds are placed in quarantine and tested regularly. If subsequent testing of individual herds shows active infection, further testing may be postponed pending the use of vaccination; otherwise all

reactors are identified and sent for immediate slaughter. Vaccination may continue at the Chief Veterinary Officer's discretion.

3. A provisionally-free Area requires that the prevalence (number of reactors as a percentage of the breeding animals in the area) must not exceed 0.2 percent. All infected herds are placed in quarantine and testing started. All reactors are identified and slaughtered. Vaccination is prohibited except in special circumstances. All herds must be tested before the area qualifies.

4. A Free Area is one in which all herds have been tested, and in which there is no evidence of the disease. Herds that have shown evidence of the disease within the previous five years must have a negative test within the year prior to the declaration. Abortion investigations are carried out in areas 2, 3, and 4 above.

Detailed techniques for the performance of diagnostic tests are kept up to date by a working party of laboratory officers which meet once a year. This party consists of one or more representatives from each principal state veterinary laboratory, along with representatives from the central government and the CSIRO. The research organization (CSIRO) is in contact with the other interested parties at all stages of the organization of the campaign.

The tests used for monitoring infection are the milk ring test (MRT) and the buffered brucella antigen or Rose Bengal test (BRT). The MRT is carried out on all milk and cream received from producers. The samples are taken from the holding tank on the farm and are tested at the dairy. Because large dairy herds are uncommon, the problem of excessive dilution of the milk sample seldom occurs. Samples of blood are taken at abattoirs and are subjected to a RBT and positive samples are re-tested by the complement fixation test (CFT).

For eradication testing in infected herds, all breeding cattle over six months of age are required to be tested at intervals of 30 to 60 days until a clean test is obtained, after which the intervals between tests are lengthened. The blood samples are first subjected to a screening test (RBT) which is always done in the laboratory. The technique of the RBT as used in Australia has already been described in a previous paper (Alton 1977 - Development and Evaluation of Serologic Test to Detect Brucellosis - this symposium).

Blood samples positive to the RBT are re-tested by the CFT which is considered to be the definitive test. It is believed that the CFT is the most accurate test available for the diagnosis of bovine brucellosis. We fail to isolate *Brucella abortus* from a substantial proportion of CFT reactors. In order to detect the vast majority of infected animals it is necessary to use a testing procedure that will give a substantial number of false-positive reactions. We believe that the RBT gives very few false-negative reactions.

The CFT technique that is standard for Australia is a micro-system that can be completely automated. The details have already been given in a previous paper (Alton 1977). Almost all the state veterinary laboratories have fully automatic equipment for performing this type of CFT.

Before the agreed standard diagnostic tests were introduced, a workshop was organized and attended by laboratory personnel from each state to familiarize everyone with the technique of the micro-CFT and with the operation, care and maintenance of the machinery available for automating the work. Serum samples are distributed to the state laboratories at frequent intervals to check on the sensitivity of the diagnostic tests.

Standard techniques have been worked out for a number of other diagnostic tests that may be useful in special circumstances such as the serum agglutination test and the anti-bovine globulin test. A micro-technique has been worked out for this latter test for use in the micro-titer system which allows more tests to be carried out per operator than the standard technique. The anti-bovine globulin test is a very sensitive procedure but we do not yet know how to interpret the results. We feel that we may need to establish a second testing regime for problem herds, i.e. those that do not soon become brucellosis free on routine testing. The Attwood laboratory, which is a Victoria (State) diagnostic laboratory, has developed a radio-immuno-assay method that may be useful despite its complexity, need for radio-active isotopes and a scintilation counter.

The handling of data is a very important part of any disease eradication program and we are fortunate in Australia in having the help of the Veterinary Epidemiology and Preventive Medicine (VEPM) Unit at the University of Melbourne. Drs. Morris and Roe of this unit have established a detailed program for an Australian Brucellosis and Tuberculosis Information System. They have produced three reports setting out proposals in some detail for the Australian Bureau of Animal Health. There are some alternatives proposed but what is likely to be adopted is something like the following. Each diagnostic laboratory will have a mini-computer and there will also be a larger central computer in Canberra. There will be eighteen testing laboratories throughout Australia and information will be transmitted on flexible discs to Canberra and "the machine."

The computer at the laboratory will handle such information as vaccination records, records of milk ring tests, and abattoir traceback results. The computer will also handle the results of diagnostic tests carried out in the laboratory. The District Veterinary Officer (DVO) will receive the results in the form of a computer print-out and in this way we hope to decrease the time that elapses between bleeding cattle and slaughtering reactors. The computer will provide an efficient filing system for the DVO, keep current the records of the state of progress in each herd, and assist in program planning.

Records of sequential test results on individual cattle will be kept for approximately 2-3 percent of the herds and these results will be used to evaluate the effectiveness of the various procedures being used. The VEPM Unit already has a disease model for brucellosis epidemiology with which they are able to project into the future and thereby make predictions about the likely effect of various alternative courses of action. Personnel operating this model are, however, conscious of the fact that the accuracy of the predictions is dependent on the accuracy and relevance of the information that goes into the computer. Obviously as the campaign proceeds and more data relevant to different conditions becomes available, the accuracy of the predictions will improve. Use of the model has already allowed some interesting predictions to be made, such as:

1. The premature cessation of vaccination will be epidemiologically dangerous;
2. A small increase in the efficiency of the diagnostic tests used is likely to increase the efficiency of the process of eradication; and
3. A certain tempo of testing needs to be maintained to prevent the eradication program from becoming static at a certain low level of prevalence.

Summary

The national program to eradicate brucellosis from Australia commenced in 1966. One Australian state is now brucellosis-free and another almost brucellosis-free. Test and slaughter, the final phase in the eradication program, is about to begin throughout Australia. A target date of 1984 has been set for the whole of Australia to achieve provisional freedom from brucellosis (0.2 percent prevalence).

References

Alton, G. G. 1977. Development and Evaluation of Serologic Tests to Detect Brucellosis. International Symposium on Bovine Brucellosis. Texas A&M Press, Diagnosis Section.

Slatter, W. 1977. Experiences with Brucellosis Under Range Conditions in Australia. ibid. Management and Prevention Section.

The National Brucellosis Program of France

Michel Plommet

Even though it is an unpleasant fact, the French must admit that in France the control of bovine brucellosis is a failure. There are 970,000 cattle herds in France and in 1974, 345,000 (35 percent of total) were examined for brucellosis; 258,000 (75 percent of those examined) were found to be free of brucellosis. We, therefore, estimate that 25 percent of the herds are infected. The prevalence, by herd, varies considerably from one region to another. By department (a department corresponds to a large county and there are 100 in France), the prevalence rate ranges from five percent in Britanny to 75 percent in Normandy. As a comparison, Denmark successfully eradicated brucellosis in 1957.

In 1966, the first national program was started in France. It was improved in 1973. The program was successful in some departments, particularly in Britanny. However, failures, i.e. no improvement, were noted in other areas, especially those departments in central France and above all in Normandy.

In France there are 17 million adult cows on 973,000 farms - 13 million used for milk production and 4 million beef cattle (primarily Charolais breed). The average herd, therefore, has a mean of 18 cows. The average size of herds managed by individuals who depend on cattle as their sole source of income is higher and is increasing fast. The average is anticipated to reach from 40 to 50 cows in 1985. However, in some regions there are many small herds (one to two cows) belonging to factory workers, and prophylaxis represents a particular and difficult problem in these areas.

Dairy cattle are concentrated mainly in the western (Britanny, Normandy, Charentes) and eastern parts of France (Lorraine, Franche Comté, Savoie). Beef cattle are located principally in the central (Auvergne, Limousin) and southwestern departments (Aquitaine).

The Ministry of Agriculture is charged with the responsibility for the control of animal diseases through the Veterinary Service, which includes civil servants working either in the central services of the Ministry of Paris or in the departments where a director is responsible for prophylaxis. In each department there is a Diagnostic Laboratory that also has responsibility for control of vaccines and antigens.

The Veterinary Service is normally represented by veterinary surgeons in private practice and they are remunerated for these professional services by the government. Because many veterinary surgeons are not interested in the prophylaxis of brucellosis, there is presently a tendency toward the use of government personnel to provide these services to the farmer. Milk ring tests are carried out by different laboratories (agricultural and dairy organizations) in charge of milk analysis and the results are transmitted to Veterinary Service.

Veterinary research is mainly carried out by the National Institute for Research in Agriculture (I.N.R.A.) which is supported by the Ministry of Agriculture. Research is also conducted by the Diagnostic Laboratories of the Veterinary Service and in the Schools of Veterinary Medicine.

Prophylaxis programs are formulated by the responsible members of the Veterinary Service after consultation with expert committees. The committees include specialists from the I.N.R.A., from medical research groups, from educational establishments, and from the Veterinary Service plus representatives of breeder organizations. The expert consultation system is not entirely satisfactory because the technical aspects of a program are not separated from the political aspects. Rather than recommending correct technical solutions, these committees usually serve as mechanisms to achieve political compromises.

The 1966 Program

The French control program against brucellosis consists of two parts, each of which is inspired by a different philosophy. These two parts, sanitary police and collective prophylaxis, were completely separated in the 1966 program but were combined to some extent in 1973.

The first part, or Sanitary Police, is inspired by the traditional prophylaxis against the important communicable diseases and consists of the isolation and destruction of the infected foci. The defensive measures of the Sanitary Police are imposed by law. The starting point is the statement of abortion by the farmer and the veterinary surgeon. If the abortion is recognized as due to Brucella: 1. the farm is put under quarantine and 2. the cow in question has to be killed within 30 days. The quarantine prohibits the selling of animals except for slaughtering. The quarantine will be cancelled after the appropriate measures imposed by law (slaughtering of positive animals or vaccination of all the animals) have been applied.

The measures of Sanitary Police impose very heavy constraints that the farmer generally tries to avoid by not reporting abortions. These measures are, at this time, without any real efficiency. The prescribed measures for the cancellation of the quarantine are merely administrative and, therefore, the herd is not free with any degree of certainty from brucellosis.

The second part of the program or Collective Prophylaxis aims at the progressive reduction of infection foci. The 1966 program was deeply influenced by the success of the anti-tuberculosis program. It appeared to be possible to transpose a test and slaughter policy of cattle by replacing tuberculin sensitization with seroagglutination tests. In order to avoid vaccinal interferences with the diagnosis, vaccination was discouraged.

The main points of the 1966 program were as follows (Figure 1):

1. Diagnosis of brucellosis by seroagglutination - blood samples were collected twice a year from all adult cows. If all were negative the herd was declared brucellosis-free.
2. In herds not considered as free, different policies were applied depending upon:
   a. infection rate;
   b. the obligation of the farmer to adhere to the regional program;
   c. the decision made by the farmer and the veterinary surgeon to conduct a policy of total slaughter, partial slaughter, or no slaughter but systematic vaccination during several years.
3. An attempt to educate individuals to insist on blood sampling and purchase only animals negative to brucellosis tests.

This program included many serious errors clearly visible to specialists but not to those charged with its application.

1. The facts were ignored that brucellosis is a disease that does not always cause abortion and sometimes has long periods of latency. Therefore, diagnosis on an individual basis has only limited value to the herd.

	1966	1973
Diagnosis		
Milk Ring Test	..	Once per month
Serum agglutination test - twice per year	30 I.U.	80 I.U. 30 to 80 → CF or RBP*
Bacteriology after abortion	Stamp **	Stamp and culture (placenta and milk)
Vaccination		
Strain 19 and 45/20	Free but discouraged	Compulsory - heifers; also H 38 vaccine
Removal of Cows to Slaughter	Brucella abortion; Positive serum agglutination if registered;	Brucella abortion; Positive serum agglutination if registered in some areas, all cows in other areas;
Education	Purchase of replacements Declaration of abortion Necessity of blood sampling	

*Serums with 30 to 80 I.U. of agglutination are tested by supplemental tests; CF = Complement Fixation; RBP = Rose Bengal Plate (Card)

**Stamp = Microscopic examination of placental cotyledons after staining

Figure 1. Comparison of Brucellosis Control Programs in France

The insistence on blood sampling of individual cattle made farmers believe the serologic tests were good guarantees.

2. The lack of epidemiologic surveys to locate free herds that could be used as a source of replacement stock for herds after elimination of infected animals made restocking very uncertain.
3. The lack of a coherent vaccination policy led to confusion and many farmers stopped vaccinating. Therefore, the disease reappeared in areas where it had previously disappeared.
4. The education of farmers concerning the communicability of the disease and the measures to eliminate it did not take place. In fact, the insistance on government indemnity for the slaughter of infected cows made many farmers believe that brucellosis was a natural plague that cannot be avoided and that the government has to pay for the resulting prejudice.
5. The methods of diagnosis, including serologic agglutination tests and identification of Brucella by microscopy alone, were not precise enough.
6. Too many vaccines were authorised. The efficiency of each vaccine was not always proved and insufficient quality control of successive batches of proved vaccines was exercised.

The 1973 Program

The 1973 program was proposed to correct the main mistakes. Nevertheless, the program is still insufficient - in particular as far as the education of farmers and its method of application are concerned. The main points of the program are as follows:

1. Bulk-milk ring tests are conducted one a month. This measure makes up for the errors of sampling individual cows and, therefore, diagnosis is based on the herd results. The identification of free herds becomes automatic.
2. Compulsory vaccination of heifers except in areas with a low rate of infection. The vaccine is supplied free of charge.
3. Education of farmers is improved. The transmission processes has begun to be better known. However, there still remains a lot to do in order to make up for former errors.
4. The program is applied to the whole country.
5. Methods of diagnosis have been improved; agglutination is no longer the only test applied; and identification of Brucella by culture procedures is spreading.
6. The number of authorized vaccines has been reduced to those that have proved effective in a test carried out

The following points are considered deficiencies in the program:

1. Only 50 percent of the heifers have been vaccinated in 1975. It is difficult to transition from a policy of discouraging vaccination to one of mandatory vaccination. This transition is made even more difficult because certain persons in the Veterinary Service are not convinced themselves of the good reason for such a change. The limit concerning the infection rate under which vaccination is no longer compulsory is too high. It varies with the regions, but is around five percent. One percent would be more realistic. Therefore, new outbreaks of disease are quite frequent.

2. Authorized vaccines belong to the following three types (Figure 2):

HEIFERS (COMPULSORY) — Strain 19 or 45/20 or H 38
↓
(2 INJECTIONS 2-3 MONTHS APART)

COWS — 45/20 | H 38 (Infected Herd)

PRIMARY	RECALL	PRIMARY
↓	↓	↓
2 INJECTIONS	1 INJECTION AFTER PRIMARY (Strain 19, 45/20 or H 38)	2 INJECTIONS

Figure 2. Brucellosis Vaccination Program in France - 1973

Living vaccine - strain 19; killed vaccine composed of bacteria in smooth phase - H 38; killed vaccines, bacteria in rough phase - 45/20. The decision on the type of vaccine and the method of administration is made by the veterinary surgeon. For each of the three types, there are several different commercial brands, and, therefore, slight differences. The quality control of successive lots of vaccine is quite difficult and expensive. The number of authorised vaccines should be reduced in order to carry out a better control of each lot. This may be easy, since the vaccines are purchased by the government.

3. Very often the milk ring tests results are badly employed; correct results are not reported; communication of the results to the farmers is delayed and the study of regional epidemiology from the data of the ring test is not performed.

4. Prophylaxis is compulsory, but the program is not always followed exactly. Some veterinary surgeons, thinking that they are no longer involved and needed, have lost interest in the program.

The Future

The stated deficiencies will have to be corrected in order to get satisfactory results. Probably in less heavily infected regions, eradication will be attained within five years. Yet, in the more heavily infected regions, Normandy for instance, where the cattle density is very high, or in the mountain regions of central France, where the beef cattle are half wild, considerable effort will have to be expended for many years in order to achieve eradication. Maybe not before the year 2000.

As I see it (which is not the viewpoint of the responsible members of the Veterinary Service) we should principally back up the prophylaxis by well performed generalised vaccination, and focus on the education of farmers rather than the measures of administrative coercion and slaughter. These test and slaughter measures are quite expensive, not well accepted by the farmer, and terribly discouraging because apparently they never end.

Conjunctival vaccination with live strain 19 gives, according to our experiments (Plommet and Fensterbank 1976), the following results:

1. A short lived serological response in both adults and calves.
2. A clearly better protection than that afforded by vaccination by the subcutaneous route because a second inoculation is possible six months later.

In addition, this vaccination method is economical because, being performed within a wide range of age (4-10 months and

10-16 months), it requires only two visits by the veterinary surgeon per year. It seems to me that such a vaccination would be a very effective means in heavily infected areas. It would be possible to erase many of the years previously forecast to achieve eradication of brucellosis in France.

The diagnosis by blood sampling remains a dangerous operation that farmers and veterinary surgeons in beef cattle areas refuse to perform twice a year. Following the work carried out in California by Dr. Elberg and his team, and by Dr. Lois Jones at Wisconsin, our laboratory at Nouzilly has experimented with the protein antigen (Brucellin) and its product - delayed hypersensitivity. Dr. Fensterbank has studied the use of this test for the diagnosis of bovine brucellosis. The results are quite encouraging and new experiments are being carried out. I think that before long it will be possible to use the skin test for the diagnosis of *Brucella* infection which will make prophylaxis easier and more efficient.

References

Dhennin, L. 1973. Résultat de l'étude comparée de sept vaccins antibrucelliques. Bull. Acad. Vétér. 46:171-190.

Plommet, M., and Fensterbank, R. 1976. Vaccination against bovine brucellosis with a low dose of strain 19 administered by the conjunctival route: III, Serological response and immunity in the pregnant cow. Ann. Rec. Vétér. 7 (to be published).

The National Brucellosis Programme of the Republic of Ireland

Brendan Cunningham

In the Republic of Ireland there are some seven million cattle kept in 200,000 herds. For the purposes of brucellosis eradication some three million are defined as "eligible" animals, viz. females over twelve months of age and bulls over nine months of age.

Following the Attestation of the State under the Bovine Tuberculosis Eradication Programme in 1965, brucellosis received priority on the Animal Health Programme. A country-wide survey was carried out in 1964 using the milk ring test (MRT) on churn samples of milk from some 102,000 herds - 85 percent passed the test, twelve percent failed and three percent were suspect.

There are 26 counties in the State and these form administrative areas in which the progressive Area-Eradication of Tuberculosis had been carried out. There were 18 District Veterinary Offices administering the program in 26 counties and it was decided to pursue the eradication of brucellosis also on a progressive (County) area-eradication plan.

The results of the 1964 MRT survey indicated that herd-prevalence in the Northwest counties was as low as 1.5 percent and gradually increased to some 45 percent of herds in the worst of the Southern counties. The Southern counties are engaged almost entirely in intensive dairying; in the West many young store cattle are reared and in the Midlands and East of the country the cattle are finished for slaughter. Thus, there is a lot of movement of cattle.

Eradication commenced in 1966 in five Northern and Western counties. The first county was pronounced Accredited Brucellosis-Free in 1968. With the progress of time more counties were brought into the Clearance Area. At the present time six counties are Accredited Brucellosis-Free; seven are in the Clearance Area and are almost ready for certification and the other 13 counties are taking part in a Pre-Intensive Control programme.

Each herd has an official herd number. Each animal must be officially recorded and identified as soon as practicable after birth by:

1. An official "tamperproof" steel ear tag carrying a county letter and individual number - placed in the left ear, and;
2. An identity card carring its tag number, breed and colour, sex, age, the herd number, and dates of vaccinations, and tuberculosis (TB) and brucellosis tests. The entries are signed by the veterinarians certifying them.

If a TB reactor occurs in a herd all cards are withdrawn until the herd is cleared. Similarly, in a Clearance or Accredited Area, they are withdrawn if a brucellosis reactor occurs. The colour of the card indicates the status of the herd of origin of the animal, e.g.

1. Blue - Free of tuberculosis; No brucellosis status; All steers have blue cards.
2. Yellow - Brucellosis Clearance Area - herd clear on last test.
3. Pink - Accredited Brucellosis Free Area - at least three clear tests.

No bovine animal may be offered for sale without its identity card and test certification must be "in date".

Legislation

Orders are made as required under provisions of the Diseases of Animals Act 1966 (A consolidation of relevant acts from about 1874). Such orders regulate Declaration of Clearance Areas, Movement Controls, Control of Vaccination, General Provisions, Declaration of Brucellosis Disease-Free Areas, etc.

Diagnostic Tests

The basic test is the Serum Agglutination Test (SAT); < 30 international units (i.u.) is negative; 30 to < 60 i.u. is inconclusive and ≥ 60 i.u. is positive. Serum from animals in the inconclusive category are subjected to the Complement Fixation Test (CFT) and classified as negative if < 20 European Economic Community (E.E.C.) units or positive if ≥ 20 E.E.C. units. Antigens are prepared from *Brucella abortus* strain 99. No vaccinal tolerances are allowed in either the CFT or SAT.

The Milk Ring Test antigen contains 4 percent by volume of packed cells stained by haematoxylin and is adjusted to World Health Organization (WHO) standards. The test is carried out on one ml samples of fresh milk at 37.5°C for one hour. For churn or bulk samples interpretations are either negative (- ; +) or positive (++ ; +++; ++++). When carried out on individual animals the milk under test is diluted ten-fold with negative milk before testing.

Eradication Procedures

General permission for vaccination is withdrawn 12 months before test and slaughter commences. Limited use of vaccine may then be made only by official Veterinary Inspectors in approved circumstances. Each eligible animal in a Clearance and Accredited Area is blood tested annually. The completed operation being termed a "round" of testing.

Reactors are branded, valued at market value, purchased by and removed by the Department of Agriculture for slaughter. The herd is "locked-up", identity cards taken up and no eligible animals may be brought in or sold (except under special license to a slaughtering plant) until the herd reattains the status of the area. At this stage the identity cards are reissued.

Occasionally in some herds this process can take years; can result in gradual erosion of the productive herd to an uneconomic size and also can eradicate the farmers. We have seen many instances in which the number of reactors removed in a three year period has exceeded the number of eligible animals originally in the herd, and the disease was still present. The economic cost to the state has been such that it would have been more economical to put a State Veterinary Officer in residence on the farm with the sole duty to manage it - all that for a 150 cow herd! In more recent years we have very successfully used K45/20A vaccine as a diagnostic aid (using the anamnestic test). Whether the vaccine has any prophylactic effect is rather immaterial, because reinfection in herds treated in this way has been remarkable so far by its absence. In fact, many of us working in the field would now question the logic or economics of tackling any problem herd without the use of K45/20A vaccine.

The standard procedure in reactor herds is to retest at intervals of 60 days following removal of reactors and disinfection. Occasionally, if gross infection is present, one might slaughter out the entire productive herd, but we now tend to use vaccine wherever we judge that it will decrease losses of either stock or money. In one series of infected ("breakdown") herds in a clearance area it was shown that by using K45/20A vaccine one could spare 67 percent of the animals in herds that should otherwise have been slaughtered out (Cunningham and O'Connor 1971).

From ten years of close association with difficult eradication situations in the field I would say we have been conservative, possibly to a fault, in being slow to use K45/20A vaccine in circumstances where it could have been of great benefit. By this I am not advocating blanket vaccination, or even the liberal uncontrolled use of vaccine. In particular, when the vaccine in use is K45/20A vaccine one can selectively restrict its use to particular situations, such as in "problem" herds or large infected herds. There are no contraindications to its use in adult, pregnant or lactating females.

There are certain duties imposed upon owners. They are required: to keep accurate and complete herd records; to isolate reactors pending removal; to cleanse and disinfect contaminated areas and to notify the District Veterinary Officer of any abortions. Animals introduced into a herd in a Clearance Area must meet statutory requirements and be isolated from the herd for at least six weeks (dry stock), and in the case of pregnant females until they have passed blood tests three weeks after calving.

There are penalties for non-compliance or negligence (e.g. the owner may be excluded from benefits of other official programmes or may be required to slaughter animals at his own expense).

The Pre-Intensive Control Scheme

This programme was devised essentially to reduce the "pool of infection" in our intensive dairying areas where the prevalence of the disease was high.

It had been noted that strain 19 vaccine had been used

liberally in this area from 1950 to 1965. In spite of this, prevalence of brucellosis in the area, as a whole, remained at about 30 percent, although abortions were quite well controlled. Thus it appeared that vaccination on its own could be expected to control abortions but not to reduce the prevalence of brucellosis. K45/20A vaccine had been in widespread use in the area from 1965 to 1973 but its use allowed only the control of abortions and more or less enabled us to maintain the level of prevalence at 30 percent in spite of increasing herd sizes and increasing intensification.

Previous experience in one county had impressed upon us that it was most unwise to commence a test and slaughter policy in a dairying area with a disease prevalence of 30 percent. Briefly, it was a good way of eradicating farmers without having a worthwhile effect on the disease. Thus a programme had to be devised which would embrace the following parameters.

1. Require an improvement in hygienic management within herds. This was helped by framing a programme in which practicing veterinarians became involved as advisers to their farmer clients.
2. Require the vaccination of breeding cattle - particularly their home-reared heifer replacements. (A free vaccination service was provided).
3. Utilize a simple test which would not lead to overkilling - for this purpose the MRT was chosen. Underkilling was desirable in the early stages of control, and it was accepted that "as a rule, infected cattle which are not pregnant no longer transmit the disease, but that the principal danger lies in the infected pregnant animals" (Van den Born and Vervoorn 1965).
4. Provide an incentive to farmers to dispose of reactors as soon as it was economically feasible to do so.

Headage grants and a terminal cash bonus are provided.

5. The branding of reactors so that they could not be offered for sale on the open market. And
6. Establish a status of "MR-negative herd" which would facilitate the buying and selling of animals of a minimal status.

With these objects in mind the Pre-Intensive Control Programme was framed and rather than my attempting to paraphrase it I am attaching the official leaflet on the programme (See Addendum I).

References

Cunningham, B., and O'Connor, M. 1971 Vet. Rec. 89:680-686.

ADDENDUM I

PRE-INTENSIVE BRUCELLOSIS SCHEME

1. This Scheme is intended to help herdowners who wish to remove brucellosis reactors from their herds in advance of area eradication.

2. A herdowner interested in the Scheme should apply to his local District Veterinary Office (DVO) veterinary surgeon or creamery for an application form. If he wishes to participate in the Scheme he should send the application form duly completed to the DVO.

3. Herdowners participating in the Scheme must help reduce herd incidence of the disease by maintaining a system of good herd management and hygiene, including

(a) Isolating all females at calving or abortion while such animals show any uterine discharge.

(b) Isolating all reactors which are more than 5 months pregnant.

(c) Planning a phased removal of reactors.

(d) Purchasing only such animals as are indicated in paragraph 10.

(e) Disinfecting all isolation boxes, stalls, etc. where calving took place. Disinfection of all contaminated material and proper disposal of such materials.

(f) Calling in his Veterinary Surgeon immediately if an animal aborts.

(g) Availing of the free Breeding Heifer Vaccination Scheme.

4. (a) Where an approved bulk milk ring test proves positive the owner will arrange with his Veterinary Surgeon to Milk Ring Test individually all the lactating animals in his herd in order to identify the reactor animals. Samples should not however be taken.

(i) in the period of 7 days following calving

(ii) where there is obvious mastitis or

(iii) where a cow is producing less than one gallon of milk daily.

Tests may not be applied after 31 August in any year except with the specific agreement of the District Veterinary Office.

(b) If, however, the herdowner is supplying milk to a creamery with suitable laboratory facilities he may by arrangement with the creamery, submit individual samples, which must be taken from all lactating animals in his herd, with the exception of those specified at 4(a), for testing at the creamery under veterinary supervision. Any reactors to this test will require to be independently milk sampled and tested by a veterinary surgeon or at the creamery under veterinary supervision.

(c) If a herd has not been included in a Department's or Creamery's bulk Milk Ring Test the owner will arrange with his Veterinary Surgeon to bulk test and/or individually Milk Ring Test all the lactating animals in his herd.

(c) Where in any year a herdowner has additional animals for testing he must have each of the lactating cows in his herd individually milk-tested at least once in that year, at a stage when not less than 75% of the cows are in milk.

5. First individual reactor identification tests must normally be carried out when 75% of the cow herd is in lactation.

6. If in the case of a herd accepted for participation in the Scheme an animal aborts and appropriate documentary evidence of tests as required at (a) and (b) hereunder to indicate that the abortion was due to brucellosis is furnished to the DVO within 3 weeks of the abortion of the animal may qualify for a grant:

(a) in the case of an animal vaccinated (primary or booster) within the previous 12 months, the test of a blood sample in addition to material for smear or culture (e.g. foetus, placenta or milk) or

(b) in the case of an animal not so vaccinated the test of a blood sample or material for smear or culture as specified at 6(a).

7. The herdowner will allow any reactors in his herd to be punched by the Veterinary Surgeon who carried out the individual Milk Ring Test and will hand over to him for transmission to the DVO the relevant identity cards in respect of reactor animals. In the case of animals individually sampled by the herdowner the identity cards will be handed over when the suspected reactor animals are being milk sampled by the Veterinary Surgeon but punching will not be carried out until the reactor result is confirmed.

8. Reactors may be disposed of only to a registered Meat Plant and if more than five months pregnant must be isolated from the

rest of the herd pending removal. N.B. It is essential before any reactor is removed to a Meat Plant that the DVO be notified of the date of removal and the name of the Meat Plant concerned. The DVO will then issue a permit for the removal. Grants will only be paid in respect of reactors moved in accordance with such permit.

9. Milk Ring tests may be carried out as frequently as necessary for the purpose of identifying individual reactors. Animals already adjudged reactors may not be retested except in the circumstances set out at 4(b) or with the Department's permission. The qualifying tests for final payment (as indicated in para. 12) will normally be two consecutive clear herd tests carried out at an interval of not less than three months between the first and final tests; the first test being not earlier than 3 months from the date of the removal of the last individual reactor. Where the Department so requires it may specify more than two consecutive clear tests. At least 75% of the cow herd must be in lactation at each qualifying test.

10. Herdowners who join the Scheme may bring into the herd only such eligible animals as have either (i) come direct from a herd which has passed two successive Milk Ring Tests; (ii) come direct from a Brucellosis certified herd or a herd in the Brucellosis Free Area or from a clear herd in the Clearance Area; or (iii) have passed a brucellosis blood test or milk test within 14 days prior to entry. In the case of bulls only animals which comply with conditions at (ii) or (iii) may be brought into the herd.

Where animals are moved into a participating herd the owner shall within seven days of the movement, forward to the DVO one or other of the following documents:--
In the case of animals at (i) the form of WARRANTY.
In the case of animals at (ii) the relevant movement permit and
In the case of animals at (iii) the appropriate 14 day test certificate.

11. The fees for all tests other than those carried out by officers of the Department are payable by the herdowner.

12. Provision for grants payable in respect of reactors sent for slaughter under the Scheme:--

£40 per reactor at slaughter

and

(a) £20 per animal slaughtered if herd has had at least 2 consecutive clear tests as mentioned at paragraph 9 within 3 years of identification test

or

(b) £10 per animal slaughtered if herd has had at least 2 consecutive clear tests as mentioned at paragraph 9 within 4 years of identification test.

IT IS IMPORTANT TO NOTE THAT GRANTS ARE NOT PAYABLE TO HERDOWNERS WHO FAIL TO AVAIL OF THE DEPARTMENT'S FREE BREEDING HEIFER VACCINATION SCHEME OR WHO FAIL TO CONTINUE IN THAT SCHEME EACH YEAR IN RESPECT OF ELIGIBLE ANIMALS IN THEIR HERDS.

The scheme is for heifers 12 months and over. The first inoculation must be given while the animal is maiden and the second inoculation at an interval of not less than 6 weeks and not more than 12 weeks. Vaccinated heifers must be identified by a special A.V. ear tag inserted in the left ear on completion of the second inoculation. A booster dose is essential after 12-18 months. Cost of latter dose to be borne by herdowner.

13. Herdowners participating in the Scheme will be required to undertake to use only (a) bulls in applicant's own herd which have passed a blood test, (b) bulls in herds which are at least of twice clear Milk Ring status, or (c) A.I. Service for animals in their herds. The Department may subject any bull in a participating herd to an appropriate blood test for Brucellosis and if the animal proves to be a reactor require its removal for slaughter. In such circumstances compensation will be paid at full market value subject to the maximum applicable under the Department's B.T.E. Scheme.

14. The acceptance of any application under the Scheme is entirely at the Department's discretion. The Department can accept no liability other than the provision of official free tests in accordance with the Scheme and the payment of grants for reactors where the requirements of the Scheme and any instructions or directions by the Department's officers in the matter, are fully observed and the herd has been accepted as officially clear. Applicants will also be required to comply fully with the provisions of any Scheme in operation for the purpose of disease eradication in cattle or any other Scheme under which grants are payable by the Department or any statutory requirements under the Diseases of Animals Act (1966) or the Livestock Breeding Act 1925.

A Veterinary Inspector or authorised officer of the Department, or a Veterinary Surgeon operating under the Scheme, may at all reasonable times:--

(i) enter on any land or premises of an applicant for the purpose of examining, testing, marking or punching animals or taking samples for the purposes of this scheme and

(ii) he may require the herdowner or his representative to give any assistance that may be reasonably necessary.

15. The terms of the Scheme including the value of the grants may be varied by the Minister at any time and the operation of the Scheme may be suspended or discontinued at any time.

16. The Minister's decision on the acceptance of any application under this Scheme or in respect of any provision of the Scheme shall be final.

17. Advisory leaflets on the control of brucellosis are available at DVOs.

Herdowners are advised in their own interest to have at least two tests of the individual cows in the herd carried out in a lactation period in order to identify and control additional reactors particularly those which are pregnant and liable to abort.

BRUCELLOSIS

THE INFECTED HERD

A herd which contains infected animals presents a threat to clean animals and to adjoining herds. If the number of infected herds is not reduced, this prolongs introduction of eradication. An incentive scheme is now available. Its object is to assist owners in removal of reactors. Copies are available from the District Veterinary Office or from a Veterinary Surgeon. The owner who decides that he will not take action and who waits for a compulsory scheme is unwise. Eradication may not be introduced in some counties for a number of years. During that time the disease may spread. An abortion storm may hit a herd. The neighbour who decides that he will take no action now, is not a good neighbour. Owners of clean herds expect cooperation from owners of positive herds. This means an effort to control and eliminate brucellosis.

What steps should an owner take?

1. Ask a Veterinary Surgeon to identify positive animals. He will take milk samples.
2. When results of tests are available, the owner should discuss the scheme with his Veterinary Surgeon.
3. If the owner decides to participate, he should obtain an application form from the Veterinary Surgeon or the local District Veterinary Office.
4. The Veterinary Surgeon will ear punch each infected animal and arrange future tests.

During the period between identification of reactors and a herd passing two consecutive milk ring tests, there are many points which must be taken into consideration.

1. PREGNANCY

Pregnant reactors may abort. Should this occur, over 90% of infection is shed. Unless the owner takes precautions, the entire herd will become infected. Adjoining herds may become infected. Isolation is therefore essential. This is particularly important when cows or heifers reach five months of pregnancy. In some cases, onset of abortion may be noticed. Springing occurs or a discharge is seen. Regular inspection is therefore important. This applies particularly to beef herds where calvings and abortions may take place in the open. Calvings should also take place in isolation. An infected cow or heifer may calve at full term and spread millions of brucella abortus bacteria. Reactors aborting or calving at the silage face are a certainty to spread brucellosis.

2. ISOLATION

If loose boxes are not available, group isolation in a 'Tie Up' arrangement is satisfactory. Paddock isolation is also satisfactory. This should take place away from the boundaries of nearby herds and away from the byre.

3. DISINFECTION

During isolation after calving or abortion, disinfection is essential. Isolation should continue until discharges cease. This usually takes a few weeks. Discharges and contaminated material e.g. bedding, should be effectively disposed of and not allowed to come in contact with the breeding herd. Any approved disinfectant is effective.

If disinfection is to be effective, it must be thorough. Disinfection procedure should be carried out as follows:--

(a) Before removal of manure or other material, spray or saturate with an approved disinfectant.

(b) After removal the parts must be thoroughly scraped and scrubbed with a 4% solution of washing soda (one pound to two and a half gallons of warm water).

(c) The parts must be sprayed with an approved disinfectant.

4. ABORTION

Abortion should be notified to a Veterinary Surgeon. If abortion occurs at pasture, breeding stock should be removed from the field and every effort made to locate and dispose of the foetus and afterbirth. The site of abortion should be sprayed with an approved disinfectant and straw burned on it. The field should be free of breeding stock for two months in the growing season and three months in the non-growing season.

5. MANURE AND SLURRY

Manure should be stacked and not used on grazing land for 12 months. It may be used on tillage or meadowland after 6 months. Slurry should not be used for 3 months. The owner should not dispose of manure or slurry for use in a herd which is brucella free.

6. MACHINERY

Brucellosis may be carried on farm machinery and equipment. The owner of a clean herd should be informed of infection before borrowing or hiring machinery or equipment.

7. DOGS, FOXES

Spread may also take place by dogs, foxes, rats and other vermin. The owner has a responsibility to control mechanical carriers.

8. FENCES

Fences should be kept in good repair. Infected animals may transfer infection to an adjoining farm.

9. SALES

It is a condition of the scheme that reactors are marked and sold to factories. If an owner does not participate in the scheme it is important that he does not sell brucellosis to another herd owner.

10. TRANSPORT

Transport for reactor disposal should not be used for brucellosis free animals until thorough cleaning and disinfection is carried out.

11. PURCHASES

Owners participating in the scheme must ensure that they do not reinfect their herds by purchasing infected animals as replacements.

12. VACCINATION

Vaccination is a valuable aid in control. It is not a cure for infected animals. The use of vaccine must be supported by good farm hygiene and management, if satisfactory results are to be achieved. This simply means that wide-spread use of vaccine and no attention to abortions or infective calvings, will not result in success. If the germ known as the brucella abortus is allowed jungle law in the farmyard and on pastures, no known vaccine will alter that situation. Vaccine is as good as the support which a herdowner gives it.

DEPARMENT OF AGRICULTURE AND FISHERIES

JUNE 1973

The National Brucellosis Program of Mexico

Jaime Arturo del Rio

The National Brucellosis Program in Mexico was inaugurated in 1971. Four stages were planned to implement the program.

Stage I. - Prevalence of Disease and Extension Activities

Due to the lack of information about the problems of the disease in the Republic, the Department of Animal Health conducted a serologic survey of the cattle that were to be exported in 1968 and 1969.

After analyzing the results obtained, the Department of Animal Health decided to begin control of brucellosis in selected areas. This program was designed to obtain more information about the disease in these areas and also to disseminate information about the program.

Stage II. - Disease Control Programs

In the present stage of the program the work is developing principally under two different plans.

1. The first optional program has been the traditional approach to disease control. It encompasses the following parameters:
   a. Test and slaughter of reactor animals.
   b. Test and quarantine of reactor animals.

c. Vaccination of female calves between three and six months of age with Brucella abortus strain 19 vaccine.

2. The other optional program consists of a voluntary mass vaccination of calves from three to six months of age using Brucella abortus strain 19 vaccine.

At the present time, brucellosis control programs are employed in parts of 227 municipalities (counties). These counties represent 26 states of the Republic which is 9.5 percent of all counties in Mexico. There are 2,133 cattle herds (dairy, beef, and dual purpose) that contain a total of 549,979 cattle currently under the program. A total of 114,373 female calves have been vaccinated. The prevalence of brucellosis in these cattle is 4.4 percent. A total of 235 herds have been declared disease-free. These disease-free herds contain 46,676 cattle. Disease-free revalidation of 170 of these herds has been made which accounts for 72.3 percent of total certificates granted.

In conjunction with the control program activities, disease surveillance is being practiced in slaughter houses, pasteurization plants, and milk collection routes to identify the focal points of infection in an area. Animal economic losses attributed to brucellosis in Mexico are estimated at $376,773,210.00 -- ($26,221,856 U.S. Dollars). These economic losses are the result of abortion; milk losses; replacement costs and losses resulting from reproduction problems.

The factors that have influenced the success of the program in certain areas that should be mentioned include the following:

1. The "non compulsory" nature of the program favorably attracted some herd owners to solicit information and enter into the program.

2. The courtesy and high professional ethics of technical personnel working in the program.
3. The favorable results of the program has been a recommendation for a greater number of cattlemen to enlist in the program each day.
4. The collaboration of other government institutions such as the Secretary of Health and Assistance, Public Education, Secretary of Water Resources, Secretary of Land Reform, and the Federal Bank have collaborated in dissemination of information about the program in zones where no personnel of Animal Health are assigned. For example the Federal Bank requires that cattle purchased on credit be free of brucellosis and that the applicants for credit enter in to the brucellosis control program.
5. The social, economic, and culture levels of some of the owners of the cattle. Some progressive cattlemen applied their own initiative to enter in the program, thus increasing the enthusiasm of other cattlemen to enter into the program.
6. The service of the program is free. The herd owners pay nothing for the service except the cost of production of the vaccine used.

The factors that have tended to delay and retard the program in some zones should also be mentioned. These include:

1. The lack of human and material resources needed for the continuity and complete development of the program.
2. The voluntary nature of the program.
3. The lack of economic resources that would permit indemnity payments to the owners of cattle sent to slaughter.
4. The lack of sufficient biological products (vaccines and antigens) in the amounts and at the precise times

needed.

5. The lack of an identification system to control movement of infected animals from one part of the national territory to another.
6. The social, economic, and culture level of some herd owners makes it difficult to extend and correctly execute the program.

Stage III. - Vaccination

In order to increase the effectiveness of technical personnel in the program, some aspects of the program have been combined. We should mention the following:

1. The program has begun to intensify vaccination of female calves from three to six months of age using Brucella abortus strain 19 vaccine in areas with a high prevalence of infection.
2. All the new herds entering the program must accept the vaccination plan. However, each herd will be tested once in order to know its infection status. We consider this to be the most convenient system for the control of brucellosis in our country, because it is cheaper and more practical.
3. We are making the necessary arrangements with some state; establishing agreements between the state governments and the Animal Health Department and instituting a unique identification system for vaccinated calves.

state; establishing agreements between the state governments and the Animal Health Department; and instituting a unique identification system for vaccinated calves.

4. The regulations for the program are being incorporated into the new Animal and Plant Health Law of Mexico, which will provide us with the necessary legal basis to declare the program as a public benefit and change it to a compulsory program in those areas where this is needed.
5. At the end of the present year an official laboratory for production of biological products for animals will be operating and will supply to the program the vaccines and antigens needed to carry out the program.
6. We have started to intensify mass vaccination of female calves between three and six months of age in the Southeastern states of our country (Yucatan, Campeche, Quintana Roo, Chiapas and Tabasco). This project is expected to take seven years (calculated productive life of our dairy cattle). After this period of time we will be able to estimate the effectiveness of the vaccination. Then we will decide whether to eradicate the disease or continue the vaccination program.
7. In the future we will apply for international credit in order to complete the massive vaccination program against brucellosis in the country and to progress to the eradication stage.

Stage IV. - Eradication

We consider a national system of animal identification essential to a successful brucellosis program. But also, we consider it very important to have the necessary buildings for controlling the slaughter of reactors and cattle movements. For this reason the Animal Health Department of Mexico has established a national system of animal identification, composed of letters and numbers on an ear tag which provides the following information: state, county and the animal number.

We also have an identification system for vaccinated calves. The legend in the right ear contains the following information: state, year and the code of the technician who performed the vaccination. In the inferior border of the same ear an inverted "V" is cut. The location of this V designates the trimester of the year when the vaccination was performed, so we can identify a vaccinated calf at a long distance without looking at its tattoo. We need this information in order to know what diagnostic criteria we ought to follow.

Infected cattle are being identified by a fire letter - "B" on the right jaw.

The National Brucellosis Programme of Britain

W. J. Brinley Morgan

The eradication of bovine brucellosis in Britain is expected to reach its final stages in 1980 when the last areas will be declared as Compulsory Eradication Areas so that by around 1982-84 the whole country will be expected to be *Brucella*-free.

Although a start at eradication was made before 1939 it was not until 1967 that an official Brucellosis (Accredited Herds) Scheme (BAHS) was started, aimed at identifying and then maintaining disease free those herds believed to be *Brucella* free or nearly so (Simpson 1968). This voluntary scheme had been preceeded by a vaccination programme based on the use of strain 19 vaccine which was first introduced in 1944 and by the National Survey of Brucellosis conducted in 1960-62 (Leech et al. 1964).

The BAHS was replaced in 1970 by the Brucellosis Incentives Scheme (BIS) - again a voluntary scheme but with certain changes introduced; for example in the method of compensation and the introduction of the Rose Bengal plate test (For complete description see addendum I - Brucellosis Incentives Scheme Conditions and Rules). In 1971 compulsory area eradication was started in three selected areas. Further eradication areas have been added with firm plans to cover the whole country by 1980 (Figure 1). At present, 67 percent of the herds containing 66 percent of the testable animals are subject to eradication measures.

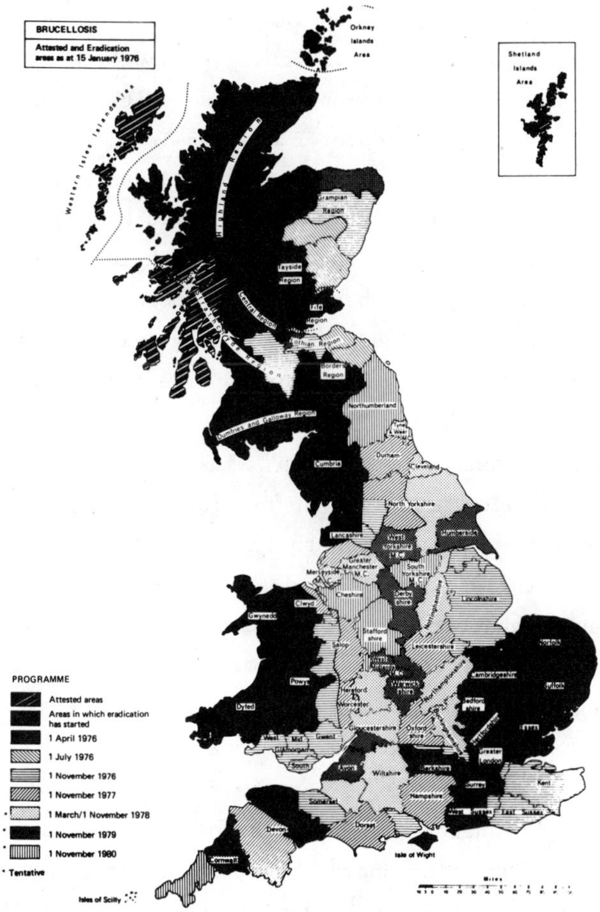

Figure 1. The Progess of and Schedule for Brucellosis Eradication in Britain

From the introduction of the BAHS in 1967 to date a number of changes have been made (Morgan and Richards 1974). Their introduction in part being the result of experience, research and development work and, in part, imposed by changing circumstances. These include such inevitable changes as increase in the size of herds, often with reduced facilities for isolating animals, for observing animals for signs of impending abortion (or oestrus detection), husbanding animals in close proximity in yards, mixing animals of various ages and stages of pregnancy, the sharing of equipment, and economic factors.

One very obvious example of changes is in the use of Milk Ring Test (MRT). When the BAHS was introduced, the MRT was used as a "pre-registration" test in dairy herds by submitting churn or "group" milk samples to the MRT every three months. After three successive negative herd MRTs the herd was then subjected to an "official" herd blood test of all eligible animals; if it passed, the herd was then registered. The collection of the milk samples was done by officers of the department and, if churns were not used, then "group" milk samples had to be prepared by pooling milk from up to six cows. The increasing numbers of herds that changed to the use of bulk tanks to store the milk for the whole herd, and the increasing cost of sending someone every quarter to collect churn milk (when available) or to supervise the collection of milk from each quarter of each cow and pooling the milk from six cows to produce an artificial churn sample forced us to look at alternatives. The only practical alternative was to use the bulk tank sample but to increase the frequency with which samples were collected. Since 1971 the Milk Marketing Boards have, on behalf of the Ministry, been doing monthly MRTs on bulk milk on all herds selling milk to the boards. This has enabled the department to monitor the status of Brucella-free herds as well as to identify herds with successive negative bulk MRTs so as to encourage the owners to join the voluntary scheme.

In view of the increasing size of herds and the consequent greater dilution factor where milk from one infected cow could be diluted with that from 50 or more negative cows, it is natural to ask how effective has been the programme of the monthly bulk MRT. It has been found that in 64 percent of herd breakdowns, the first indication of infection was the result of the monthly bulk MRT. This figure, of course, only relates to herds subject to monthly MRT, and excludes e.g. non-dairy herds. Somewhat surprisingly there was little difference as regards numbers of reactors disclosed in relation to herd size and the result of the MRT.

Another basic change has been in the detail of tests used to take into account advances made in diagnostic methods. In 1970 when the original BAHS was replaced by the BIS, two important changes were introduced. The first was the payment of incentives once a herd became accredited (based on milk output or per capita in non-dairy herds). The second was the introduction of the Rose Bengal plate (RBP) test as a screening test on all blood samples of eligible animals in the herd before becoming accredited to repace the three MRTs (see Table 1). After three successive negative herd blood tests a herd was declared _Brucella_-free but the subsequent monitoring was by a monthly MRT for dairy herds and an annual blood test in the case of non-dairy herds. All eligible heifers (more than 12 months for non-vaccinates and more than 18 months for vaccinates, as well as bulls over six months of age) were subject to an annual blood test. All abortions must be reported - the aborting cow being isolated and subjected to examination on the day of abortion and again 14 days later if the results of the first tests are negative. The results of herd blood tests are stored in a computer and preliminary results are proving to be interesting and reliable e.g. the early indications of a herd breakdown.

These three herd blood tests before registration have put a heavy load on the method of collecting blood samples, their identification on the farm, their testing and identification in the laboratory, and the correct collation of the test results to

Table 1
BRUCELLOSIS INCENTIVES SCHEME

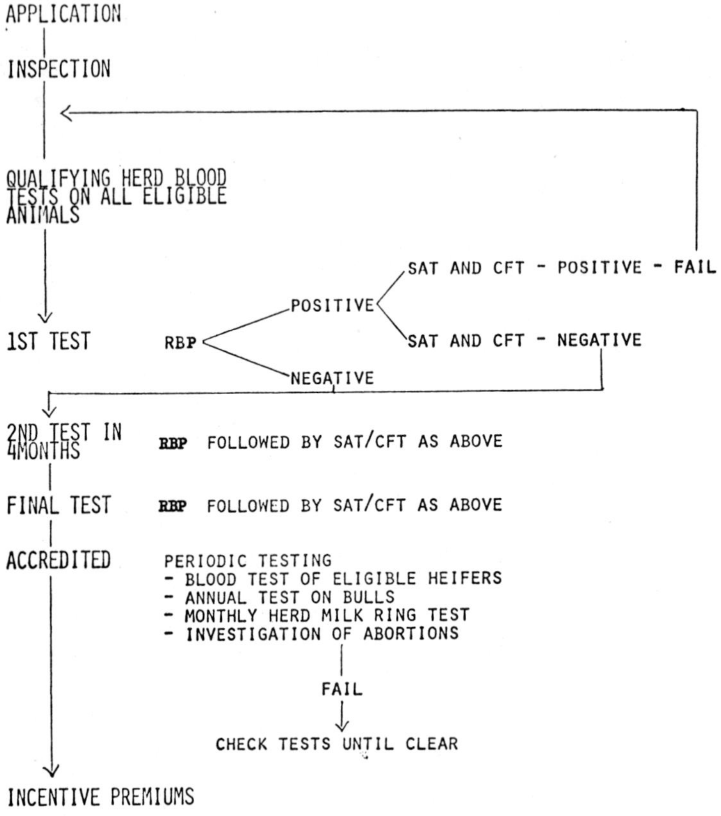

THROUGHOUT, ALL ABORTIONS TO BE NOTIFIED AND TESTS MADE WHILST ANIMAL IN ISOLATION. THESE INCLUDE: BLOOD TEST OF DAM, MILK CULTURE, AND CULTURE OF VAGINAL SWABS.

the individual animals in the division offices.

Because of the intensive testing of individual animals e.g. herd blood tests, abortion inquiries, the frequent movement of animals between herds and for shows, etc., it is now essential to have a permanent and easy means of identifying individual animals. This is required in order to enable the often detailed tests done at laboratories to be correctly related to individual animals at farms so that the right animals are recognised as reactors and thus removed from the herd.

From the beginning of the eradication campaign work a conscious decision was made to attempt to mechanise, as far as possible, the routine tests in order to reduce human error in the identification of samples, in reading the tests, and in collating the test results. As discussed in my first paper (Diagnosis Section) we have been successful in mechanising the RBP test by the use of the Autotape system (Gower et al. 1974) and the routine serum tube agglutination tube test (SAT) has been successfully mechanised using the SATAS machine so that we are now being equipped to handle large numbers (around five million) of sera annually at three central points (Weybridge, Worcester and Lasswade).

As mentioned earlier, the first indication of infection in breakdown herds is a reaction to the monthly MRT on bulk milk in about 64 percent of cases, whereas abortion inquiries are the first indication in around 10 percent. This has lead us to revise the nature of the tests done following initial abortion inquiries and these now consist of a blood sample from the dam for RBP (and SAT/complement-fixation test - CFT - if the RBP is positive), cultural examination of colostrum, and a vaginal swab. Under certain well-defined circumstances in which the herd history is well-established, a second abortion inquiry may not be made if the results of the first inquiry are negative. However, a second inquiry is certainly essential in infected herds or those in which the history is not well established since in a proportion of cases the results of the first inquiry may be negative but the results of the second inquiry 14 days later may be positive.

We were also conscious that as the eradication programme gained momentum and whole areas became virtually Brucella-free we would have to look critically at our vaccination policy as regards both vaccines (strain 19 and 45/20). With the current Brucella situation in Britain it is still official policy to encourage farmers in all areas to vaccinate their calves with strain 19 but there are two main factors that must now be taken into account. These are European Economic Community (EEC) regulations as regards "Officially Brucellosis-free" whereby to qualify inter alia, no Brucella vaccines may be used or have been used in the preceeding three years. Therefore, Brucella-free herds that are exporting animals to Europe may well decide in the future not to use any Brucella vaccine. However, brucellosis-free herds that wish to supply replacement animals in our own current eradication areas would be well advised to supply protected, i.e. vaccinated animals.

The other factor is the so-called "problem heifer" reactor. We first became aware of the extent of this problem following the introduction of the RBP test and the reduction in the age of the first testing of official vaccinates from 24 to 18 months in 1970. Heifers at around 18 months of age often in otherwise apparently Brucella-free herds reacted to our serological tests along the following lines: RBP positive, SAT around 30 - 100 international units; and CFT around 2/4 - 4/20. Repeated tests in these animals over the succeeding four to six months often resolved the status of these animals with the CF test eventually reaching "pass" levels, less than or equal to 1:4. The tests invariably reached pass or negative levels in the same order, namely - SAT, followed by RBP, followed by CFT. However, the status of many animals was not resolved after repeated testing and, in the end, after many months of having been in isolation such animals had to be recognised as reactors and slaughtered. We estimate that around 0.5 percent of heifers vaccinated with strain 19 vaccine eventually become "problem" vaccinates (within the meaning described above). We have purchased about 20 such heifers that were pregnant and kept them in isolation at the laboratory until they calved. Extensive investigations have not led to the isolation of *Brucella* after calving nor at post mortem examination afterwards.

Quite recently it has been noted that some "problem" vaccinate heifers suffer some degree of lameness, particularly of the stifle joint. In some cases which have been investigated joint fluid has contained high levels of *Brucella* antibody although, as yet, we have not had unequivocal results as regards the isolation of *Brucella*.

Although there are reports in some countries, notably in the USA, that some animals can become permanently infected with and excrete strain 19 organisms, this has not been our experience in Britain.

One of the difficult decisions that will have to be made fairly soon is the timing of the phasing out of the use of *Brucella* vaccines. If the use of vaccines is phased out too soon it could delay final eradication in certain herds. If it is phased out too late it would certainly delay herds becoming "Officially-free" under EEC regulations, and the cost both of making and administering the vaccine and of "problem" reactors could be greater than any benefit that could be derived.

The 45/20 adjuvant vaccine became available in Britain in 1967 and guidance was given by the Department as to circumstances under which it could be used (Anonymous 1967; Morgan and McDiarmid 1968). With widespread use of strain 19 in Britain, the superimposition of 45/20 vaccine caused reactions, especially to the CF test, to persist for up to 18 months. Even in animals not previously vaccinated with strain 19 vaccine, post 45/20 reactions could still (perhaps exceptionally) persist for up to 12 months or even longer (MacKinnon 1963). For these reasons the use of 45/20 vaccine was not allowed in herds participating in voluntary schemes (the Brucellosis Accredited Herd and the Brucellosis Incentives Schemes) nor was its use allowed without permission in any herds for a period of 18 months before an area became declared a Compulsory Eradication Area.

There are some areas in Britain with a very high cattle density and also with high levels of infection. These are the last areas scheduled for compulsory eradication. However, in order to reduce the level of infection in these areas and to make it feasible to introduce compulsory eradication measures in 1980 a 45/20 vaccination programme was started earlier this year (the programme being financed by the State). The use of the vaccine under these circumstances is only allowed if there is evidence of infection in the herd; this usually means after a herd blood test has been done and reactors disclosed. The use of 45/20 vaccine in adult cattle is not a departure from existing policy of brucellosis vaccination; it is still official policy to use strain 19 vaccine in female calves between three and six months of age.

The success of our programme, as of any other programme, has depended on and been influenced by a number of factors. These have depended on a sense of purpose and energy by farmers, veterinary surgeons, doctors, administrators, and regulatory professional staff. The programme has been influenced by direct experience in the field and by a willingness by all parties to be prepared to listen and, where needed, to modify. Where results of research work have indicated that better, quicker, or more effective methods are available, these have had to be evaluated and, if proved successful and opportune, they should be introduced. There is a real danger that too much so-called research activity and a demand for every new test to be introduced can seriously delay progress by detracting resources from the main objective. Too much rigidity can be just as counter-productive as too much flexibility.

The serious economic and inflationary pressures which, to some degree or other, have afflicted many countries also have serious implications for any national programme, and brucellosis eradication has been no exception. There have been, on the one hand, pressures to increase spending and, on the other, pressures to reduce spending. In the end, sensible compromises have to be reached. As an example, the top valuation limit of compensation for slaughter of reactors was £240. With time, this figure became unacceptable to farmers and agreement was reached to raise the limit to £400. Any considerable delay on this could have delayed the whole progress of eradication.

Summary

The present programme in Britain consists of a voluntary scheme (the Brucellosis Incentives Scheme) and Compulsory Area Eradication. The last areas for compulsory eradication are scheduled for 1980 so that by 1982 the country should be virtually brucellosis-free. As of March of this year there were 106,664 herds (67 percent of the total) subject to eradication measures and these contained some 4.4 million testable animals which represent 66 percent of the total testable animals. Changes have been made since the programme began in 1967; these have consisted of changes caused by economic and management factors as well as those arising from results of well tried and well tested advances in research. In all circumstances it is essential to maintain dialogue between the parties involved - the farming community, veterinary surgeons, state regulatory staff, research staff and administrators. The overall approach should neither be too rigid nor too flexible.

References

Anonymous. 1967. Agricultural Departments of Great Britain: Joint statements. Vet. Rec. 81:2921.

Gower, S. G. M.; Wright, E. C.; Davies, G.; Morgan, W. J. Brinley; Hopkinson, W. I.; Gibbs, D. F.; and Bennet, E. J. 1974. Vet. Rec. 95:544.

Leech, F. B.; Vessey, M. P.; Macrae, W. K.; Lawson, J. R.; MacKinnon, D. J.; and Morgan, W. J. B. 1964. Animal Disease Surveys No. 4. London: HMSO.

Morgan, W. J. B., and Richards, R. A. 1974. Vet. Rec. 94:510.

Morgan, W. J. B., and McDiarmid, A. 1968. Vet. Rec. 83:184.

Simpson, J. W. 1968. Vet. Rec. 82:11.

ADDENDUM I

BRUCELLOSIS INCENTIVES SCHEME - CONDITIONS AND RULES

CONDITIONS

SECTION I FOR ALL HERDS

Observation of Rules

1. The Accreditation Rules must be observed unless written exemption from a particular Rule has been obtained from the Department.

Liability

2. The Department shall not be liable for expense, loss or damage arising out of any requirement under the Scheme.

Minister's decisions final

3. The decision of the Minister shall be final on:

   (a) acceptance of premises, herds and individual animals into the Scheme and retention of a herd on the Register;

   (b) whether an animal is deemed to be a reactor for purposes of the Scheme;

   (c) interpretation of the Conditions or the Accrediation Rules.

Applications

4. Applications must be rendered to the Department in writing:

   (a) on the prescribed form for entry into the Scheme;

   (b) for movement or other permits so as to reach the Department at least three days before the operative date of the permit.

Testing

5. Where a herd is accepted for the Scheme, and the Accreditation Rules are observed, the Department will undertake free of charge all tests on the herd that may be required to obtain its registration, to confirm its continued freedom from brucellosis and to clear up any case of re-infection. All other necessary tests (eg where a non-accredited animal is moved in under permit) must be arranged and paid for by the owner.

Disclosure of test results

6. Where the Department or its agents undertake tests under the Scheme the results may be disclosed to the owner's veterinary surgeon, to

the Milk Marketing Board concerned and to the Medical Officer of Environmental Health in England and Wales or to the Chief Administrative Medical Officer in Scotland.

Withdrawal from Scheme

7. An owner may withdraw his herd from the Scheme at any time.

Re-admission following withdrawal

8. Re-admission to the Scheme will be at the discretion of the Minister. It will not be permitted when the owner of a herd which is:

(a) in an eradication or attested area withdraws from the Scheme. Such a herd will automatically become subject to compulsory eradication measures;

(b) not in an eradication or attested area withdraws from the Scheme, following the disclosure of reactors to tests carried out under the Scheme, until the reactors have been slaughtered.

Slaughter of reactors

9. Reactors slaughtered under the Accreditation Rules will be exempt from the levy of Meat and Livestock Commission payable under Section 13 of the Agriculture Act 1967.

Registration

10. Provided the Scheme Conditions and Accreditation Rules have been observed, a herd participating under this Scheme will be entered on the British Register of Brucellosis Accredited Herds on completing the qualifying testing programme required by the Department.

Change of ownership

11. Where ownership of an accredited herd changes, any future entitlement to incentives or compensation:

(a) will pass to the new owner provided he undertakes to comply with the Scheme Conditions and Accreditation Rules, and provided the herd concerned remains a separate entity on the same approved premises;

(b) will be determined by the Minister in all other cases.

Penalties

12. Any breach of the Accreditation Rules may lead to withdrawal of the herd from the Scheme or, in the case of an accredited dealer, to withdrawal of his permit.

13. In accordance with Section 106(7) of the Agriculture Act 1970 and Section 7(1) of the Diseases of Animals Act 1950, any person who knowingly or recklessly makes any false statement for the purposes of obtaining for himself or any other person any payment under this Scheme shall be liable on summary conviction to a fine not exceeding £100 or imprisonment for a term not exceeding three months or both.

Representations

14. Where the Minister proposes to withdraw a herd from the Scheme and the owner will be so informed in writing and given an opportunity to make representations. Similar facilities will be accorded to an accredited dealer if the Minister proposes to withdraw his accreditation permit.

SECTION II FOR HERDS AFTER REGISTRATION AS ACCREDITED AND DURING INCENTIVE PERIOD

Payment of incentives

15. Incentive payments applying to an accredited herd participating in the Scheme will be made during the incentive period of 5 years as follows:

(a) in the case of a dairy herd to the person registered as the milk producer by a Milk Marketing Board; and in the case of a beef herd to the person entitled to receive Hill Cattle Compensatory Allowances or Beef Cow subsidy;

(b) in the case of a dairy herd with effect from the first day of the month following accreditation; and in the case of a beef herd normally from the next qualifying day for Hill Cattle Compensatory Allowances or Beef Cow subsidy as appropriate;

(c) in the case of a beef herd on those animals which are eligible for Hill Cattle Compensatory Allowances or Beef Cow subsidy or by such arrangements as may be approved when this subsidy ceases, as appropriate.

Loss of incentives on withdrawal from Scheme

16. Entitlement to milk incentives will cease at the end of the month in which a herd is withdrawn from the Scheme and eligibility for beef incentives will cease immediately.

SECTION III FOR HERDS AFTER EXPIRY OF INCENTIVE PERIOD

Reactors compensation, valuation and slaughter

17. If an animal fails a Scheme test for brucellosis and is classed as a reactor or the disease is confirmed by other means, the Department will arrange for the animal to be valued, collected and slaughtered and for compensation to be paid at 75 per cent of the market value as an accredited animal up to a maximum payment of £300 per animal.

Ascertainment of value

18. The value of any reactor slaughtered by the Department will be ascertained by agreement between the owner and the Department or by a professional valuer appointed by agreement between the parties. Valuer's fees will be paid by the Department. Failing agreement on the appointment of a valuer the valuation will be made by a valuer nominated at the request of the Department by the President of the Royal Institute of Chartered Surveyors in England and Wales or in Scotland by the President of the Institute of Auctioneers and Appraisers. The value fixed by any of these methods will be final and not subject to appeal.

Carcase Receipts

19. The Department will retain the proceeds from the sale of the carcase of any reactor slaughtered for which compensation is payable subject to any sum in excess of the compensation paid being repaid to the owner after deduction of any reasonable expenses incurred by the Department.

Slaughter by herd owner

20. The herd owner may make his own arrangements, subject to the approval of the Department, for the slaughter of a reactor and disposal of the carcase in which event the Department will not arrange for valuation and compensation will not be payable. The owner may retain the receipts from the sale of the carcase.

Re-admission following withdrawal

21. If a herd is withdrawn from the Scheme after expiry of the incentive period the owner may apply for re-admission to the Scheme if the herd is not then situated in an eradication or attested area. Following restoration to the Register the herd will be eligible for compensation for reactors as in Condition 17.

SECTION IV APPROVAL OF MARKETS, AGRICULTURAL SHOWS AND DEALER'S PREMISES

Markets etc

22. Where the Department is satisfied that the Accreditation Rules will be observed, and that the safeguards implicit in those Rules will be secured, it will be prepared to approve:

(a) a market, or a separate section of a market, for the sale of animals from herds within the Scheme; special sales recognised by the Breed Societies; and holding premises if so requested;

(b) an Agricultural Show, or section of an Agricultural Show, for the exhibition of animals from registered herds;

(c) dealer's premises for registration under an accrediation permit.

ACCREDITATION RULES

PROTECTION OF THE HERD

THE OWNER SHALL:

Fencing, isolation

I. provide and maintain:

(a) boundary fences/walls which, to the satisfaction of the Department, are calculated to keep his herd within approved premises and to prevent contact with other cattle;

(b) such premises/facilities as the Department deems necessary for isolating animals, having regard to the type of herd and the management system.

II. take all possible precautions to keep his herd within the approved premises and to ensure that it does not come in contact with non-accredited cattle; and notify the Department of any straying or other accidental contact with non-accredited cattle.

Prompt notification of abortions etc

III. inform the Department immediately he suspects that an animal has aborted or has calved prematurely (ie less than 271 days after service or insemination); and keep the animal in isolation and, where possible, retain the foetus and placenta, until otherwise instructed by the Department.

Precautions against contamination

IV. comply with any written notice from the Department requiring:

(a) isolation of any animal, or any contaminated material or article;

(b) disposal of any infected material by burial or incineration;

(c) cleansing and disinfection of any specified part of the premises;

(d) prevention of access by animals to specified land and buildings;

(e) any other reasonable action necessary to safeguard the herd or limit the spread of infection.

Cattle movements

V. ensure that no cattle (other than steers over six months of age) are moved on to the approved premises except under the authority of a permit issued by the Department; and that any animals moved under such a permit are transported, and where appropriate, isolated and tested, in accordance with the conditions of the permit.

Dairy products

VI. ensure that no milk or dairy by-product (unless boiled, sterilised, pasteurised or in powder form) is brought on to the premises without a permit issued by the Department.

FACILITIES AND ASSISTANCE

THE OWNER SHALL:

Testing

VII. notify the Department in writing of the results of any private test or examination related to brucellosis conducted after entry to the Scheme; and submit copies of the relevant test certificate or laboratory report to the Department.

Assistance

VIII. provide all necessary facilities and assistance to enable an officer or authorised agent of the Department to inspect animals, premises and records and to take samples and to remove for slaughter animals eligible for payment of compensation; and furnish such information as may reasonably be required for the purposes of the Scheme.

Identification of animals

IX. permit the Department to paint, stamp or clip or otherwise identify any animal in the herd for the purposes of the Scheme; and he shall not permit the obliteration, or duplication, of such a mark.

DISPOSAL OF REACTORS

THE OWNER SHALL:

Isolation of animals

X. immediately isolate any animal not passing a blood or cultural test carried out by or on behalf of the Department.

Slaughter by herd owner

XI. if the herd is not eligible for compensation terms and unless otherwise instructed by the Department:

(a) have the animal removed for slaughter under arrangements specified or approved by the Department within twenty-one days of notification of the test results;

(b) accept that the udder, uterus and genitalia of the slaughtered animal are subject to surrender to the Local Authority Meat Inspector;

(c) furnish to the Department, within twenty-eight days of receipt of the failed test result, an approved form of certificate confirming slaughter of the animal.

Slaughter by Department

XII. if the herd is eligible for compensation terms and unless otherwise instructed by the Department, agree to the Department arranging for the animal to be valued and slaughtered

Owner's option to arrange slaughter of a reactor

XIII. if he so wishes elect to make his own arrangements for the slaughter of an animal that would otherwise be eligible for compensation and in such event the requirements of Rule XI will apply.

RESTRICTIONS ON VACCINATION

THE OWNER SHALL:

Vaccination

XIV. ensure that no bovine animal in the herd is vaccinated against brucellosis except under the provision of the Free Calf Vaccination Service, or under such other conditions as the Department may approve.

HERD RECORDS

THE OWNER SHALL:

Nature of records

XV. maintain a herd record in an approved form giving the following details in respect of each bovine animal in the herd in addition to particulars of movement required by the Movement of Animals (Records) Order 1960:

(a) identification, breed and sex;

(b) date of vaccination with brucella vaccine;

(c) date on which it was served or artificially inseminated (if appropriate);

(d) date on which it calved or aborted (if appropriate);

(e) date of birth, death or disposal;

(f) any calving abnormality such as stillbirth or retention of the placenta for twelve hours or more after calving.

Approximate dates under (b-f) shall be acceptable only where the system of management makes precise dates unobtainable.

Preservation of records

XVI. retain the records in Rule XV for not less than three years from the time the entry was made.

SUPPLEMENTARY RULES FOR ACCREDITED DEALERS

AN ACCREDITED DEALER SHALL:

Accredited dealers

XVII. operate under an accreditation permit issued by the Department; and as a business concerned specifically and exclusively with transactions in accredited cattle.

XVIII. provide and maintain premises (for which the dimensions and design are in a plan approved by the Department) in which:

(a) pregnant animals or any newly calved animals within 14 days of calving are accommodated only in buildings and concrete yards capable of being cleansed and disinfected;

(b) there are adequate loose boxes;

(c) there are adequate facilities for disposal of afterbirth;

(d) any resident stock are of accredited status and are kept completely separate from the dealing section.

XIX. ensure complete cleansing and disinfection:

(a) of vehicles before transporting individual animals or batches of stock;

(b) of the entire premises other than pasture at least once a month or following an abortion due to brucella or other evidence of brucella abortus.

XX. isolate calving animals in loose boxes.

XXI. maintain adequate records of transactions and of dates of cleansing and disinfection of the dealing premises.

GENERAL

In Eradication and Attested areas

XXII. The foregoing Rules will apply generally but will be subject to the provisions of:

(a) The Brucellosis (Area Eradication) (England and Wales) Order 1971 (as amended) or The Brucellosis (Area Eradication)(Scotland) Order 1971 (as amended);

(b) the relevant eradication or attested area Order.

MINISTRY OF AGRICULTURE, FISHERIES AND FOOD

DEPARTMENT OF AGRICULTURE AND FISHERIES FOR SCOTLAND

The National Brucellosis Program of Canada

G. R. McKeown

I appreciate this opportunity to briefly outline Canada's brucellosis eradication program.

There are approximately 15 million cattle in our country with herds varying in size from 100 to 1000 or more animals.

The first step towards brucellosis eradication in Canada was taken in 1950 with the establishment of the Federal-Provincial Calfhood Vaccination Program. At that time, it was estimated that the national level of infection was nine percent. Under this program the Federal Department of Agriculture purchased the vaccine and the Provincial Veterinary Services administered the program and distributed the vaccine to the veterinary practitioners. We have only permitted the use of *Brucella abortus* strain 19 vaccine in our vaccination program. The brucellosis calfhood vaccination program was successful in reducing the national infection rate from approximately nine percent in 1950 to 4.5 percent in 1956.

With the ultimate goal of total eradication, the next step was the introduction of a test and slaughter program. This program was commenced in 1957 under the authority of the Federal Animal Contagious Diseases Act. Testing was mandatory, infected herds were quarantined, and reactors uncovered using the serum agglutination test were ordered slaughtered with the Federal Department of Agriculture paying compensation to the owners. The compensation rates have been revised from time to time. Currently, the maximum rates are $450 for purebred cattle and

$200 for grade cattle. In addition to the compensation, the owner receives the meat salvage value of the carcass.

Under the test and slaughter policy, Brucellosis Control Areas were established throughout the country, with all eligible cattle being submitted to the serum agglutination test conducted at a federal laboratory. When the infection rate was reduced to below one percent of the cattle population and five percent of the herds, the area was certified for a period of three years. When the infection rate was below 0.2 percent of the cattle in the area and one percent of the herds, the area was designated as Brucellosis-Free and certified for a period of five years. Of the 687 Brucellosis Control Areas in Canada, all have reached certified area standing and 514 of these areas have achieved Brucellosis-Free Area status.

About 1960, the Health of Animals Branch introduced two surveillance procedures, namely, the brucellosis milk ring testing (MRT) and the market cattle testing (MCT) programs. These programs, which are being carried out across the country on a continuing basis, have proved to be effective in locating infected herds and have reduced the volume of on-farm testing required to recertify areas.

Under the MRT program, our inspectors collect milk and cream samples at least three times a year from each herd shipping milk or cream. These samples are collected at receiving depots and in some provinces at the central milk testing laboratories. Negative test results are credited to the herd, but where a reaction is disclosed, the herd of origin is traced, investigated and submitted to a brucellosis blood test.

In the MCT program, female cattle over 24 months of age marketed for slaughter are identified with plastic type backtags at the first point of assembly. Our inspectors collect blood samples from these animals at the time of slaughter and forward them to a federal laboratory for testing. Similarly, in this program, negative results are credited to the herd. If a reaction is encountered, the herd of orgin is blood tested.

During the past three years there has been an increase in the incidence of brucellosis in a few provinces. As a result, we have reviewed all aspects of our program and although we concluded the program was sound, it was felt that some modifications were necessary. We are now collecting blood samples from a herd that shows any evidence of a titre on the MRT test. Previously, on the reading of the test, only a reaction of 2+ or greater was considered significant.

We have also emphasized the need to test all herds adjacent to infected herds. In addition, we have lengthened the period of time a herd remains under quarantine, and it is now necessary for an infected herd to pass negative 30-day and 90-day retests before the quarantine is released. For some time, we have been ordering the slaughter of the calf-at-foot of a reactor cow.

Our veterinary epidemiologists study the pattern of the infection in each problem herd. In these herds, we make use of supplemental tests. From our experience, it has been found that it is preferable to depopulate a herd where the disease is firmly established or where it is not possible to readily eliminate the infection by testing procedures and other control measures. In areas where it appears the disease is not being contained, we perform a serum agglutination test of all the herds. On the retest of some infected herds, we use the agglutination test and the complement fixation test in parallel and remove reactors to either or both tests.

It has been our experience that in most instances herds become infected when an owner unknowingly buys a brucellosis-infected cow. Through news releases, we have informed owners of precautions to take in order to keep their herds free from brucellosis, and stress the importance of testing all cattle at the time of purchase and again before being added to the herd.

Since many replacement cattle are purchased at community auction markets, we have expanded our testing program at these markets.

Recognizing that the total eradication of brucellosis could not be accomplished in conjunction with mass calfhood vaccination, and with the national infection rate below two-tenths of one percent, the Health of Animals Branch began de-emphasizing calfhood vaccination a few years ago. As a result of the increase in the incidence of brucellosis, the question of vaccination has been thoroughly discussed and considered. At this stage in our eradication program, we feel that the disadvantages of the vaccine outweigh the advantages and, accordingly, we are continuing to de-emphasize the use of the vaccine. Consideration is also given to the removal of the vaccination interpretation in the reading of the test except perhaps for young animals.

In conclusion, we are confident that with the diligent application of our control and eradication procedures and the continued co-operation of the livestock industry and veterinary profession, brucellosis can be eradicated.

The National Brucellosis Program of the United States

Paul Becton

The Cooperative State-Federal Brucellosis Eradication Program has been in existence in the United States since 1934. This program has always been based on the belief that brucellosis can and should be eradicated from the livestock population. This position has been reconfirmed by the livestock producer, regulatory officials, and the scientific community on numerous occasions over the years.

The program has not always been operated at a level that could achieve eradication. In the early days it was primarily an effort to selectively reduce the cattle population because of drought conditions in this country. However, several states saw this as an opportunity to reduce the losses due to brucellosis by increasing their efforts and did make progress toward eradication.

By 1940, 209 counties in 17 states had achieved modified accredited (certified) status in recognition of progress made in reducing the level of brucellosis. To qualify, they reduced their infection rates to less than five percent of the herds and to less than one percent of the cattle. In 1942, North Carolina became the first state to achieve modified certified status. In 1934 and 1935 the reactor rate in the adult cattle population tested was 11.5 percent. By 1937 the reactor rate had decreased to five percent and it reached a low of 2.4 percent of cattle tested in 1941.

The U. S. Department of Agriculture began supplying a

standardized *Brucella* antigen to the state laboratories in 1939. This was a significant change, each state previously had been producing their own antigen, which resulted in test discrepancies. Following extensive laboratory evaluation and field testing, strain 19 vaccine was introduced and used in 39 states in 1941.

During and following World War II, eradication efforts were reduced considerably and in some states very little was done other than supporting the efforts of individual owners whose herds had become infected. There was also some increase in the use of strain 19 vaccine. Due to decreased resources and effort in the program, the number of reactors among cattle tested increased to five percent by 1946. There was an increase in cattle numbers in the United States during this time, which contributed to the increased incidence of brucellosis as more cattle were being moved and introduced into existing and new herds.

In 1947, the United States Livestock Sanitary Association, a national organization of industry and regulatory representatives, recognized that brucellosis should be treated as a national problem and recommended the adoption of the first Uniform Methods and Rules for the Eradication of Bovine Brucellosis. These rules were approved by the Department of Agriculture and serve as a guideline for the eradication of the disease on a herd, area, state, and national basis. The rules have been revised from time to time to meet the changing needs of the program.

In 1952, the milk ring test (BRT) was adopted for use in the national program. The procedure provided the means for frequent screening of dairy herds at a low cost. In fiscal year 1971, 0.3 of one percent of the herd milk samples were positive compared to 26 percent positive in 1954. Thus, in 1971, dairy cattle blood testing activities were concentrated on the 0.3 percent suspicious herds; thereby, almost eliminating the blood testing of BRT negative herds.

By 1954, livestock producers throughout the country had become extremely concerned over the losses due to brucellosis because of the increased incidence of this disease. In the fall of 1954, additional funds were made available and plans developed for an all-out effort to eradicate brucellosis. This involved state-by-state planning and support of the program to find and eliminate this disease. The basic thrust at that time was down-the-road area testing with quarantine and retest of herds found to be infected. Reactors were identified and removed for slaughter. Calfhood vaccination with strain 19 was encouraged and in some states vaccine was administered at a very high effective level and did contribute to the eradication effort. Some states moved ahead faster than others. Included in the front runners were some states that initially had a very high level of infection.

By the time the area testing had been completed and all of the states had attained a modified-certified status, approximately 30 states had also achieved certified-free status. These were the states that started early and never stopped working. Some of these states were certified free by the time other states were just starting a program.

During the early and mid-1960's, changes were taking place in the overall approach to finding the disease. As states became modified certified, area testing every three years gave way to a continuous surveillance program. In addition to the BRT, a sampling procedure for the beef cattle industry was developed which involves the collection of a blood sample from animals being marketed for slaughter (market cattle identification or MCI). The cow is identified with a backtag and a blood sample collected at slaughter. The purpose of this program is to identify positive animals and trace them back to the herd of origin so that the infection may be eliminated at that point. It also furnishes information regarding the prevalence of the disease within the population. The MCI includes the negative tests on breeding cattle in modified certified areas for recertification statistics.

Another dimension has been added to this surveillance program in some states by testing all eligible animals in the livestock market including those being sold for slaughter. This procedure has increased the coverage and effectiveness of the market cattle testing (MCT) program. The procedure has identified infected animals earlier in the marketing process at a time when exposed animals can also be identified and removed from the marketing channels before being sold as breeding animals. This procedure is desirable in the more heavily infected states where it is necessary to increase the capability of finding the disease. The MCT program has been very effective in monitoring the total population for brucellosis in areas where the number of infected herds is low. It has done this without requiring the assembling of negative herds of cattle for testing.

There are some weaknesses, however, in this procedure. The major weakness is that a livestock producer must sell a diseased animal before we find the herd to be infected. Also, the identification system is not infallible; for example, we have livestock dealers who purchase animals from several different farms and the animals are subsequently taken to a market for sale. It is entirely possible that all of the animals at the time of sale will be identified to the dealer rather than to the herd of origin. Consequently, if an infected animal is located by use of samples collected at slaughter, it is difficult if not impossible to determine the exact herd from which the animal originated.

Another problem with this procedure is that owners who wish

to do so can give inaccurate information concerning the herd of origin in cases where they own more than one farm or if they have cattle located on more than one premises. Another concern is that this procedure allows us to deal with and communicate only with the producer whose animals are found to be reactors. As a result of this, we have decreased our information efforts with the negative herd owners. This I believe has created a serious lack of information concerning the status of the disease and information needed by cattle owners concerning the danger or threat of this disease entering their clean herds.

During the past few years we have renewed efforts to inform cattle owners concerning brucellosis, and certainly much progress has been made in this direction. Another change in the program which occurred during the mid-1960's was a decision to deemphasize calfhood vaccination with strain 19 vaccine even though much credit had been given to strain 19 vaccine for the progress that had been made. One primary factor in this decision was that lingering titers were causing diagnostic problems in the cleaner states. It was also thought by program planners at that time that the opportunity for exposure to brucellosis had been diminished to the point that the cost for continued vaccination at a high level was not justified.

The role of strain 19 vaccine in the eradication program has been reevaluated by the U. S. Animal Health Association and the U. S. Department of Agriculture. We are encouraging calfhood vaccination in high incidence areas and in other areas that may sell cattle into high incidence areas. We are requesting federal funds to support vaccination in states where this support is needed and requested.

During the late 1950's and early 1960's, the complement fixation (CF) and several supplemental tests were developed to aid in the differential diagnosis of brucellosis. These supplemental tests included the acidified plate antigen (APA), rivanol, mercaptoethanol (ME), and heat inactivated tube (HIT), which destroy or inhibit certain classes of antibody which may be present in the serum and are used by veterinary epidemiologists to identify the primary class of antibody in the serum as an aid in interpreting the probable status of an animal.

In 1958, we initiated epidemiologic studies on brucellosis problem herds. In order to effectively work with these problem herds, veterinarians were selected for additional academic and field training so that they could better understand the use of supplemental testing procedures, immunology, and in more specific ways, how brucellosis behaves in unusual herd situations. This has continued to be an intricate part of our program.

In 1963, the brucellosis card test was adopted as an official brucellosis test for swine. The card test was modified for use in testing cattle and was adopted as an official test in 1966.

The program today can best be summarized by briefly discussing each of the activities.

1. Surveillance

a. The brucellosis ring test (BRT) is conducted at least three times a year in each dairy herd. All eligible animals are blood tested in herds found to be positive on the BRT. When reactors are disclosed on the blood test, the reactors are tagged, branded, and removed from the herd for slaughter. The herd remains under quarantine and is retested until the infection is eliminated.

b. The market cattle testing program is the procedure for screening the beef cattle population at slaughter and at livestock markets to find infected herds. Reactors disclosed are traced to the herd of origin and the herd tested and handled in the same way as a suspicious dairy herd.

c. Another procedure being used to find infected herds

is the community area test. This is usually done in areas which have been cleaned up and infection has been reintroduced or other areas where the disease seems to be spreading faster than normal surveillance methods will find it.

2. Epidemiology

Epidemiology could be considered part of the surveillance system. Each newly found infected herd is studied in an attempt to find how it became infected and whether or not infection has moved from that herd to other herds. In this way other herds are often identified which should be tested.

3. Indemnity

Federal funds are made available to indemnify owners of reactor cattle which are disposed of for slaughter in keeping with program requirements and regulations. Many states also pay indemnity. At the present time, the maximum federal indemnity is $100.00 for registered animals and $50.00 for nonregistered. In certified free states and states nearing free status, indemnity is also paid for cattle in badly infected herds which are depopulated.

4. Calfhood Vaccination

Strain 19 vaccine is still used rather extensively in some parts of the country. It is not being used enough in the areas with the greatest need for it. We are actively encouraging the official vaccination of calves and have plans to support this part of the program more.

Summary

The program has been in effect for many years, a very large amount of money has been expended, and untold hours of work have gone into this effort. What has it done for the cattle owner? What progress has been made toward eliminating brucellosis from the livestock population in this country? The answers to both questions are tied together. Roughly 40 years ago, area testing was revealing that 11 percent of the cattle were infected. No records show the infected herd percentage. About 20 years later when we began the accelerated program, the same type of area testing was revealing only a 2.6 percent cattle infection rate. Even with this reduction, the infected herd rate was 14.4 percent. Last fiscal year, our cattle infection rate was less than 0.7 of one percent (0.67), and our infected herd rate was just over one-half of one percent (0.54). Another way of saying it could be - each infected herd owner would have 26 others to keep him company in his misery if there had been no accelerated program.

Economic losses to the livestock owner due to brucellosis have been reduced many-fold. In the late 1940's it was estimated that brucellosis was costing the livestock producers in this country $100 million each year due to decreased milk production and fewer calves. Today losses due to brucellosis are estimated to be a little over $20 million annually. Considering the purchasing power of today's dollar, the decrease in losses is even more significant.

Progress in reducing the incidence of brucellosis has not been the same in all parts of this country. Some areas are virtually free of the disease while other areas still have many infected herds and additional infected herds are being located. This indicates that the disease continues to spread in these areas. It is important to remember this as we briefly consider the factors which made progress possible.

One factor has been program procedures based on the best information available concerning brucellosis. The program procedures have been reviewed periodically and changed as new information and new techniques indicated.

Another important factor has been the availability of public funds and personnel to carry out the necessary procedures.

When resources have been less than adequate, progress has slowed down or stopped altogether.

A major factor has been owner acceptance of the required program procedures in spite of the inconveniences, cost and additional work it has created for them. The states which have not made as much progress did not get into a complete eradication program as early as other states. Also, the beef cattle industry has expanded much faster in these Southern states. During this growth period, there has been an increase in herd size and in the movement of breeding animals. Both of these factors have added to the difficulty of eradication. Another reason for slowed progress in recent years has been the necessity to direct resources to handle several emergency situations; hog cholera, exotic newcastle (VVND), and Venezuelan equine encephalomyelitis (VEE), for example.

As we look ahead to completing this task of eradicating brucellosis, the owner's acceptance of program procedures is becoming increasingly important. This is due to larger herds, increased labor costs, and inconveniences caused by the program. It is the responsibility of the scientific community and the regulatory agencies to furnish the cattle owners with enough information to make the correct choice regarding what is best for the industry. Given this kind of information, I am confident the industry will choose to eradicate brucellosis rather than to live with it and pass the problem on to future generations.

National Programs Discussion

DR. ARCHIE I. FLOWERS (Texas A&M): I will briefly summarize what was said and then I will give the speakers an opportunity to respond. It appears to me that there is an almost universal agreement that in heavily infected areas vaccination is a preliminary tool that must be considered. Once the disease incidence level is reduced in a given area, the time of discontinuance of vaccination seems to be a problem that is not easy to solve. There is a lack of universal agreement concerning this but the availability of additional diagnostic tests today will probably alter this. We may be able to vaccinate older cattle than we have in the past without complicating the interpretation of our diagnostic tests.

We have talked about changes in programs but, in general, the various programs are similar with some minor differences. It is obvious that in the highly intensive livestock production areas of Europe there is a better system for control of movement of cattle and for animal identification. These problems have not been satisfactorily solved in the United States. One of the questions the speakers were asked to respond to was the necessity of a system of permanent individual animal identification in an effective brucellosis control program. If I have interpreted correctly, those speakers that responded indicated that a system of animal identification was a necessity. This was certainly a part of the Irish program, where an identification card must be presented with each animal at the time of sale.

The eradication program in the United States and the problems we are encountering are similar to those of Australia and, to a certain extent, those of France. With this brief summary and the little time that we have, I would like to ask if our speakers have any comments that they would like to make or questions they would like to ask?

DR. BRINLEY MORGAN (Weybridge, England): May I make a comment. We also have an identification system for all animals. This information is in my paper but I failed to mention it. The identification system is based on a county number, a farm number, and an individual animal number. We think this is essential for traceback of origin of infection, not only for brucellosis and tuberculosis, but also for foot and mouth disease as well. We believe that it is essential to have an animal identification system.

DR. FLOWERS: Dr. Morgan has stated that he feels that an identification system for all animals is necessary for disease control. Would any of the other speakers care to comment?

DR. GODFREY ALTON (Victoria, Australia): I'm afraid I neglected to apply myself to this question. In Australia we think that this is highly desirable, but this has not been achieved in the ranching areas. For abattoir traceback it is essential to be able to identify animals that go to slaughter.

DR. FLOWERS: Dr. Alton agrees with Dr. Morgan and Dr. del Rio from Mexico has previously stated that this was one of the things that they felt was essential. Any other comments?

DR. DEL RIO (Mexico City, Mexico): I want to make only one comment. I forgot to mention the tests we are using in Mexico.

Routine tests include the milk ring, plate, slow tube and card tests. The supplemental tests we are using include complement-fixation, mercaptoethanol, rivanol and Coombs antiglobulin tests.

DR. FLOWERS: Are there any questions or comments from the other speakers? Are there questions from the floor?

ANONYMOUS: Dr. Cunningham mentioned that reactors are appraised and purchased by the state. What sort of appraisals are made and what prices are paid for reactors?

DR. CUNNINGHAM (Dublin, Ireland): The state pays normal market value of the cattle up to stated limits for pedigreed and commercial cattle. I think that at the present time the upper limit of these prices is being reviewed up, but on all commercial cattle it is the actual market value. Occasionally someone might be hard hit with very valuable and pedigreed cattle, where the upper limit may not be sufficient.

ANONYMOUS: By market value, do you mean slaughter market value?

DR. CUNNINGHAM: No, the market value of the animal is judged as the price the animal would make in normal sale to a purchaser who is unaware that the animal was affected with brucellosis.

DR. FLOWERS: We probably have time for one more question and then I need to turn the meeting over to Dr. Clarke. Any other questions? I hate to wrap it up; it is a shame to be in this big of a hurry to end a meeting as important as this. I'd like, on behalf of the University, to thank our speakers and those who participated in the Symposium. I do feel too, as some of our speakers have stated, that with this openness and willingness to discuss the problems, we can proceed with a satisfactory program. We appreciate your participation. Dr. Clarke, would you like to make some comments?

DR. CLARKE: I would like to second what Dr. Flowers and others have said in thanking the speakers and the audience for their active participation. If you will permit me, I would like to specifically recognize the members of the Symposium Committee who have been involved with getting this program together over the last several months. I would particularly like to ask Dr. Dick Crawford if he would stand and be recognized as the fellow who has done an awful lot of the work. Dr. Charles Boyd, whom you had as one of your session moderators, was in charge of arranging the banquet. With Dr. Crawford was Dr. Richard Hidalgo who helped put the questions together, worked on the international travel and was very active in putting the overall Symposium together. Dr. Warren Kilpatrick helped with many of the arrangements. Mr. Richard Hall was helpful in recording of the sessions which will enable us to put the proceedings together. Dr. Archie Flowers is the fellow you are either in love with or mad at because of transportation arrangements. I can assure you that he has made many a round trip around here in the last few days. I would like to personally take this opportunity to thank each and every one of these people for helping us pull it off. Thank you all for coming.

APPENDIX

Speakers' Affiliations and Addresses

Godfrey Alton, M.R.C.V.S., B.Sc., D.V.M.S.

Animal Health Research Laboratory
CSIRO, Private Bag #1
Parkville, Victoria
Australia, 3052

Jaime Arturo del Rio, D.V.M.

National Supervisor of Brucellosis Control
Dr. Mora #5 - 7º Piso
Mexico 1, D.F.
Mexico

Paul Becton, D.V.M.

Director
National Brucellosis Eradication Program
Veterinary Services
USDA
Hyattsville, Md. 20782

Brendan Cunningham, M.R.C.V.S., B.V.Sc., Ph.D.

Chairman
Department of Veterinary Pathology, Bacteriology and Parasitology
Veterinary College of Ireland
Ballsbridge, Dublin 4, Ireland

Frank A. Hayes, D.V.M.

Director
Southeastern Cooperative Wildlife Disease Study
Department of Parasitology
College of Veterinary Medicine
University of Georgia
Athens, Georgia 30602

Lois M. Jones, Ph.D.

Research Associate
Department of Veterinary Science
University of Wisconsin
Madison, Wisconsin 53706

G. R. McKeown, D.V.M.

Chief
Eradication Programs
Contagious Disease Division
Health of Animals Branch
Canada Department of Agriculture
Ottawa, Canada

Margaret Meyer, Ph.D.

Professor
Department of Epidemiology and Preventive Medicine
School of Veterinary Medicine
University of California, Davis
Davis, California 95616

W. J. Brinley Morgan, M.R.C.V.S., B.V.Sc., Ph.D., D.Sc., Dip. Bact.

Deputy Director
Central Veterinary Laboratory
New Haw, Weybridge
Surrey Co., England

Claude J. Nelson, D.V.M., M.P.H.

Senior Staff Veterinarian
Cattle Diseases
APHIS/USDA
Hyattsville, Maryland 20782

Paul Nicoletti, D.V.M., M.S., Dip. A.B.V.P.H.

Regional Epidemiologist
Veterinary Services
USDA
Gainesville, Florida 32608

Donald E. Pietz, D.V.M., M.P.H.

Chief, Diagnostic Reagents
Veterinary Services Laboratory
USDA
P. O. Box 70
Ames, Iowa 50010

Michel G. Plommet, D.V.M.

Director of Research
Pathology of Reproduction Laboratory l'INRA
Novzilly, France 37380

Winthrop C. Ray, D.V.M., M.S.

Chief Staff Veterinarian
National Brucellosis Eradication Program
APHIS/USDA
Hyattsville, Maryland 20782

William J. Slatter, B.V.Sc.

Veterinarian
Brunette Downs
Northern Territory, Australia